# THE
# DOCTORS
## OF THE
# WARSAW
# GHETTO

**The Holocaust: History and Literature, Ethics and Philosophy**

**Series Editor**
Michael Berenbaum (American Jewish University)

# THE
# DOCTORS
## OF THE
# WARSAW
# GHETTO

## MARIA CIESIELSKA

**Edited by Tali Nates, Jeanette Friedman,
and Luc Albinski**

**With forewords by Michael Berenbaum
and Luc Albinski**

**Translated from the original Polish
by Agata Krzychylkiewicz**

BOSTON
2022

Library of Congress Cataloging-in-Publication Data

**Names:** Ciesielska, Maria, 1971- author. | Krzychylkiewicz, Agata,
  translator.
**Title:** The doctors of the Warsaw Ghetto / Maria Ciesielska ; translated
  from the original Polish by Agata Krzychylkiewicz.
**Other titles:** Lekarze getta warszawskiego. English
**Description:** Boston : Academic Studies Press, 2022. | Series: The
  Holocaust: history and literature, ethics and philosophy | Includes
  bibliographical references and index.
**Identifiers:** LCCN 2021053644 (print) | LCCN 2021053645 (ebook) | ISBN
  9781644697252 (hardback) | ISBN 9781644697269 (paperback) | ISBN
  9781644697276 (adobe pdf) | ISBN 9781644697283 (epub)
**Subjects:** LCSH: Getto warszawskie (Warsaw, Poland) | Jewish
  physicians--Poland--Warsaw--Biography. | Holocaust, Jewish
  (1939-1945)--Poland--Warsaw. | World War, 1939-1945--Medical
  care--Poland--Warsaw. | Jews--Persecutions--Poland--Warsaw. | Jewish
  hospitals--Poland--Warsaw--History--20th century. |
  Jews--Medicine--Poland--Warsaw--History--20th century.
**Classification:** LCC DS134.64 .C5413 2022  (print) | LCC DS134.64  (ebook) |
  DDC 940.53/1853841--dc23/eng/20211102
LC record available at https://lccn.loc.gov/2021053644
LC ebook record available at https://lccn.loc.gov/2021053645

ISBN 9781644697252 (hardback)
ISBN 9781644697269 (paperback)
ISBN 9781644697276 (adobe pdf)
ISBN 9781644697283 (epub)

Book design by Lapiz Digital Services
Cover design by Jacqui Morris

Published by Academic Studies Press
1577 Beacon Street
Brookline, MA 02446, USA
press@academicstudiespress.com
www.academicstudiespress.com

# Contents

# Acknowledgements

Thanks to the Johannesburg Holocaust & Genocide Centre for its strong support in publicizing the story of the Warsaw Ghetto doctors and supporting the publication of an English-language version of Dr. Maria Ciesielska's book. One of these Warsaw Ghetto doctors, Dr. Halina Szenicer-Rotstein, is honored with a memorial plaque, put up even before the Centre was officially opened in March 2019, which greets every visitor who walks up the stairs from the basement parking. Since its opening, the Centre has provided a forum for well-attended presentations on the fate of the Warsaw Ghetto doctors as well as providing guidance and financial support for the translation and editing of the book.

A special word of thanks needs to go to Tali Nates, the founder and director of the Centre, who enthusiastically supported this book project from her very first meeting with Dr. Maria Ciesielska in Warsaw in 2018. Tali spent countless hours on the draft of the book, editing it line by line, and her contribution to the ultimate product is immense. It would not have seen the light of day without her support.

Professor Michael Berenbaum's passionate interest in the book was evident from the outset; from that hot summer day in 2018 when Tali first described the book project to him as we walked from Auschwitz to Birkenau during the March of the Living. We are very grateful for his support and the wonderful foreword, which he has contributed.

We are deeply indebted to Agata Krzychylkiewicz, a retired associate professor of Russian literature and civilization at the University of South Africa, who took on the arduous task of translating the book from Polish. Her passion for the book, which, amongst many other topics, covered the fate of the mother of her good friend, Wanda, was always touchingly evident.

We would like to thank Jeanette Friedman for the many hours of work she spent editing the book and ensuring it was in a form that could be successfully published in the United States.

Most of all, we would like to thank Dr. Maria Ciesielska, who devoted years of her life to the research of the most detailed and painstaking kind in order to bring the story of the Warsaw Ghetto doctors alive and save it from the oblivion that it would otherwise have suffered. Maria was also deeply involved in checking and double-checking the English version of the book in order to ensure that the inevitable errors and omissions were weeded out prior to publication. We are deeply grateful to her for her immense work of restorative justice; by the most detailed form of documentation, she has made remembrance and commemoration possible for future generations.

Luc Albinski,
January 23, 2021

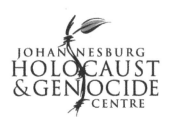

# Foreword
## by Michael Berenbaum

Dr. Maria Ciesielska's *Doctors of the Warsaw Ghetto* is a book rich in detail. I read it three times: when it was translated into rough English—before it was condensed and edited—the first draft of the major edit, and the galleys that became this book. Each time, I learned something important, something different. It is not an easy read but it is one that forces us to confront fundamental issues of humanity, ethics, and survival.

Having committed myself to writing the preface, I decided to offer readers a "map" to assist them in understanding Ciesielska's highly detailed and exacting research and how those statistics and lists are the heart-rending description of the reality the doctors and their patients faced in Warsaw before and during the Holocaust.

Historians of the Holocaust struggle to decide whose history to write. Which stories should they tell? Is it the history of how Jews were killed? That is telling German history and the history of its allies, collaborators, and enablers. That is what we call perpetrator history, in which their victims appear precisely as the perpetrators want them to appear—as targets deprived of their identities and agency. How Jews were killed is just part of the story. If we tell the stories of the killers, we must also focus on their victims—who they were, why they were chosen, and how they were separated from the societies in which they were more or less integrated, and how they were enslaved and murdered.

Ciesielska tells the story of how Jews lived under horrific conditions, struggling under circumstances not of their doing. She writes of physicians, nurses, and pharmacists who did what they could to sustain a medical system under conditions the Germans designed to methodically kill them and their patients, one step at a time.

Under German occupation of Poland, Nazi leaders generally had no interest in the health of the Jewish population. But they were keenly interested in preventing epidemics that could endanger German personnel or get beyond the ghetto walls and afflict the general population. In the latter case, it was feared that the disease might infect German troops and civilian personnel making German occupation deadly for the occupiers.

In 1941 a typhus epidemic hit Warsaw hard. The ghetto wall did not prevent the epidemic from spreading to the Aryan side, especially since many Poles and Germans were going back and forth from one side to the other. German assistance to the hospitals, pharmacists, physicians, and health services of the ghetto was motivated by a desire to contain epidemics—most especially, the typhus epidemic. But the measures put in place were not designed to enhance the well-being of the captive Jewish population.

Healthcare professionals, many of them leaders in their respective fields, worked under conditions of deliberate deprivation. Proper medical supplies were incredibly scarce; the populations they were serving were starving and living under horrifying conditions. Food was inadequate, sanitation was primitive, water was scarce, and treating patients was challenging, to say the least. One in ten Jews died in 1941. Two percent of the population died from disease and despair in each of the first seven months of 1942 just before the Great Deportation. (Had there been no such deportation, one in four inhabitants of the Warsaw Ghetto would have died that year without a bullet being fired or a train transporting them to Treblinka.) Doctors numbed themselves to the numbers they lost and conditioned themselves against getting too involved with those they could not treat and those too far gone to treat at all. They found their only solace in patients they saved and dared not ask themselves the questions: *From what? For what?*

Rachel Auerbach, one of the few resistance fighters to survive the Ghetto Uprising, ran a soup kitchen in the ghetto. She was a sensitive observer of her own situation and of the people she served. In February 1942, a mere five months before the Great Deportation, she wrote in her diary:

Death's new, pithy balance sheet. What else could I be writing about in the context of my work in the soup kitchen? It has slowly dawned on me that all the work of our charitable institutions should be called death by installments, meting out death in installments. We finally have to come to terms with the fact that we are incapable of saving anyone from death, since we have nothing to do it with. We can only put off death, stretch out death, but not prevent it. I have not managed it through my work with a single person, not one!

We are powerless, we are working in a vacuum. The only outcome of our work may be the fact that the whole ghetto will not die out all at once, that death is regulated in some way, that we can more or less keep up with burying the bodies. We are incapable of changing anyone's fate.

As you read about these medical professionals, try to imagine their despair. They were dealing with people no longer capable of going to the soup kitchens. Their wards were the anterooms to death.

Most Holocaust memoirs are written in three essential chapters: *before, during,* and *after.* This work, while not a memoir, is no exception. The structure of Ciesielska's work follows that familiar pattern. *Before* is a comprehensive history of the medical profession in Poland; its training of doctors, its major institutions, and the essential professional organizations; its specialties, and subspecialties. Because she is dealing with Jewish doctors, she grapples with the distinct obstacles they had to overcome to become doctors.

Some of the restrictions placed upon would-be Jewish medical students in Poland were like those American Jewish medical students faced in the 1930s. Others were not. A quota system restricted the admission of Jews into Polish medical schools. Polish nationalists wanted to Polanize the profession. American readers will not intuitively understand that Polish nationality was linked to Roman Catholicism, and policies were promoted by nationalists to exclude Jews, even those whose families had lived in Poland for centuries.

Because interest in becoming doctors was so high, many Jewish students did an end run around the restricted admissions in Poland getting their training and degrees in other countries, often earning more advanced and prestigious degrees. Ironically, when they returned to Poland, they had higher status than their peers, warranted by their advanced training. Polish physicians who were antisemitic but committed to getting the best treatment for their patients might, however reluctantly, refer patients to Jewish specialists.

The students who were finally admitted still suffered humiliations such as the "Jewish Bench"[1] initiated by nationalist students who sought to confine Jewish students to segregated seats. Defiant Jewish students who were proud chose to stand rather than sit in "the back of the bus" and be shamed. Some professors were inclusive and had liberal leanings, so they ignored the "Jewish Bench" because to them it was morally repugnant. For others it was a matter of integrity: no matter the political currents in their universities, they would not enforce the "Jewish Bench" or permit students to stand. A few Roman Catholic students stood in solidarity with their classmates; many more would not. Eventually, administration and faculty gave in to the antisemitic students so as to keep the peace.

Jewish students were also rejected because they could not produce bodies for autopsies, which are crucial for training in medical schools. Jewish tradition prohibits autopsies except when required by civil law or when it can immediately save an identifiable person's life, so few Jewish bodies were offered to science. In retaliation, Jewish students were prohibited from training on Polish Christian corpses. No Jewish corpses meant no training for Jews.

Some Jews understood that being Jewish was a handicap and were anxious to rid themselves of that inconvenience, so they converted just to make it possible to advance their careers. There were similar situations in prewar twentieth-century America. One of the greatest American Judaic scholars wrote in Harvard's *Menorah Journal* in 1923, "Some are born blind, some are born lame, some are born Jewish." The sense that being Jewish was a condition to be avoided if one wanted to succeed was far more widespread than one might assume today. For those less committed to Jewish tradition, less tied to their Jewish family or to the Jewish people, conversion was a way of assimilating and participating in

---

1   A practice of obligatory separation of Jewish and non-Jewish students, manifested concretely in the former being seated on the left of the lecture hall, and the latter on the right.

one's chosen profession and in the greater society with fewer obstacles to advancement.

Such "former" Jews were not universally accepted. They were in a state of what one today might call "conditional Polishness." After conversion, one might still be considered a social Jew, with the benefit of official conversion that diminished most legal and ethnic forms of discrimination. Until the Germans arrived.

When the Germans invaded Poland—and every other country—they imposed the Nuremberg Laws of 1935, defining Jews by race and not by identity or religion in occupied territory. Converts once again found themselves legally defined as Jews. There was no escape. And once Jews in Poland were confined to ghettos, converted doctors suddenly found themselves ghettoized precisely among the people they wanted to avoid. Betrayed by the Germans and often by their Polish colleagues, they in turn found themselves considered traitors by many of the Jews they treated. The loss of status was dramatic, their sense of alienation acute.

Those who converted for faith rather than advancement were in an even more problematic situation. Still, one of the last buildings in the Warsaw Ghetto to survive was a Roman Catholic Church frequented by racially Jewish but religiously Catholic priests, nuns, and devout parishioners. Ironically, the residents of the ghetto respected the converts of faith much more than they respected the converts of convenience.

The more the doctors wrapped themselves up in their professional identities, the more they were insulated from the social currents of the world around them. As Robert Jay Lifton has demonstrated, doctors are trained in *doubling*, as they divide their personality into the physician-self and the non-physician self. This makes it possible for a doctor who is also a loving father to tell parents that their child is about to die, or for a male gynecologist to examine a beautiful woman while remaining fully professional.

This *before* the war period was important to what happened *during* and *after* it. Because Jewish doctors trained with their non-Jewish colleagues and worked with them when in residence, in hospitals and in practice, they knew the difference between colleagues who were hostile, those who were timid, and those who might be willing to help them survive. Such knowledge, such cultural fluency, empowered them to seek cooperation or shelter during the Holocaust—and even after the Warsaw

Ghetto Uprising, when they hid on the "Aryan" side. Yet, because they were in contact with non-Jewish colleagues and patients, they were easy to spot and identify when they were on the Aryan side. They were more easily outed, betrayed, and/or blackmailed.

To fully understand Ciesielska's depiction of the Holocaust, one must consider the four years of German occupation as a series of stages, two preceding ghettoization and then the multiple stages of manipulating conditions in the Warsaw Ghetto itself. The first stage was the siege: Poland was under German assault from the West and Soviet assault from the East. At that time, medical practice for Jews and non-Jews alike meant going to the front or finding that your city had become a front, to do triage, functioning under wartime conditions with very limited resources, when soldiers and civilians were under unrestrained attack—and the Germans were bombing hospitals. The second stage was the period between occupation that commenced on October 1, 1939 and ghettoization, which began in October 1940 and was completed by mid-November. Jews were barred from treating non-Jews and segregation and discrimination became a way of life. The third stage was the period of the ghetto, which is the heart of this book.

A word about Jewish and German perceptions of the ghetto: in retrospect—but only in retrospect—we understand ghettoization was an interim measure. For the Germans, it was a way to segregate and isolate the Jews until they decided what to do with them. For the Jews, ghetto was a way of life, which they were forced to survive until . . . [u]ntil what?

*At first, neither Jew nor German knew what "until" would be.* The Jews hoped that they would live in confinement until Germany lost the war or came to its senses. *Iberleben*, to outlive them, was the strategy of Jews incarcerated in the ghetto. I am of the historical conviction that when Jews were ghettoized in German-occupied Poland, the Germans were not yet clear as to how they would handle these massive numbers of Jews. In retrospect, we see the ghetto as a place to confine the Jews until the decision was made to annihilate them—no small achievement considering how many Jews were in Poland—and a place to keep them while they built the means of their destruction, the killing centers.

The timing was swift. Thirty-seven-year-old Odilo Globocnik received his instructions from Heinrich Himmler to build death camps in October 1941. Chełmno became operational on December 7 and

Bełzec came along in the winter of 1942. Sobibor began operating in the spring and Treblinka did so in the summer of 1942. In less than fifteen months, most Polish Jews were murdered, only a remnant remained in hiding or in Lodz.

And yet it would be a mistake to regard ghettoization as one process. In Warsaw, ghettoization was announced on Yom Kippur 1940. The ghetto was closed in November after being surrounded by an eleven-foot high wall. Thirty percent of the population of Warsaw was confined to 2.6 percent of the city's space.

There were six stages to Jewish life in the Warsaw Ghetto, and each is reflected in the dilemmas the doctors faced and in the delivery of medical care.

The first stage was the process of moving in when everything was in turmoil, personally and professionally. There was a difference between the personal and institutional turmoil. Because the ghetto was established in a run-down and impoverished section of Warsaw, and because many physicians were economically better off, many had to find a place to live, and their hospital had to move into the ghetto or cope with the dramatic change of staffing as non-Jewish doctors and nurses had to leave, as did non-Jewish auxiliary personnel. Jewish doctors, whether by race or religion, were forced to move into the ghetto—or hide. Those who were intermarried faced a crisis regarding the fates of their spouse: separate or stay. And what of their children, considered *mischlinge* in Nazi speak? By law they were mixed breeds, but often they considered themselves as socially and culturally assimilated Poles. Institutionally, some hospitals were forced to relocate; many medical offices were forced to move into the ghetto with their valuable, lifesaving, medical equipment. Maria Ciesielska describes the efforts to move medical equipment and to set up hospitals while coping with this stressful, desperate situation. She also describes the thefts and confiscation of life-saving equipment.

The second stage was settling in for an indefinite future with little known about what that future might bring. The only thing that was certain was that the next day would be worse, and it always was. The goals of everyone in the ghetto, physicians included, were stabilization and survival.

The third stage was the period when rumors about deportation took hold and everyone began to sense that the end was near. The pressure on every ghetto inhabitant was intense, life and death hung in the balance. Where will they send us? What will that mean? To medical personnel, the issue was both professional and personal. What does a doctor do with his or her family? Will they be exempt? What does a physician do with his or her patients? Some operations were performed to facilitate hiding, a *nose job* to reduce the stereotypical Jewish nose, or, more importantly, reversing the circumcision of men and boys enabling them to pass as non-Jews. Medical ethics were even more challenged from now on. Triage took on a whole new meaning. They had to choose who would live and who would die.

The fourth stage was the period following the Great Deportation, which occurred on the Jewish calendar between Tisha B'av and Yom Kippur, between July 23 and September 21, 1942. At least 265,000 souls were deported from Warsaw to Treblinka. There was no selection at Treblinka. All were condemned to death. Perhaps less than one person in a thousand, a carpenter or a jeweler, or some other useful worker, would be chosen to work in the camp. Maria Ciesielska paints a vivid picture of some of the heroic medical personnel—physicians, nurses, pharmacists, and lab technicians who could produce scarce and necessary drugs when possible and provided them for patients who needed to be sedated to make their end or the journey to the end more bearable and less painful.

Like the Jewish Council, the *Judenrat*, doctors were forced to compile lists, to decide who shall live and who shall die. From one perspective, this act condemned some to die, from another perspective, it was an act of rescue. We are not equipped to offer moral judgment, certainly not facile judgment, which the author poignantly resists. But we must note what was done.

There was a hospital overlooking the *Umschlagplatz,* the deportation point. A few could be offered a haven, but only a few. They had to be hidden. Ambulances came into the site with patients, a few could be offered a place to hide for the return trip, taken from the mouth of the beast. Who to choose, how to choose? Some nurses and doctors saved children, even infants, left by loving mothers who knew that this was the end, and that abandonment offered their beloved child a chance to survive, even if it offered no guarantees.

It would take a poet of great talent to depict their anguish, their courage, their loss. Maria Ciesielska is a scientist and a historian, she presents the facts tastefully, accurately. It is the reader who must find a way of understanding such acts, such mothers. Literary historian Lawrence Langer eloquently and precisely described these as choiceless choices "which do not reflect options between life and death, but between one form of abnormal response and another. Both imposed by a situation that was in no way of the victim's choosing."

The fifth stage was the time between the *Grossaktion*, the Great Deportation, and the start of the Ghetto Uprising on April 19, 1943.

At the time, no one could imagine a positive future. It was assumed that if one worked and one's work was deemed useful, one might live a bit longer. Medical personnel had to adjust again, less assured of a distinct status, less equipped to continue their work. Desperate as all were desperate, anxious as all were anxious, they sought to find a way to survive and plan what to do not *if* but *when* the ghetto was destroyed.

The sixth stage was the Uprising, which began on a day unlike any other day during the Holocaust. For Himmler and the Nazis, this was the eve of Hitler's birthday. What better way to celebrate than to give him a *Judenrein* (Jew-free) Warsaw as a gift? For the Jews, it was the eve of Passover, the night that celebrates the Exodus from Egypt and the joy of freedom. The Seder ends with the chant of hope: "Next Year in Jerusalem." It was recited from the deepest abyss of exile. In Bermuda, an international Conference was held that would offer little hope to the refugees. More importantly, as far as the Allies were concerned, was to try and appease those pressing for concrete action. In Belgium, a young Jewish medical student held a red lantern on the side of the railroad tracks, and halted the twentieth transport from Malines to Auschwitz, opening the doors and allowing some to escape for freedom. In Warsaw, Ukrainian troops and their German masters gathered to deport the Jews—the final deportation—while young Jewish fighters fielded two fighting forces—one right-wing Revisionist and the other left-wing Zionist and Bundist. Even with the enemy at the gates, Jews could not unite to resist the enemy, but they chose to battle, the few against the many, the weak against the strong. This was their last stand, their proclamation of Jewish honor. It began on April 19 and continued until SS-Gruppenführer Jürgen Stroop blew up the Tłomackie Street Synagogue, Warsaw's Great Synagogue, and reported to his superiors, "the Jewish Residential Quarter of Warsaw is no longer." He burned the ghetto to the ground.

Dr. Ciesielska's history tells how Jewish doctors, pharmacists and nurses, men and women of diverse ages and background, lived through each of these stages.

We should be aware that medical ethics were developed from the sins of Nazi physicians. A new set of ethics was born from the behavior, or rather, from the misbehavior of Nazi doctors. The Nuremberg judges proclaimed ten principles of medical ethics, foremost among them the right of the patient to be informed and to consent to their treatment.

Many have written of the disintegration of Jewish life in the ghetto, the breakup of the family, growing divisions, victims turning one against the other. Physicians were part of this bleak picture, but this depressing description is incomplete; there were exceptions, important exceptions. As a religious Jew, I read the weekly portion of the Torah each week. That includes the story of Joseph, the prince of Egypt, who had been sold by his Israelite brothers. Joseph called his youngest son Efraim, "for the Lord has made me fruitful in the land of my oppression." And Ciesielska presents us with models of moral behavior that must be emulated and taught to those training to be doctors, nurses, and pharmacists so that they can learn not just what not to do but, more importantly, what they should do. Here are examples that inspired this seasoned reader.

Nazi doctors exploited their patients, performing experiments on them. Because they regarded their "patients" as subhuman and their lives as disposable, they did not care if the patients would live or die, suffer or heal. Josef Mengele, MD, PhD, experimented on twins and most especially on children. These were models of what never to do.

But there were others who did care. Some Jewish doctors were fruitful in the land of their oppression.

Ciesielska shows how the Warsaw Ghetto doctors observed the impact of hunger on their patients and kept meticulous records. When the ghetto burned, they did what they could to save those documents, they had them placed in milk cans as part of the famed *Oyneg Shabbes Archive* of Emanuel Ringelblum and his colleagues who wanted future generations to understand the ghetto from within. They studied the impact of typhus epidemics and both traditional and improvised ways of containing it so that their postwar publication enabled other physicians to heal malnourished patients or treat those suffering from the pangs of hunger and typhus.

With too few medical personnel to provide for the needs of the ghetto, innovation was also required. As a form of resistance, Warsaw Jewish doctors created courses for medical students, nursing students, pharmacy students, and anyone who cared to attend the classes. This is how they partially alleviated the personnel shortage. They modeled their curriculum on how they were taught and did so well at it that the Warsaw University honored their credits after the war. It seems incredible, but some physicians began their training in the ghetto and completed it at the University. Their ghetto professors were able to maintain their dignity and productivity even inside the ghetto walls.

Courage took many forms in the ghetto, not just armed resistance. On August 6, 1942, the Germans struck against the children's institutions in the ghetto. Dr. Janusz Korczak, who was the Doctor Benjamin Spock and Mr. Rogers of Poland, ran an orphanage in the ghetto. Well-respected and well-connected, he knew deportation meant death. He lined his children up in rows of four. The orphans were clutching flasks of water and their favorite books and toys. One hundred and ninety-two children and ten adults were counted off by the Germans. Korczak stood at the head of his wards, a child holding each hand. One child carried the flag of King Matt, and the other, a Star of David set against a white field. They marched through the ghetto to the *Umschlagplatz*, where they joined thousands of people waiting in the boiling August sun. There was no shade, shelter, water, or sanitary facilities. There were none of the cries and screams usually heard when people were forced to board the trains. The orphans walked quietly in their rows of four. One eyewitness recalls: "This was no march to the train cars, but rather a mute protest against the murderous regime . . . a process the likes of which no human eye had ever witnessed." Korczak was offered a way out of the ghetto for himself, but not for the children. The teacher would not abandon his students, the physician his patients. He was with his children to the end. All were gassed at Treblinka.

Ciesielska writes that less dramatic but no less valiant were the acts of Dr. Halina Szenicer-Rotstein, near the end of the Great Deportation:

On September 12, all patients and remaining hospital personnel boarded the boxcars. Even those who had "tickets" and stayed in the hospital on Stawki Street to tend to their patients to the very end were also deported. Among them was Dr. Halina Szenicer-Rotstein who, despite being permitted to leave the *Umschlagplatz*, chose to accompany her patients. Dr. Adolf Polisiuk remembered that "she went to a wagon voluntarily, to be with those needing her help; this is how she understood her duty. To many such a gesture seemed abnormal, for the will to survive was so strong. Her behavior was very poignant in its heroism."

You will read of her act three times, here, in the preface, in the foreword by her grandson, and again in the text. Repetition should allow you to remember her name: Dr. Halina Szenicer-Rotstein. Humility should empower you to remember the majesty of her deed.

No good deed goes unpunished. The cruel and corrupt commander of the Jewish Police was approached by a young nurse who timidly asked whether personnel had to accompany the children. "Korczak showed you the way," he answered.

Noble doctors do not abandon their patients, rabbis their congregants, teachers their students. There are other reports from the Great Deportation of physicians who injected their patients to ease their pain, to facilitate their deaths, of doctors boarding the train voluntarily, knowing that they were taking leave of the world. Not every doctor or nurse can be a hero but when they are, we must remember their names, revere their deeds.

*The Warsaw Ghetto Doctors* tells us how medical personnel lived in the ever-present shadow of death. In *extremis veritas*, there are truths that are made most manifest by extreme situations. Doctors in the Warsaw Ghetto lived and died in these extremes.

Dr. Maria Ciesielska has given us a tool by which to understand their truths.

Michael Berenbaum,
American Jewish University
Los Angeles, CA, USA

# Foreword
## by Luc Albinski

The phone rang one evening in Johannesburg in 2016. When I answered, the excited voice of an eighty-one-year-old Holocaust survivor, my mother, greeted me. "I have just been contacted by a researcher who is writing a book about the doctors in the Warsaw Ghetto," she exclaimed. "She wants to meet with us to hear our story." It was at that moment that a relationship formed between our family and Dr. Maria Ciesielska.

Soon afterwards, my mom sent me Maria's article, which had recently been published by the Eleonora Reicher Institute of the Medical University of Warsaw. Its lengthy title: "To Care for Children on Their Way and Beyond—History of Female Doctors from the Warsaw Ghetto Who Stood with Their Patients until the Very End," was arresting; its tragic import clearly telegraphed. My eyes darted to the abstract where, momentarily, I found the name of my grandmother, Dr. Halina Szenicer-Rotstein. My heart missed a beat. Thanks to Maria's painstaking research I was about to read for the first time English account of my grandmother's life and of her tragic sacrifice. Skipping over the sections on her peers, I jumped to the two paragraphs on Halina. I was soon overcome with emotion, teary as I read the second paragraph:

> As recalled by Dr. Adolf Polisiuk, Dr. Rotstein received the so-called number of life and could attempt to rescue herself. Instead, however, she ". . . voluntarily entered the wagon with her patients considering it her duty to do so."
>
> Dr. Makower described her actions in the following way: "How calm was this woman, perhaps just a little younger than me (a mother of four whose husband was God knows where in

the USSR), in the middle of unparalleled uproar and the general anxiety in the hospital! When it became clear that the heads would leave the hospital. . . Dr. Rotstein did not hesitate and took everything under her control. . . The children walked by themselves, with only some of them being carried away in arms. Adult patients were usually transported on stretchers. This was horrible, incomparably more horrible than a procession of healthy people walking towards their demise."

I hurriedly forwarded the article to my aunts, uncles and cousins. The cousins who now received Maria's article were the same ones who had daringly broken family taboos to tell me two decades earlier, when I was barely into my twenties, about my heroic Jewish grandmother. For two decades, a short paragraph in Henryk Makower's Polish-language book, *A Diary from the Warsaw Ghetto*, had constituted the only published record concerning my grandmother that I had been shown. To fill in the gaps, my mother and I had commissioned a Warsaw-based researcher, Wiesław Tomczak, to scour public archives and old Polish newspapers for more information about the Rotstein family.

Maria's Polish-language book, *The Doctors of the Warsaw Ghetto*, was a godsend. It provided us with fascinating detail about Dr. Halina Szenicer-Rotstein. We learnt about Halina's work in the first-aid wooden cabin on the *Umschlagplatz*. We learnt how, every time the cattle wagons departed, she and Nurse Fryd would collect twenty to thirty babies abandoned by their terrified parents on the railway platform. We learnt about Halina's last-ditch attempts to keep the Stawki Street hospital going; how she carried out operations to treat victims of gunshot wounds, how she protected the hospital's meager inventories posting a guard to ensure the food was not stolen. Most importantly, we learnt how she remained at her post after many of her colleagues had left for the Aryan side, deciding on September 12, 1942, to depart to Treblinka with her patients rather than to seek to save herself, abandoning her "life ticket" and her four children who had by then been smuggled out of the ghetto.

Dr. Maria Ciesielska lists seventy-four Catholic doctors who risked their lives and those of their families to help Jews, often their professional peers, to escape the ghetto and hide on the Aryan side. Some of these Catholic doctors belonged to Żegota, an underground resistance organization that was tasked with assisting Jews. Amongst these were two, Dr. Trojanowski and Dr. Radlińska, who helped to save Halina's four children, one of which is my mother, Wanda. Without them I would not be here today writing these words.

To cite Paul Auster, "the truth of the story lies in the details" and in the hundreds of pages of meticulous detail. Maria, a practicing family physician, who did the research in her spare time, succeeds in conveying the truth about the extraordinary courage and resilience of the men and women constituting the Warsaw Ghetto's medical corps who faced daily horrors of murder and deprivation with, in many cases, an almost super-human resolve. They formed part of a group of more than 831 doctors in the ghetto who ran the *Judenrat*'s Medical Council, the ghetto's three hospitals, eighteen pharmacies, medical laboratories, and emergency healthcare services. They staffed charitable organizations such as TOZ but also in a few cases provided medical services to the Jewish Police. They organized a successful underground medical university and nursing school. Maria explains how this remarkable cohort of dedicated doctors found, in the midst of the agony of the ghetto, the spiritual wherewithal to conduct medical research on hunger disease and typhus for the benefit of future generations.

Maria's book has been important for dozens of families who survived the Shoah and who are attempting many decades later to pick up the shards, connect the dots, and understand, imperfectly, the tragedy experienced by their grandparents and great grandparents. To illustrate this point, Maria told me of an unforgettable encounter with one second-generation survivor who experienced a tremendous sense of closure when he learnt whilst reading her book about the awful fate of his grandfather, hitherto unknown, one of the few doctors in the ghetto to have starved to death.

Maria had become interested in the fate of the doctors in the ghetto after watching a docudrama about Adina Blady-Szwajger, a novice ghetto doctor forced to kill her young charges to save them from murder by the Nazis, which was movingly performed by Adina's daughter, Alina. She spent years in the archives researching a book which, whilst ultimately an award-winner in Poland,[1] was initially self-published, a testimony to

---

1   The Maria i Łukasz Hirszowicz Award from the Jewish Historical Institute (2018).

Maria's burning desire to ensure that the stories be told, that the tragic sacrifices of the ghetto doctors not be lost in the ashes of time.

Following a republication of Maria's book in Poland, which received excellent reviews, Tali Nates, the founder and director of the Johannesburg Holocaust & Genocide Centre (JHGC), and I resolved to ensure that a more widely accessible English-language version of the book was published. We approached my mother's close friend and retired academic from the Russian and Slavic Studies Department at the University of South Africa, Agata Krzychylkiewicz, to do an English translation for which we are most grateful. The English-language version was then sensitively edited by Jeanette Friedman and by Tali.

Tali taught me that memorialization is a form of justice. In the pursuit of justice, with Tali's encouragement and support, a plaque with Halina's name was commissioned at the JHGC. This book is a continuation of the same pursuit. In this regard, we are deeply grateful to Maria for her outstanding work of scholarship born of a deep sense of empathy with her professional peers from an earlier generation. The Żegota doctors, moved by empathy, reached out across the wall to help their Jewish colleagues in their moment of greatest need. Maria, a true successor to Żegota and motivated by the same empathetic spirit, has reached across the wall of forgetting to bring alive for future generations the marvelous sense of duty and sacrifice that animated the doctors in the Warsaw Ghetto. May they never be forgotten!

Luc Albinski,
Johannesburg, January 23, 2020

A strange dualism characterized the Warsaw Ghetto,
on the one side—certain death and the futility of any endeavor,
on the other—actual work, no matter that it was Sisyphean and hopeless.*

*    Account by Mojżesz Mieczysław Tursz (Thursz), "Jak kształtował się sanitariat w ghetcie warszawskim," YVA O.3/438.

# Preface

Thousands of memoirs have been written during the years since the Second World War ended, tens of thousands of eyewitness testimonies have been recorded, and countless studies have been conducted and published about the Warsaw Ghetto. That notorious ghetto was the 1.3-square-mile area in the middle of one of Poland's major urban centers, Warsaw, where the Germans imprisoned more than half a million Jews between 1940 and 1943 and sent most of them to die in the gas chambers of Treblinka and Auschwitz. But little has been written about the medical care and doctors in the ghetto and how healthcare organizations worked under such terrible conditions, probably because original source materials are scarce.

The title of this study is *The Doctors of the Warsaw Ghetto*. Whilst this study refers exclusively to doctors, rather than to other medical staff, the contributions of nurses or support personnel are not ignored. There are references to the heroic deeds of nurses tending to their emaciated patients—especially those who, without hesitation, rendered assistance on the *Umschlagplatz*, the train platform where the cattle cars came to carry the Jews to Treblinka and their deaths.

This book is the result of a multifaceted examination of the fate of doctors who worked in the Warsaw Ghetto, and an analysis of their fight against epidemics and hunger. Central to these efforts were the ghetto hospitals and the measures that the organized Jewish community (the *Judenrat*), and the Health Council affiliated to it, put in place to prevent and combat epidemics.

There is also information on pharmacies operating in the ghetto. And though the pharmacists could only supply the bare necessities, the doctors and pharmacists shared a common goal of working for their patients' benefit. Considering the circumstances, we will not evaluate the correctness or legitimacy of treatments undertaken, because diseases in the ghetto were primarily related to hunger and seemingly never-ending outbreaks of typhus. The basic methods for treating those illnesses would have been adequate diet and improved sanitary conditions—conditions that could not be met and did not exist in the ghetto.

In principle, the study is limited to the period during which the Warsaw Ghetto existed, from November 1940 until the Ghetto Uprising in April 1943. The focus is on institutions within the borders of the ghetto—excepting the hospital at 109 Leszno Street administered by the *Judenrat*. We also show the career paths medical professionals in Poland had to follow and how changes driven by antisemitism gradually affected the professional standing of Jewish doctors in the interwar period. Our goal is to demonstrate that Jewish doctors in the Warsaw Ghetto created a professional healthcare system in extreme circumstances—a system in which hospitals and polyclinics functioned under horrific conditions, while, at the same time, clandestine medical training and scientific research took place.

These are some of the questions this study strives to answer, not necessarily in this order:

- How was the healthcare system for the Jewish population organized after the outbreak of the Second World War and how did it change after the gates to the ghetto were closed in 1940?
- How many doctors worked in the ghetto, and what was their fate?
- How were polyclinics in the ghetto organized to provide help for outpatients?
- Were hospital departments established in the ghetto?
- How were treatments provided in existing healthcare institutions?
- Were doctors involved in tasks other than their primary duties, for instance, participating in underground education programs or research?

We describe the professional position of Jewish doctors in the period of the Second Polish Republic; the course of their studies during the interwar period; the steps they took to achieve professional accreditation, including their academic titles and degrees, and the process of granting recognition to a degree from a foreign university (nostrification)—with attention paid to the barriers impeding Jews from accessing medical education, and in some cases their conversions to Christianity.

We also discuss the organization of civil administration and healthcare in Warsaw during the first months after the outbreak of the Second World War. Many Jewish doctors participated in defense-related activities during 1939 and were taken prisoner by the Germans or the Soviets. We also focus on conditions in Jewish hospitals in Warsaw when the war broke out, and the care system that the Jewish religious community established and other Jewish community groups implemented.[1] Included is a history of how the Jewish Medical Chamber was established along with an analysis of its role in Jewish self-governing structures.

We describe the healthcare system in the ghetto and how it tried to combat epidemics, including officially recognized training courses presented by a de facto underground medical school. We also examine the scope and aims of non-hospital institutions involving doctors, including medical commissions, polyclinics for employees in the Jewish Police, casualty departments, the Department of Hospitalization, the Chemical and Bacteriological Institute, and the Central Health Council.

In addition, we analyze the work done by doctors in the Warsaw Ghetto hospitals: the Czyste Jewish Infectious Diseases Hospital, the Bersohn and Bauman Children's Hospital and its affiliates. Highlighted are the medical personnel's research on typhus and hunger sickness, along with the doctors' involvement in the deportations and its aftermath. We reveal the fate of several doctors who went into hiding on the Aryan side, as well as a number of those who were deported to the death camps.

The author expresses her gratitude to the chair of the Department of Social Sciences of the Medical University of Silesia in Katowice, Dr. hab. Anna Marek, and the chair of the Institute of History at Rzeszów

---

1   *Gmina wyznaniowa żydowska* (kehillah, Hebrew קְהִילָּה "congregation") was a form of Jewish community organization; it refers to a congregation which is internally coherent, has certain regulatory structures and a governing body to safeguard the community's identity and enforce its laws. This form of organization was regulated not only by the Jewish law but also by the Polish law defining its privileges and the degree of its autonomy.

University, Prof. Dr. hab. Wacław Wierzbieniec, who kindly proffered critical comments and helped with the research.[2]

This heavily edited translation is based on a substantially revised second edition of the Polish original and has been edited as a narrative for general English-reading audiences.

---

2 *Habilitacja* is a postdoctoral degree that qualifies one for a professorship (here abbreviated to "hab.," which indicates the holder of such a degree).

# Chapter 1

# Introduction to the Jewish Community in Poland

The largest Jewish community in Europe, the second largest in the world after the one in America, lived in Poland between the world wars. A 1921 Polish national census counted 2.86 million Jews in a population of 27.2 million; a decade later the Jewish population had risen to 3.1 million in a country of 31.9 million people. Spurred by industrialization in the nineteenth century, Jews moved to the cities. By the late 1930s, nearly one-third of Polish Jews lived in the twelve largest cities, and forty percent lived in towns of at least 10,000 people.[1]

The Jewish economic structure was significantly different from that of their Polish peers. While most ethnic Poles were employed in agriculture, in 1931 about ninety-six percent of Polish Jews worked in non-farm occupations, mainly as artisans, traders, or small shopkeepers. Small minorities were industrialists or members of professions such as medicine or law. Jews were a significantly higher percentage in those professions than the percentage of Jews in the general Polish population. In 1931, fifty-six percent of doctors and one-third of lawyers and other legal professionals were Jewish.[2]

The Jewish population itself was a conglomerate of different levels of observance. There were Polanized Jews who considered themselves an integral part of the Polish nation. There were Bundists, secular Jews who

---

1   Karen Auerbach, "Polish Jewry between the Wars," My Jewish Learning, https://www. myjewishlearning.com/article/polish-jewry-between-the-wars, accessed February 6, 2020.

2   Ibid.

pursued the Jewish values of social justice and were treated with disdain by the Orthodox. There were Zionists, whose loyalties to the Jewish people were encompassed in a passion for the Land of Israel, preparing to physically return to Zion in the near future. The *Hasidim* were deeply religious, dreaming of the Land of Israel in the time of the Messiah, and often, only their *rebbe*, their leader, would be in contact with the powers ruling their environment—whether seventeenth-century noblemen or twentieth-century Polish politicians. Many of these miracle-working *rebbes* would also act as doctors, writing amulets and offering cures, but when it was serious, they would act as go-betweens with legitimate doctors. The *Mitnagadim*, those who opposed the *Hasidim*, were also deeply religious, and preferred little or no interaction with Polish people, but relied on professionals for medical care.

This diversity manifested itself in language differences, too, with Yiddish dialects, German dialects, and even Polish ones being spoken. City Jews, suburban Jews, and country Jews covered every degree on the circle—from total poverty in the *dorfs* (small villages) of the former Pale of Settlement (the western region of imperial Russia that permitted Jewish residency) to rich bankers in the urban centers. Between them, there was incredible difference in terms of religious observance and education.

This may seem confusing, but between the wars, there was a sense that the Jews had multiple identities, which defined how they "fit" into Polish society. Being Jewish meant one had a sense of multiple allegiances—to family, to profession, to friends and fellow Jews, to the country, to ideals and values. In the end, each individual decided where his or her allegiances lay.

Jewish doctors were a unique case because of their professional training and because they worked with non-Jews all the time, together, to save human life. They were already connected to the secular world and modernity and adjusted their religious observance accordingly. Doctors had a higher social standing, as well as greater economic opportunity, and were connected to a professional ethic, one deeply entrenched in Jewish values and best expressed in the Oath of Maimonides[3] and the Oath of Hippocrates.

---

3    Jay W. Marks, "Medical Definition of Oath of Maimonides," Medicine Net, https://www.medicinenet.com/script/main/art.asp?articlekey=7294, accessed February 11, 2020.

Despite this vast Jewish experience between the wars in Poland, and notwithstanding whichever Jewish walk of life one took, Jews felt it was hard to be Jewish. It was, they believed, a form of curse. And so, some professionals who wanted to get ahead in life and provide better lives for their families converted. This was particularly true of medical doctors. Many decided their main allegiance was to their patients.

When Józef Piłsudski ruled Poland in 1926–1935, life was better for the Jews because there were no pogroms during his time in office. Under his administration, citizens were judged by their loyalty to the state, not by nationality, and many assimilated Jews were able to define themselves as "observers of the Mosaic tradition." However, Polish nationalist movements, like *Endecja* and the National Radical Camp, were openly antisemitic and pumped up antisemitism in the public sphere, most effectively outside the urban areas.

When Piłsudski died in May 1935, Polish Jews were devastated[4] and the situation for Jews deteriorated. In Grodno, antisemitic incidents led to the creation of a student self-defense group called Brit HaHayal (Soldier's Alliance) consisting of stronger Jewish youth. Polish high-school students, influenced by the *Endecja movement*, bullied their Jewish peers. The teachers were usually afraid to intervene. Jewish children often fell victim to antisemitic incidents on their way to or from school.[5] Further academic harassment, anti-Jewish riots, and semi-official or unofficial quotas (*numerus clausus*) introduced in 1937 in some universities cut in half the number of Jews in Polish universities in the late 1930s. From 1935 to 1937, seventy-nine Jews were killed and five hundred injured in antisemitic incidents.[6]

The Jewish community was the largest minority in the country but one without a homeland or ambitions for Polish land. It was not as assimilated or connected to the secular and Christian populations around it as were the Jews in Western Europe. There was no interest among Catholic Poles in allying with the Jews in the battles against Nazi Germany, and the Jews themselves, who were, in general, poorer than

---

4   Timothy Snyder, *The Reconstruction of Nations: Poland, Ukraine, Lithuania, Belarus, 1569–1999* (New Haven, CT: Yale University Press, 2003), 144.

5   Joseph Marcus, *Social and Political History of the Jews in Poland, 1919–1939* (Berlin: Walter de Gruyter, 1983), 20.

6   "The History of David-Gorodok Village," sec. 4, Tripod.com.

most of the population, were divided in numerous ways that prevented them from seriously organizing themselves against a common enemy—the Germans.[7]

Because of the antisemitism, pogroms, and discrimination sweeping Europe, as well as difficult economic conditions, by the late 1930s, many Jews were basically indigent, except for those few urban Jews who were industrialists and major merchants. By 1937, Catholic trade unions restricted memberships to Christians only, leaving Jewish doctors and lawyers adrift. Civil service jobs were gone, and Jews were "pensioned" out or fired. In July 1939, *Gazeta Polska*, the unofficial organ of the Polish government, wrote: "The fact that our relations with the Reich are worsening does not in the least deactivate our program with regard to the Jewish question—there is not and cannot be any common ground between our internal Jewish problem and Poland's relations with the Hitlerite Reich."[8]

7   Celia Stopnicka Heller, *On the Edge of Destruction: Jews of Poland between the Two World Wars* (Detroit, MI: Wayne State University Press, 1993).

8   Quoted in Heller, *On the Edge of Destruction*.

# Chapter 2

# The Medical System in Prewar Poland

In the eighteenth century, Poland was divided between Prussia, Austria, and Russia and did not regain its independence for 126 years, until the end of the First World War in 1918. To manage public health, the Polish government had to unify Prussian, Austrian, and Russian healthcare systems, which became the purview of the Ministry of Health, Social Care, and Protection of Work in 1918.[1] Józef Piłsudski, the chief of state, appointed Witold Chodźko as under-secretary of state for the Ministry in December 1918. The Ministry's first mission was to teach the general public basic hygiene and how to prevent the spread of communicable diseases or epidemics.

The Ministry was modeled after the German "Bismarck" system, similar to the healthcare system in America—a combination of private and public insurers. Employers and employees contributed jointly to the *Kasa Chorych* (sickness fund) through payroll deduction, but only wage-earning workers (fourteen percent of the population) benefitted.[2] There was no universal healthcare coverage in Poland before the Second World War: such privileges were limited to small groups of white-collar

1   Paul Puchta, *Polish Healthcare System in Transition—Perceptions of the Old and New Systems* (Main Campus CORE Scholar Master of Public Health Program Student Publications, Wright State University, Detroit, MI, 2014), accessed February 6, 2020.
2   M. Cichon and C. Normand, "Between Beveridge and Bismarck—Options for Health Care Financing in Central and Eastern Europe," *World Health Forum* 15, no. 4 (1994): 323–328, http://www.ncbi.nlm.nih.gov/pubmed/7999215.

workers and government employees. Health insurance premiums were generally paid by employees and, to a certain extent, by large employers. The state did not finance healthcare, with benefits solely dependent on premiums paid by the workers.[3]

In 1924, Józef Piłsudski dissolved the Ministry of Health, dividing its functions between the Healthcare Department of the Ministry of Internal Affairs, the Ministry of Labor and Social Care, the Ministry of Religious Beliefs and Public Enlightenment, the Ministry of Transportation, and other entities.[4] Post-1930, the healthcare institutions were placed under the umbrella of the Ministry of Social Care. The distribution of prophylactics, aimed to combat sexually transmitted diseases and epidemics, and the treatment of the sick became the responsibility of local autonomous authorities, while the *Kasa Chorych* was subordinated to departments in the Ministry. In 1934 the sickness fund system was transformed into *Ubezpieczalnie Społeczne* (social insurers) in order to cut costs, and health insurance was canceled for most rural workers.[5]

In Warsaw, these functions were performed by the Department of Hospitalization and Public Health in 1919–1923, and then by the Department of Social Care and Hospitalization. In 1925, the Department of Social Care and Hospitalization established healthcare centers. In 1934, it merged with the Department of Public Health, and outpatient municipal healthcare was reorganized.[6]

The first medical chambers appeared in Poland already during the partition, in the Austrian and the Prussian parts.[7] Nevertheless, fully functioning self-governed Polish medical institutions were established only once Poland regained its independence. Such medical chambers

---

3   Puchta, *Polish Healthcare System in Transition* .

4   E. Więckowska, "Instytucje Zdrowia Publicznego w II Rzeczpospolitej—organizacja, cele, zadania," *Przegląd Epidemiologiczny* 54, no. 34 (2000): 418.

5   M. Paszkowska, "Finansowanie systemu opieki zdrowotnej w wybranych państwach UE, *e-Finanse* 1 (2006).

6   Z. Podgórska-Klawe, "Warszawa i jej instytucje medyczne w latach 1820–1951," in *Towarzystwo Lekarskie Warszawskie 1820–2005*, ed. Z. Podgórska-Klawe, part 1 (Warsaw: Towarzystwo Lekarskie Warszawskie, 2005), 99; K. Brożek, "Ruch na rzecz podnoszenia kwalifikacji zawodowych polskich lekarzy w latach 1805–1952, Towarzystwa i kursy," *Medycyna Nowożytna* 10, nos 1–2 (2003): 63.

7   T. Nasierowski, *Świat lekarski w Polsce. II połowa XIXw. i pierwsza połowa XX w. Idee, postawy, konflikty* (Warsaw: Okręgowa Izba Lekarska w Warszawie, 1992), 23–32.

were formed in 1921 on the strength of a decree.[8] Permanent representation on, and direct self-governing authority over all medical chambers in the country, were in the hands of the Supreme Medical Council based in Warsaw. It consisted of representatives from the Polish provinces who gathered for the first time on June 9, 1923, to elect the leadership of the Supreme Medical Council.[9] The Supreme Medical Council, an autonomous institution representing doctors, played an essential role during salary negotiations with the Ministry of Labor. Apart from the representatives of the Supreme Medical Council, members of the Association of Doctors of the Polish State, the Union of Doctors in *Kasa Chorych*, the Association of Doctors in Social Insurance in Warsaw, and the directors of *Kasa Chorych* all participated in these talks.

Initially, seven medical chambers were created: in the city of Warsaw, the provinces of Warsaw and Białystok (merged into the Warsaw-Białystok Chamber in 1922), Łódź, Poznań-Pomerania, Lviv (Lwów), Kraków, and Lublin.[10] By order of the minister of Home Affairs, the Vilnius-Nowogród Medical Chamber was formed in 1925, and the Silesian Medical Chamber in 1934. In June 1923, Dr. Jan Bączkiewicz, a long-standing activist in the Association of Polish Doctors and member of the Warsaw Medical Society, was elected the first president of the Supreme Medical Council. He served two terms, 1923–1928. Witold Chodźko was elected for the third and fourth terms (1929–1934), and Prof. Mieczysław Michałowicz was elected for the fifth term (1935–1939).

The Warsaw-Białystok Medical Chamber was comprised of the capital city Warsaw and the Warsaw and Białystok provincial chambers.[11] The respective presidents were doctors Leon Babiński, a general practitioner,

---

8   Ustawa o ustroju i zakresie działania Izb Lekarskich z dn. 2 grudnia 1921 roku, Dz.U. RP no. 105, pos. 763.

9   P. Kordel, *Geneza, struktura i funkcjonowanie samorządu lekarskiego w Polsce w latach 1989–2009* (Doctoral thesis supervised by Prof Dr. hab. Michał Musielak, Institute of Social Studies, Department of Health Sciences, Karol Marcinkowski Medical University, Poznań, 2012), 26.

10  Rozporządzenie Ministra Zdrowia Publicznego z dnia 15 marca 1922 r. o przedmiocie utworzenia Izb Lekarskich. Rozporządzenie Ministra Zdrowia Publicznego z dnia 22 września 1922 roku o przedmiocie zmiany rozporządzenia o utworzeniu Izb Lekarskich.

11  T. Szkudaj, "Izba lekarskaWarszawsko-Białostocka w zbiorach specjalnych Głównej Biblioteki Lekarskiej," *Medycyna Nowożytna* 5, no. 2 (1998): 118.

Jerzy Bujalski, a surgeon and gynecologist (killed in Auschwitz), and Władysław Szenajch, a pediatrician.

On the strength of a directive issued in 1938 by the then minister of Social Care, Marian Zyndram-Kociałkowski, dentists were included in the formal healthcare system, and the territory of Poland was divided into four provincial medical and dental chambers.[12]

One of the tasks assigned to medical chambers was to compile detailed lists of all doctors residing and working in their region. They were overseen by each chamber and employed in the public, self-governed, social insurance, and private sectors. With the help of health departments at the provincial offices, which issued permits for the right to practice to doctors and district doctors, the lists became more comprehensive. Every new arrival was duty-bound to register before being included in the list of chamber members. The responsibilities of regional chambers included fixing consultation fees, even for private medical practice.

## Doctors in Prewar Poland

In 1919, there were 4,300 practicing doctors registered in Poland.[13] Between 1921 and 1935, the number of medical doctors more than doubled, while the general population grew by twenty-three percent. In 1938, there was one doctor for every 448 patients in the capital (only Kraków and Lviv had higher ratios).[14] As a consequence of healthcare deprivation and unhealthy conditions, Poland experienced high adult mortality rates of 13.9 per 1,000 individuals and high infant mortality rates, 139.2 per 1,000 live births during this prewar period.

By 1939, according to the official registry of doctors before the outbreak of the Second World War, there were 12,592 doctors in Poland.[15] In

---

12 Ustawa o ustanowieniu izb lekarsko-dentystycznych; DzURP no. 34, pos. 296.

13 Brożek, "Ruch na rzecz podnoszenia kwalifikacji zawodowych polskich lekarzy," 36.

14 E. Więckowska, *Lekarze jako grupa zawodowa w II Rzeczpospolitej* (Wrocław: Wydawnictwo Uniwersytetu Wrocławskiego, 2004), 48.

15 *Urzędowy spis lekarzy*, Ministry of Social Care (Warsaw, 1939) states that the total number of doctors in Poland was 12,592 persons, and that there were 3,686 dentists. Brożek, "Ruch na rzecz podnoszenia kwalifikacji zawodowych polskich lekarzy," states that in 1945, in Poland, for a population of 23.6 million citizens (one doctor per 3,052 people), there were 7,732 registered doctors. During the war the medical

Warsaw, there were 2,815 doctors and 1,422 dentists registered. Warsaw doctors were, as a rule, employed at one of twenty-three hospitals in specialty departments or at clinics affiliated with Warsaw University, at eleven medical centers and casualty departments, in private practice, or in polyclinics.

## The Education of Doctors in Poland

During the Second Polish Republic, doctors were educated under the supervision of the Ministry of Religious Beliefs and Public Enlightenment at medical faculties of state universities in Warsaw, Kraków, Lviv, Vilnius, and Poznań. When the University of Warsaw reopened in 1915, its Medical Faculty included the Department of Pharmaceutical Studies, which became an independent faculty in 1926.

On October 18, 1920, the minister of Religious Beliefs and Public Enlightenment issued a regulation regrading medical courses at state universities, which defined their range and duration.[16] As a rule, studies lasted five years plus one trimester (sixteen trimesters in total, each ten hours a week), with three trimesters counting towards one course. Initially, these studies were divided into two parts: general and specialized. Each part ended with two final examinations, called the first and second *rigorosum* (oral examinations).[17] The first oral exam, offered after an aspirant completed the initial five years of study, had to be passed within a year. Participation in clinical studies was possible only after a candidate passed the first exam. The second was purely clinical in nature.

From December 2, 1921, regulations were put in place to control the right to practice medicine, and only persons complying with those regulations could call themselves "doctors."[18] They had to hold Polish citizenship, have a medical diploma, complete a one-year internship, and be of

---

community suffered tremendous losses: close to forty percent of Polish doctors died or were murdered in the years 1939–1945.

16  DZ. U. RP no 22, pos. 141. The principles of admission are defined by the act of July 13, 1920 concerning academic institutions, DZ. U. RP, no. 72, pos. 494, inclusive of subsequent codicils.

17  D. Karkowska, *Zawody medyczne* (Warsaw: Wolters Kluwer Polska, 2012), 143.

18  T. J. Zieliński, "Prawo lekarskie Drugiej Rzeczypospolitej w zarysie," *Zeszyty Prawnicze* 11, no. 2 (2011): 404. The act of December 2, 1921, deals with practicing medicine in the Polish State. Dz. U. RP 1921, no. 105, point 762.

sound mind. Anyone seeking to obtain the right to practice as a medical doctor had to register with the Ministry of Public Health and submit the requisite documents, including a diploma and a certificate of completion following the one-year internship. Registration with the Ministry was paramount. It gave its holder the right to be a medical doctor with the relevant regional medical associations.

In 1928, there were more reforms regulating the duration of study and the general curriculum, specifying all activities, subjects, and the number of school hours, as well as compulsory exams (divided into seven groups). All these requirements needed to be met for a candidate to be awarded a medical diploma.[19] The exams were particularly difficult because they were held in public. After passing the final group of exams, a student received a medical diploma, opening the door to advanced studies towards the degree of Doctor of Medicine.

During the interwar period, and at the insistence of the medical fraternity, medical graduates had to undergo a one-year in-house internship. On April 1, 1929, the requirement for a two-year internship to be practiced in villages and small-town communities in order to obtain the right to be called a doctor[20] was enacted to improve professional proficiency.

At the same time, the *Sejm* (lower house of the Polish parliament) adopted legislation outlining the functioning and scope of activities of medical establishments, introducing uniform principles to define the role of these medical self-governing bodies.[21] These acts were enforced for eleven years. In 1932, the president of the Polish Republic issued new regulations, and in 1933 the *Sejm* passed legislation regulating social insurance and medical associations.[22] Among others, these regulations further clarified the exact meaning of "medical practice" and the "medical profession," as well as the principles to adhere to when awarding

---

19  See Zarządzenie Ministra WRiOP z dnia 16 marca 1928 roku w sprawie organizacji studiów lekarskich w uniwersytetach państwowych (Directive by the minister of Religious Beliefs and Public Enlightenment dated March 16, 1928, on the organization of medical studies at state universities).

20  Zieliński, "Prawo lekarskie," 409.

21  Ustawa o ustroju i zakresie działania izb lekarskich z 2 grudnia 1921 r. Dz.U. RP 1921, no. 105, pos. 763.

22  A. Baszkowski, *Od negacji po kompromis. Skutki wprowadzenia powszechnych ubezpieczeń zdrowotnych na życie zawodowe lekarzy polskich do roku 1950* (Poznań: Termedia Wydawnictwa Medyczne, 2015), 24.

professional and academic titles. A directive regulating doctorates in this field was issued in January 1932. Prior to this, universities conferred the title Doctor of All Medical Sciences only on those in professional practice.[23] From 1932, the professional title was doctor (*doktor*), while Doctor of Medicine (*doktor medycyny*) was awarded after a candidate's successful completion of his/her postgraduate doctoral studies.

At the beginning of the twentieth century, the gradual separation between distinct areas of medical specialization became evident by the emergence of specialized scientific societies.[24] Internal medicine developed narrower specializations, such as infectious diseases, dermatology (with venereology), and neurology (with psychiatry). There were (and still are) orthopedic surgeons, gynecologists and otolaryngologists (eye, ear, nose, and throat doctors), and other specializations. This was also controlled by the regulations passed in 1921.

The first body to specify the requirements for specialists was the insurance company, *Kasa Chorych*, which differentiated between the following specializations: internal diseases, neurological diseases, surgery, orthopedics, urology, laryngology, otology (diseases of the ear), rhinology, optometry, gynecology and pediatrics.[25] Candidates were obliged to present scholarly publications or the testimonials of two doctors working for *Kasa Chorych*.

Among the preferred specializations for the Jewish doctors were "non-surgical" fields such as internal diseases, children's diseases, dermatology and venereal diseases, neurology and psychiatry, and radiology. Close to forty-eight percent of Jewish doctors chose those fields, and seventeen percent selected specializations involving surgical procedures, whereas thirty-five percent did not indicate their area of specialization.

---

23 Brożek, "Ruch na rzecz podnoszenia kwalifikacji zawodowych polskich lekarzy," 70. This applied to the older universities (Warsaw, Cracow); Vilnius University was obliged to teach and award degrees in accordance with the new act issued in 1920. However, this was not so in practice.

24 H. Bojczuk, "Wykaz polskich towarzystw i zrzeszeń lekarszkich utworzonych w latach 1918–1940," *Pamietnik Towarzystwa Lekarskiego Warszawskiego* 152, no 20 (2016): 231–247. The author names 292 organizations that emerged post-independence. However, the process of defining those specializations as well as the efforts to introduce them into the medical profession started in the second half of the nineteenth century (see Bożena Urbanek, *Kształtowanie się specjalności lekarskich na ziemiach polskich w latach 1860–1914* [Warsaw: Aspra, 2010]).

25 Więckowska, *Lekarze jako grupa zawodowa*, 143.

Some doctors worked as medical professionals without completing their post-diploma training, the one-year in-house hospital internship.

In 1931, the Supreme Medical Council established a special commission to grant the right to the title of "specialist" based on a doctor's participation in training. Because the commission believed additional requirements to those already imposed on doctors would severely restrict medical professionals,[26] the commission's recommendations to the ministers used the duration of time a candidate had worked in a particular specialization as qualification for licensing. In the interim, the title "specialist" was being awarded by the ministers of Social Care and Religious Beliefs and Public Enlightenment and conferred upon approximately thirty percent of doctors.[27]

In 1934, work began on further reforms. A commission affiliated with the Supreme Medical Council, was tasked with working out reforms for under- and post-graduate students. Chaired by Witold Chodźko, the commission proposed handing over supervision of post-diploma training (the one-year internship) to medical departments at universities, public insurance companies and medical associations.[28] Discussions aimed at implementing further reforms to courses and university education were interrupted by the onset of the Second World War.

## Career Prospects of Doctors in Poland

If a medical student could make it through all the processes and get a coveted diploma, the following documents were to be submitted to the succeeding incarnations of the Ministry of Public Health before starting a professional career: a medical diploma, a certificate of fulfilment of the requirements of a one-year (and later two-year) internship at a hospital and documents confirming Polish citizenship. The Ministry would then issue a written certificate permitting the doctor to register with the regional medical chamber where his/her practice was to be located.

After receiving a permit to practice, doctors could seek employment either as so-called hired doctors (dependent, linked to a specific employer) or as independently practicing doctors. Due to the escalating

---

26  Nasierowski, Świat lekarski w Polsce, 54.
27  Brożek, "Ruch na rzecz podnoszenia kwalifikacji zawodowych polskich lekarzy," 70.
28  Nasierowski, Świat lekarski w Polsce, 55.

economic crisis, the majority of doctors tended to occupy several positions, for instance, working for *Kasa Chorych* and at their own practice simultaneously. Their full-time work in a "hired position" guaranteed them a stable income, the right to a pension, and insurance payouts in case of redundancy. In practice, some doctors working for *Kasa Chorych* were paid on a full-salary basis (from 1930, the so-called family doctors) and some were not.[29]

The best off were Warsaw family doctors who earned between 800 and 900 zlotys per month; a doctor who was head of department in a hospital would receive up to 600 zlotys, and an assistant doctor on a full pay made 300 zlotys per month.[30] The monthly salary of a district doctor was approximately 500 zlotys.[31] Official doctors (state and communal) were in a precarious financial position, paid out of state coffers and serving state employees (such as judges, public prosecutors, police and security officers) and their families. The respective provincial offices concluded agreements with such doctors for their services. As a rule, their monthly salary was slightly more than 200 zlotys. For the sake of comparison, the average monthly remuneration of a teacher was 200–300 zlotys, while an aspiring police officer earned 240 zlotys.[32] According to the *Small Statistical Yearbook* of 1937, in Warsaw, the retail price of a kilogram of bread was thirty-four groszes (a grosz, pronounced *grosh*, equaled 1/100 of a zloty), a kilogram of flour cost sixty groszes, and a liter of milk cost twenty-five groszes. A 10-kilogram bag of coal cost forty-eight groszes, while a kilogram of household soap cost 1.50 zlotys.[33]

Doctors' remuneration varied depending on the positions they held, from around 100 zlotys (for school and official doctors) to over 1,000 zlotys for high-ranking military doctors. Those who practiced

---

29 *Kasa Chorych* institutions were based on the act of June 19, 1920, which introduced compulsory insurance in case of illness. The institutions were territorial in nature, created in every county and town with a population of more than 50,000 inhabitants. Based on a directive issued by the minister of Social Care on December 30, 1933, these institutions became public insurance companies from January 1, 1934. Baszkowski, *Od negacji po kompromis*, 26.

30 Zieliński, "Prawo lekarskie," 407–408.

31 Więckowska, *Lekarze jako grupa zawodowa*, 163.

32 Data from *Mały Rocznik Statystyczny*, published by Główny Urząd Statystyczny Rzeczypospolitej Polskiej (Warsaw, 1937), 259.

33 Ibid., 234.

independently earned the most money serving in provincial practices: over half of them could count on an income of between 300 and 700 zlotys per month.[34] The highest salaries among medical specialists were paid to surgeons, gynecologists, dermatologists, neurologists, and pediatricians, and the lowest, to ophthalmologists, laryngologists, and dentists.[35]

Most doctors practicing during the twenty interwar years understood the need for a healthcare system to serve the society's destitute, yet they were not ready for the consequences of competition with polyclinics run by *Kasa Chorych*. The number of patients using private consultations steadily decreased, leading to a reduction in the income of doctors in private practice. In response to this, organizations were created to act in the name of aggrieved doctors, the two most important being the Medical Chamber and the Association of Doctors of the Polish State.[36]

## Jewish Doctors in Poland

In 1929, Marcin Kacprzak examined the registration cards at the Department of Healthcare that categorized doctors according to nationality and religion. The analysis proved problematic because it showed 11.4 percent of doctors were Jewish, while 33.5 percent professed to be adherents of Mosaic Judaism. This inconsistency existed because Jews in the former Polish Kingdom/Congress Poland of 1815–1832 considered themselves to belong to the Polish nation, whereas in the eastern part of the country being "Jewish" was equated with belonging to the nation of Mosaic Judaism. In 1928, in the province of Warsaw, 33.5 percent of doctors identified as Jewish and adhering to Judaism.[37] In 1938, B. Ostromęcki presented statistical data from various medical chambers, stating that among the doctors registered with the Warsaw-Białystok Medical Chamber, 37.8 percent said they were adherents of Mosaic Judaism, whereas Roman Catholics constituted more than sixty-two percent.[38]

---

34  Więckowska, *Lekarze jako grupa zawodowa*, 168.
35  Ibid.
36  Baszkowski, *Od negacji po kompromis*, 15.
37  Ibid., 57–58.
38  Ibid., 59.

The distribution of Jewish doctors according to specialization is found in the Old Medical Books in the Main Medical Library Archives.[39] The summary is here:

Internal diseases—27 percent
Pediatrics—10.6 percent
Gynecology and Obstetrics—9.8 percent
Dermatology and Venereal Diseases—5.7 percent
Neurology and Psychiatry—3.6 percent
Eye Diseases—3.6 percent
Laryngology—2.65 percent
Urology—0.96 percent
Radiology—0.96 percent

In the second and third decades of the twentieth century, the ratio of doctors per nationality remained fundamentally the same. However, beginning in the 1920s, Jewish doctors—converted or not—were gradually eliminated from most scientific and professional organizations because of antisemitism.[40]

---

39 All data comes from my List of Jewish doctors working and living in Warsaw in 1940–1942, members of the Warsaw-Bialystok Regional Medical Chamber (Lista lekarzy Żydów pracujących i mieszkających na terenie Warszawy w latach 1940–1942 członków Izby Lekarskiej Warszawsko-Białostockiej).
40 A. Cała, H. Węgrzynek, G. Zalewska, *Historia i kultura Żydów polskich. Słownik* (Warsaw: Wydawnictwa Szkolne i Pedagogiczne, 2000), 231.

Chapter 3

# Jewish Doctors and Antisemitism between the Wars

## Antisemitism in Academia

Soon after the end of the First World War, nationalist groups in Poland, Czechoslovakia, and Hungary attempted to introduce *numerus clausus* (quota systems) at institutions of higher learning, affecting Jews and other minorities. In 1920, *numerus clausus* was introduced in Hungary, and in Romania in 1926. The Polish academic community proposed the implementation of the quota system to regulate the ratio of Jewish students to the ratio of Jews in relation to the overall population of the Second Polish Republic (in Poznań this ratio was one percent),[1] and justified it by saying they wanted to prevent Jews from dominating certain professions.

As early as March 19, 1919, the Popular National Association proposed the creation of a committee for Jewish affairs, which would comprehensively examine the "Jewish question."[2] Because students were susceptible to nationalistic and antisemitic slogans eagerly spread by

---

1  Cała et al., *Historia i kultura*, 231; S. Rudnicki, *Równi ale nie zupełnie* (Warsaw: Biblioteka Midrasza, 2008), 137.
2  Rudnicki, *Równi ale nie zupełnie*, 136.

the National Democratic Party, they became a focal point for nationalistic propagation. Thus, All-Polish Youth, created in 1922, assembled proponents of the nationalist program. But despite their expansive politics, members of nationalist organizations were in the minority among the students, the majority of whom did not engage in politics, and only wished to be allowed to study in peace.

In his book *Equal, But Not Entirely*, Szymon Rudnicki divides attempts on the part of the nationalists into three stages:

1. In the 1920s, youth with nationalist leanings, and those in the Academic Youth Association, strove to influence students and faculty at institutions of higher learning.
2. In the first half of the 1930s, the slogan *numerus nullus* (a complete exclusion of Jews) replaced *numerus clausus*, and the battle for the "Jewish Bench" began.
3. The second half of the 1930s was characterized by the success of the newly implemented policies and intensified efforts in pursuit of keeping Jews out of universities and by the introduction of the Aryan clause.[3]

Student members of the self-help organization Brotherly Help at Poznań University joined with the Academic Youth Association and other academic fraternities to create the National Bloc and passed a resolution to ban Jews from their collegiate organizations.[4] The first city to limit the number of Jews accepted at institutions of higher learning was Lviv, where concerns were voiced about the "Jewification" of the university as early as October 1922. At the same time, they asked that those who distinguished themselves in the struggle to preserve Polish nationhood be given priority in admissions. They also proposed *numerus clausus* be implemented in accordance with the Jewish ratio to the country's entire population.[5]

---

3  Ibid.
4  Ibid.
5  A. Graboń, *Problematyka żydowska na łamach prasy akademickiej w okresie międzywojennym* (Kraków: Wydawnictwo Naukowe Uniwersytetu Mikołaja Kopernika, 2008), 134. In the years 1922/1923, Jewish students in Warsaw in all departments made up thirty-four percent of the total cohort. See Piotr M. Majewski,

We learn from Emanuel Ringelblum that when he applied to the Medical Faculty at Warsaw University in 1920, a note on his application read: "Not accepted on the grounds of *numerus clausus*."[6] In 1922, Ringelblum was registered as a student of philology—a course he completed five years later with a diploma in history. It is likely he intended to study medicine after one year, as several other unsuccessful applicants had done, but it is equally possible that his interests had changed.

The contemporary Jewish press wrote: "Practical faculties such as Medical Studies and Pharmaceutics were inaccessible, that is why someone would go with the flow and choose the semi-practical Law Faculty. However, in recent years we have noted a curious evolution. The youth enter university 'just like that . . . to obtain a certificate.'"[7] According to Warsaw University data, a quarter of applicants refused entry to the Medical Faculty would register at another faculty in the very same year.[8]

From the data I collected in the Old Medical Books Division, and the table "List of Jewish doctors working and residing in the territory of Warsaw between 1940–1942, members of the Warsaw-Białystok Medical Chamber," of the 831 Jewish doctors registered, 431 (fifty-two percent) had graduated from the Medical Faculty at Warsaw University, 38 (4.5 percent) from Vilnius, 23 (2.7 percent) from Lviv, 16 (1.9 percent) from Kraków and 4 (0.5 percent) from Poznań. Almost forty percent of the group of 831 doctors studied abroad, perhaps because of the increasingly negative attitudes towards Jewish students in Poland. Even though no official resolutions to limit the number of Jewish entrants could be ascribed to any faculty at the Warsaw University, the fact that such limitations were in place is clear from rector's reports and occasional publications.[9] These annotations and references to limitations, applicable only to certain faculties and not only to Jews, were, in practice, synonymous with *numerus clausus* directed at Jewish students.[10]

ed., *Dzieje Uniwersytetu Warszawskiego 1915–1945* (Warsaw: Wydawnictwa Uniwersytetu Warszawskiego, 2016), 143.

6  Ibid., 148.

7  Ibid., 153. Quoted from S. Szwerdszarf, "Ani 'alma' ani 'mater'. Reportaż o studentach-Żydach," *Nasz Przegląd* 20, October 10, 1936.

8  Ibid., 205.

9  Majewski, *Dzieje Uniwersytetu Warszawskiego 1915–1945*, 148.

10  Besides the Jews, there were very few other religious minorities at the Warsaw University, chiefly Ukrainians who studied Russian Orthodox Theology. The

In June 1923, the so-called "Polish majority" triumphed in the *Sejm*, which was controlled by the National Peoples' Union and the Polish Peoples' Party. A common principle of both organizations was to ensure access for Polish youth to tertiary and secondary institutions, as well as vocational schools, "in accordance with legitimate ratios among the various nationalities in the state."[11] After drafting questionnaires at tertiary institutions, parliament's Education Commission adopted a resolution limiting admission (of Jews) to universities, justifying the decision because three-quarters of the faculties called for the implementation of *numerus clausus*, either conditionally or unconditionally.[12] The proposal was rejected because it contradicted the treaty on minorities and the country's constitution—and led to objections from the Rules Committee and opposition from the League of Nations.[13]

However, in a circular issued in July 1923, the minister of Religious Beliefs and Public Enlightenment in Wincenty Witos's administration and the former president of the Peoples' National Union, Stanisław Głąbiński, instructed tertiary institutions to limit admission of Jewish students. The implementation was hampered by the so-called May Coup.[14]

In 1927, the new minister of Religious Beliefs and Public Enlightenment in Bartel's government—Antoni Sujkowski—voided the Głąbiński circular and withdrew the right of faculty boards to define admission limits. His successor, Gustaw Dobrucki, maintained a similar position, stating emphatically that Marshal Piłsudski's government opposed any such restrictions. Despite this, the National Bloc continued its attempts to restrict the admission of Jews. In the weekly *National Motto*, published in Kraków, a February 1927 article, "Injustice to Jews

---

percentage of students with non-Polish or Jewish nationalities did not exceed four percent. Ibid., 154.

11  Rudnicki, *Równi ale nie zupełnie*, 141.

12  Majewski, *Dzieje Uniwersytetu Warszawskiego 1915–1945*, 147.

13  A. Jaskóła, *Sytuacja prawna mniejszości żydowskiej w drugiej Rzeczypospolitej* (PhD dissertation supervised by Dr. Jacek Przygodzki, Faculty of Law, Administration, and Economics, Institute of State History and Law, Wrocław University, Wrocław, 2010), 68.

14  May coup (*Przewrót majowy*) was an armed coup in Poland carried out by Józef Piłsudski on May 12–15, 1926, in Warsaw. The reason for the attack was the deteriorating political and economic situation of the country, and its immediate cause, a series of cabinet crises in the years 1925–1926.

at Universities, but Actually the Numbers Say Otherwise," reported that at Lviv's Jan Kazimierz University, doctorates were awarded to twelve graduates in January of that year, ten of whom were Jews. The author cites as evidence that, in February alone, of the nine doctors promoted at the Medical Faculty of Warsaw University, six had Jewish-sounding surnames. He wrote:

> Medicine is the most expensive of all faculties. It demands absolute devotion to the field of study, so a student has no time to seek an additional income. Such studies require expensive, difficult-to-obtain books and instruments, are of the longest duration, exhausting, and require a great deal of energy. Polish youth, who are as a rule materially handicapped, avoid this faculty. Their places are taken by Jews who are either better off, materially speaking, or are supported by Jewish organizations. This singular fact needs to be pointed out. We cannot remain indifferent to a phenomenon so disadvantageous to our [national] spiritual wellbeing. We are the rightful hosts in this land, not tenants. Accordingly, we must occupy important public posts. It is not antisemitism nor is it chauvinism, but rather mindfulness that, without a Polish intelligentsia, Poland would not be Polish.[15]

On April 23, 1927, at the Conference of Rectors of State Academic Institutions, Prof. Leon Marchlewski, rector of Jagiellonian University, disclosed the university admitted only twelve or thirteen Jews for every hundred students.[16] Minister Dobrucki told him it was contrary to government policy. Ultimately, conference participants voted to reject official implementation of *numerus clausus*. But the All-Polish Youth did not give up and in May 1927, during the Fifth Assembly of the National Association of Academic Youth, the newly elected leadership was determined to demand academic and state institutions impose formal admissions quotas.

---

15  "Krzywda żydowska na uniwersytetach tylko w świetle faktycznych cyfr," *Hasło Narodowe*, February 20, 1927.

16  Rudnicki, *Równi ale nie zupełnie*, 142.

For years, this demand was raised by various collegiate bodies, and would frequently incite conflict and brawls.[17] This was aggravated at the beginning of the 1930s with almost half the representatives in so-called free professions across the country being ethnic Poles, while the other half were Jews. The remaining national minorities were a tiny percentage of the population. In the eastern territories of the Second Polish Republic, this ratio was even less favorable for Poles: among the representatives of the free professions, Jews were markedly in the majority.[18]

The nationalist *Endecja* group called this the "Jewification of the Polish intelligentsia," and accused the Jews of being partially responsible for the economic crisis in the country. In various antisemitic attacks, Jews were portrayed as opponents and exploiters, while doing away with Jewish competition was attractive to Polish manufacturers and Polish doctors.[19]

The greatest antisemitic activity at universities came from Poles inspired by Italian fascism, which captivated youths opposed to Piłsudski and his parliamentary government. In addition, there were blatant manifestations of antisemitism and efforts by the Association of Doctors of the Polish State to persuade Poles to only use Christian doctors. Polish patients, however, preferred the expertise of Jewish doctors, believing that their foreign education made them excellent specialists. Having knowledge of foreign languages and being members of international medical societies, these doctors participated in training and conferences aimed at honing their knowledge and skills.

In November 1926, Bernard Rusiecki, a representative of Catholic student organizations at Stefan Batory University in Vilnius addressed a mass rally inspired by the dearth of Jewish cadavers for study at the university. To thunderous applause and a standing ovation from hundreds of fellow students, he declared that Jews posed a danger to Christian values and that no Jewish cadavers proved the Jews were arrogant and morally deficient. "For us—Christians—a corpse represents the majesty of death.

---

17  A. Srebrakowski, "Sprawa Wacławskiego. Przyczynek do historii relacji polsko-żydowskich na Uniwersytecie Stefana Batorego w Wilnie," *Przegląd Wschodni* 9, bk. 3, no. 35 (2004): 580.

18  Ibid., 579.

19  On competition in the job market—especially in medical services professions—see Majewski, *Dzieje Uniwersytetu Warszawskiego 1915–1945*, 207, 221–222, 264, 281.

Let the Jews who have no respect for cadavers dissect Jewish cadavers. But hands off Christian cadavers! Christian corpses for the Christians!"[20]

In keeping with the tenets of Judaism, Jews could not have autopsies. They buried the dead as soon as possible. A post-mortem was permitted only if it could save the life of another, or if required under local law, but even then, intervention had to be minimal. Because various associations aligned with the Jewish religious communities carried the burden of burying homeless and indigent Jews, only cadavers of Christians found their way into dissecting rooms. Polish students considered this situation unjust, demanded corpses of Jews also be sent for dissection, and threatened to bar Jewish students from accessing the university morgue.

According to Natalia Aleksiun, antisemitic student organizations like Renaissance stepped up pressure on the cadaver issue and continued to spew antisemitic rhetoric. They demanded, in the name of fairness, that Jewish communities provide cadavers for Jewish medical students. There was already a lack of cadavers for courses in descriptive anatomy, and a call went out for any cadavers so medical students could continue their work.[21] Aleksiun notes that some historians of Polish-Jewish relations called this issue a case of "practical antisemitism," a convenient ruse designed effectively to bar Jews from medical departments at Polish universities. That included preventing Jewish students from touching Christian cadavers.[22]

As Aleksiun notes:

Analysis of the discourse surrounding the controversy suggests that there was far more at issue than merely the balance of

---

20 Natalia Aleksiun, "Students and Christian Corpses in Interwar Poland: Playing with the Language of Blood Libel," *Jewish History* 26 (2012): 327–342.

21 Aleksiun, "Students and Christian Corpses in Interwar Poland." See letters from academic authorities in 1936 requesting the assistance of local hospitals and representatives of local administrations in Warsaw, Kraków, Lviv, and Vilnius in Archiwum Uniwersytetu Jagiellonskiego (henceforth AUJ; Archives of Jagiellonian University), WL II 142, Katedra i zakład anatomii opisowej, Zwłoki ludzkie dla prosektorium.

22 Aleksiun, "Students and Christian Corpses in Interwar Poland." See also Szymon Rudnicki, "From 'numerus clausus' to 'numerus nullus,'" in *From Shtetl to Socialism: Studies from "Polin,"* ed. Antony Polonsky (London: Liverpool University Press, Littman Library of Jewish Civilization, 1993), 359–381; and Graboń, *Problematyka żydowska na łamach prasy akademickiej,* 163–167.

national and cultural hegemony within the nation's academic and medical establishments. Indeed, this single, foreseeable conflict over a restriction that Jewish law imposed on Jews inspired right-wing Polish students, journalists, and ideologues to portray Jews not only as a menace to the country's political, economic, and cultural interests but also as a moral threat to Christians in general.[23]

The antisemitic students also implied that Jewish medical students and Jewish people in general acquired a sense of religious superiority from "these denominationally biased dissections, a condition . . . perceived to endanger Christian dignity."[24]

> Thus, wielding the example of the allegedly nefarious activities of Jewish medical students, Polish activists were inspired by economic and social competition. Stirred by the rallying cry, "Christian corpses for the Christians!" they combined modern racial science with traditional prejudicial attitudes to argue in essence that any contact between Jews and non-Jews was dangerous, even after death. . .[25]

Finally, on June 26, 1926, the chair of Anatomy at the Warsaw University, Prof. Edward Loth, issued a circular stating that Jewish students could practice in dissecting rooms only if the Jewish community supplied the cadavers.[26] In effect, the regulation meant many Jewish students would be excluded from medical instruction or forced out of medical training

---

23 Aleksiun, "Students and Christian Corpses in Interwar Poland." For a general discussion of the Catholic press in the Second Polish Republic and its treatment of the Jews, see Ronald Modras, "The Catholic Press in Interwar Poland on the 'Jewish Question': Metaphor and the Developing Rhetoric of Exclusion," *East European Jewish Affairs* 24, no. 1 (1994): 49–70; Anna Landau-Czajka, "The Jewish Question in Poland: Views Expressed in the Catholic Press between the Two World Wars," *Polin* 11 (1998): 263–278; Dariusz Libionka, "Obcy, wrodzy, niebezpieczni: Obraz Żydów i 'kwestii żydowskiej' w prasie inteligencji katolickiej lat trzydiestych w Polsce," *Kwartalnik Historii Żydów* 203 (2002): 318–338.

24 Aleksiun, "Students and Christian Corpses in Interwar Poland."

25 Ibid.

26 Despite his prewar stance, during the war Prof. Loth helped organize underground education in the ghetto and saved numerous Jews, for which he was awarded the "Righteous among the Nations" medal. He was murdered during the Warsaw Uprising of 1944.

programs, a result that would have fit in well with the goals of the right-wing student organizations and political parties in the Second Polish Republic calling for *numerus clausus*.

During the 1925/1926 academic year, the first Jewish cadaver was supplied to the Faculty of Descriptive Anatomy at Stefan Batory University in Vilnius.[27] To calm an already tense situation, on October 25, 1926, the Christian organizations assembling students from all medical faculty courses penned a memorandum on the supply of Jewish corpses to dissecting rooms. They complained about the lack of Jewish cadavers, while the percentage of Jewish students was emphasized.[28] They failed. None of the petitions written to the state and university authorities bore any fruit. But during the 1926/1927 academic year, the Christian students' protests intensified.[29]

On December 17, 1926, the Warsaw University faculty senate decided that "students of the Mosaic Faith" would be allowed to participate in classes at the Institutes of Descriptive and Topographic Anatomy and Surgery only "to the extent possible" and "in accordance with the delivery of a "Jewish contingent" of corpses."[30] To calm the waters, on November 4, 1927, the university senate resolved that students would be banned from interfering in matters related to human specimens.

---

27  The table appended to Srebrakowski, "Sprawa Wacławskiego," clearly shows that prior to the 1924/1925 academic year only the corpses of Christians were available, but thereafter the percentage of Jewish bodies increased from 3.57 in 1925/1926 to 6.12 in 1931/1932. Jewish students studying medicine at Stefan Batory University in 1931/1932 made up 33.8 percent of the student cohort, which emphasizes the imbalance between student numbers and the number of corpses. See A. Srebrakowski, "Sprawa Wacławskiego. Przyczynek do historii relacji polsko-żydowskich na Universytecie Stefana Batorego w Wilnie," *Przegląd Wschodni* 9, bk. 3, no. 35 (2004): 582. The data are based on the table in "Proceedings of Activities in the Institute of Descriptive Anatomy, USB in Vilnius in the Academic Year 1931/1932; Composition (by nationality, transl.) at the University in the Years 1927/1928 and Composition at the University in the Years 1933/1934 and changes that took place in the Years 1929/1930, 1930/1931, 1931/1932, 1932/1933, Vilnius" (no date), Stefan Batory University Archives, Sygn. F.175, Ap. IA, B. 312, p. 326.

28  For more on the Jewish national minority at Stefan Batory University in Vilnius as well as the issue of corpses, see Bożena Urbanek, "Mniejszości narodowe na Wydziale Lekarskim Uniwersytetu Stefana Batorego," *Rocznik Stowarzyszenia Naukowców Polaków Litwy* 17 (2017): 47–72.

29  Srebrakowski, "Sprawa Wacławskiego," 582.

30  Ibid.

Despite this, students belonging to the Camp of Great Poland continued to call attention to the "question of corpses" as part of their anti-Jewish campaigns.[31]

According to Aleksander Rosner of the Jagiellonian University, the critical shortage of cadavers was a result of "increased concern of the family with the funeral" and the improved standard of living of the general population in villages. He wrote a secret letter to the Ministry of Religious Affairs and Education, dated April 11, 1929, asking them to tell family members of any faith if they did not claim the bodies within forty-eight hours of being pronounced dead, Polish law said the cadavers could be confiscated for use in medical schools.[32]

In the fall of 1931, protests erupted at the Jagiellonian University in Kraków and at Warsaw University. Anti-Jewish unrest continued with tacit approval from most students, academic staff and other university personnel. In November 1931, the then dean of the Medical Faculty at Warsaw University, Prof. Ludwik Paszkiewicz, gave in to the demands of right-wing students, instructing Jewish students be granted access only to the bodies of dead Jews. Ludwik Krzywicki, head of the department in the history of social systems section at Warsaw University and the Institute of Social Economics, recalled that while some professors sympathized with the brawling students, others chose to remain uninvolved.[33] His opinion was shared by his colleague, philosopher and ethicist, Prof. Tadeusz Kotarbiński.

A few organizations objected as well, including the Union of Independent Socialist Youth, Life, the Legion of the Young, the Union of Democratic Youth, and the collegiate association Wici.[34] Condemnation also came from the world of culture and journalism, from Antoni Sobański, Maria Dąbrowska and others. In February 1936, the minister of Religious Beliefs and Public Enlightenment, Wojciech Świętosławski, declared that he would not allow a "handful of politicized youth to

---

31  The question of "Jewish cadavers" was mainly on the agenda of the youth associated with the Camp of Great Poland (established in 1926). After it was disbanded, the National-Radical Camp was convened in 1934. After the split, their program with its anti-Jewish stance, was taken up by the National Radical Movement. Among its slogans were calls to free Polish culture and education from the Jews.

32  Ibid.

33  Srebrakowski, "Sprawa Wacławskiego," 267.

34  Rudnicki, *Równi ale nie zupełnie*, 149.

prevent the great majority of students from getting on with their work in a peaceful manner."[35] A year later he said that "Jewish Benches" were untenable. He lost both arguments.

The "Jewish Benches" were another attempt to alienate and dehumanize Jewish medical students. In 1937 several Polish universities accepted the ten percent cap on Jewish students, while Minister Świętosławski permitted university rectors to apply organizational measures they deemed necessary to limit escalating conflicts. University rectors held a conference in October 1937 and instituted what became known as "bench ghettos."[36] From that moment on, Jewish students were obliged to sit on designated benches, usually on the left of the lecture hall. In the Medical Faculty of Warsaw University, those were the benches with uneven numbers.[37] In *Winter in the Morning*, Zofia Bauman, a Jewish-Polish writer wrote:

> Even before I came into this world, my parents decided that, in the future, in accordance with family tradition, I would become a doctor. That much was obvious to me from my earliest years. But those plans were under threat. In the Poland of the 1930s, it was difficult for me to gain admission to study medicine. It was close to impossible for Jewish youths. Even though universities did not introduce *numerus nullus*, there was a clause limiting the number of Jews admitted to study, especially prestigious disciplines such as medicine. It seemed that the only chance of being accepted at a medical faculty was to obtain a certificate after completing a government secondary public-school education. But here, too, the same obstacle lay in wait: the number of Jewish children admitted to government high schools was strictly limited. To be accepted, one had to be very gifted and pass the entry exams with the highest marks.[38]

---

35  Ibid., 150.
36  An unconfirmed hypothesis infers that during the same conference a confidential resolution was taken to limit the number of Jews admitted to tertiary institutions. Majewski, *Dzieje Uniwersytetu Warszawskiego 1915–1945*, 148.
37  At Warsaw University, "Jewish Benches" were introduced by the rector, Włodzimierz Antoniewicz. See A. Garlicki, ed., *Dzieje Uniwersytetu Warszawskiego 1915–1939* (Warsaw: Wydawnictwa Uniwersytetu Warszawskiego, 1982), 279–280.
38  J. Bauman, *Zima o poranku* (Kraków: Znak, 1989), 16–17.

Anna Jaskóła, in "[The] Legal Position of the Jewish Minority in the Second Polish Republic," wrote that in 1922/1923 there were 191 Polish-speaking public schools, which Jewish children could attend.[39] Only a small number attended separate schools. In time, the number of Jewish children attending interfaith schools increased, while the number of single-denomination schools gradually decreased. This led to numerous objections from right-wing groups, whose followers expressed a wish to separate Jewish and Polish youths. The alternatives were private schools offering instruction in Polish. Those schools had numerous advocates in Jewish communities, since learning in the official language better equipped youth for continuing education at tertiary institutions, a goal of many.

When applying for first-year university entrance, even if Jewish candidates presented excellent grades, they would not matriculate. This is evident in the marks appearing next to each candidate's surname in the registers. Jews who applied to study medicine at Warsaw University demonstrated statistically higher average points (3.73) than Poles (3.68), in large part thanks to the contribution of female candidates (3.84 average).[40]

Youth representatives and academic staff expressed opinions on the "bench ghettos": Some saw it as an ideal solution to the Jewish question, while others harshly criticized it. The segregation of students on the grounds of faith was opposed by several professors of medical departments, among them the president of the Supreme Medical Council, Prof. Mieczysław Michałowicz, and professors Jan Mazurkiewicz, Franciszek Czubalski, Franciszek Venulet, Kornel Michejda (in Vilnius), and Franciszek Raszeja (in Poznań). At the time, Prof. Czubalski was dean of Medicine at Warsaw University, but when in 1936 he was elected as university rector, he rejected the honor following remonstrations from students.

Prof. Michałowicz officially protested the notion of "bench ghettos" on October 19, 1937. In a speech he gave in the main auditorium of the Pediatrics Department at Warsaw University, he expressed the wish to remain faithful to his Christian conscience. During another speech in the

---

39  Jaskóła, *Sytuacja prawna mniejszości żydowskiej*, 50.
40  Majewski, *Dzieje Uniwersytetu Warszawskiego 1915–1945*, 203.

Senate, he stated: "I appeal to the minister to be kind enough to remind the gentlemen professors—as I have been doing for many years—that scientific dignity is no small matter, that peace in the temple of work means more than the privilege of university extraterritoriality."[41] He was appalled by the impunity afforded to perpetrators, and incessantly emphasized that attempts to avoid meting out punishment were demoralizing.[42] When in the Pediatrics auditorium, the chairman of the circle of medical students requested that separate seating be assigned for Jews, Michałowicz replied that even though he respected the position of the rector, he personally held a different opinion. The *Endecja* press responded by demanding his removal as president, to prevent him from treating children or conducting research.[43] Church representatives, prelates Seweryn Poławski and Marceli Nowakowski, wrote an open letter expressing their support for the right-wing youths.[44] Prof. Michałowicz's adversaries claimed he is "the terrified Israel's man of providence, a modern Moses and Yeshua (*Jozue*)," and called him a "notorious Freemason."[45] Other professors who defended Jewish students were warned they would be left "without listeners."[46]

In November 1937, violent riots at Warsaw University ended with the police recapturing the Auditorium Maximum from a right-wing militia. Despite this, the perpetrators were treated leniently, with only a few ringleaders expelled while witnesses testifying against them were accused of lying and displaying pro-Communist leanings. In most cases the university management did not punish the perpetrators who used knuckle-dusters, nightsticks and razors in their brutal attacks. Prof. Hirszfeld noted: "Students lashed out at their colleagues to kill them. Professor-democrats were forced to escape through windows so as not to be beaten up by these unruly striplings, while the principals gushed

41  W. Barcikowski, "Polityk i społecznik," in *Mieczysław Michałowicz—człowiek, działacz, polityk*, vol. 1 (Warsaw: Epoka, 1972), 106.

42  M. H. Serejski, "Lekarze o humanistycznym obliczu," in *Mieczysław Michałowicz—człowiek, działacz, polityk*, vol. 1 (Warsaw: Epoka, 1972), 213.

43  Barcikowski, "Polityk i społecznik," 107.

44  Rudnicki, *Równi ale nie zupełnie*, 155.

45  Jaskóła, *Sytuacja prawna mniejszości żydowskiej*, 78.

46  Graboń, *Problematyka żydowska na łamach prasy akademickiej*, 197–198.

in speeches about their darling youths and prevented the police from re-establishing order."[47]

In December 1937, sixty lecturers from three Polish universities signed a collective protest (among them, twenty professors and six docents of the total 312 independent academic employees at Warsaw University).[48] In 1938, the rector of the Jan Kazimierz University in Lviv, Prof. Stanisław Kulczyński, refused to introduce "bench ghettos" and resigned in protest. His stance was officially supported by the remaining rectors of the Polish universities, except for Poznań. Nevertheless, on January 7, 1938, the newly appointed rector of Lviv University, Prof. Roman Longchamp de Bérier, signed an ordinance approving "bench ghettos".[49] Dr. Adina Blady-Szwajger (after the war, Świdowska), who studied during the second half of the 1930s, recalled:

> . . . I must have been in my third course [when] the "bench ghetto" started. One day, our record books were taken away and, when we got them back, there was a purple stamp inside saying: "Seating on uneven-numbered benches." Well, we did not sit down until the end of our studies. There were only two halls where we would sit—at psychiatry lectures with Prof. Mazurkiewicz, who forbade the numbering of benches, and at Prof. Michałowicz, who emphasized that he was a senator of the Polish Republic, and no inspector would order him around. A few lecturers of Jewish origin would also stand with us.[50]

In 1938, anti-Jewish policies and the Aryan clause (first initiated in Łódź in 1935) in the medical fraternity led to admission limits and Jews not being appointed to academic posts. At Warsaw University, the Association of Assistants adopted the Aryan clause by asking the rector not to appoint Jews to positions of professor, docent, or assistant.[51]

---

47 L. Hirszfeld, *Historia jednego życia* (Warsaw: Pax, 1967), 253.
48 D. Mycielska, "Postawy polityczne profesorów wyższych uczelni w dwudziestoleciu międzywojennym," in *Inteligencja polska XIX i XX wieku*, ed. R. Czepullis-Rastenis (Warsaw: Instytut Historii PAN, 1985), 328–329.
49 J. Draus, *Uniwersytet Jana Kazimierza we Lwowie 1918–1946. Portret kresowej uczelni* (Kraków: Księgarnia Akademicka, 2007), 65–66.
50 A. Grupińska, *Ciągle po kole. Rozmowy z żołnierzami getta warszawskiego* (Warsaw: Czarne, 2000), 183.
51 Majewski, *Dzieje Uniwersytetu Warszawskiego 1915–1945*, 278.

This is why many Jewish doctors converted—for the sake of job security. Similar regulations were applied at the Association of Medics at Warsaw University, where on March 8, 1938, the clause was included in its charter and barred Jews from membership. Its provisos referred to Orthodox Jews up to the third generation, regardless of gender.[52]

Tadeusz Kielanowski, a pulmonologist and phthisiologist (the care, treatment, and study of tuberculosis of the lung; today the discipline has merged with pulmonologist) who studied and worked in Lviv, wrote the following in his *Almost the Entire Twentieth Century: Memoirs of a Doctor*:

> Jews escaped the Nazi Reich wherever they could, fleeing to Poland, *inter alia*, but it was fashionable to adopt the "Aryan clause," in other words, to exclude Jews from every possible association, even from scholarly societies. At one point such a clause was even adopted by the Association of Assistants at Jan Kazimierz University, where its noble President, Marian K., was forced to inform his closest and esteemed colleagues. He chose to evade the matter, stating that he wished to kindly inform his respected colleagues that, given changes to the organizational statute, they were no longer members of their organization. Among others, such a letter was received by docent Leopold Infeld, who at the time was in North America. Later, the president showed me a card [written by Prof. Infeld], which read: "Why are you ashamed to say outright that I am a Jew?"[53]

Next came the demand not to employ Jewish doctors in state and self-governing hospitals (excluding Jewish hospitals), which was implemented across Poland, forcing Jewish doctors to go into private practice.[54] In 1931, fifty-five percent of doctors in private practice were Jews.[55]

---

52  Jaskóła, *Sytuacja prawna mniejszości żydowskiej*, 84.

53  Kielanowski, *Prawie cały wiek dwudziesty. Wspomnienia lekarza* (Gdańsk: Krajowa Agencja Wydawnicza, 1978), 106–107.

54  Data supplied by Nasierowski, *Świat lekarski w Polsce*, 170, citing J. Żarnowski, *Struktura społeczna inteligencji w Polsce w latach 1918–1939* (Warsaw: PWN, 1964), 262.

55  Ibid., 262; W. Odrzywolski, "Charakterystyka zatrudnienia lekarzy w Polsce," *Materiały Komisji Studiów TPMA* 9 (1937): 168; L. Dydyński, "Niebezpieczne zażydzenie zawodu lekarskiego," *Życie Lekarskie* 11 (1939): 170–173.

Some Jewish students opted to enter foreign universities, intending to resume their education in Poland. During the first years of the Second Polish Republic, many medical faculties were free from regulations controlling nostrification (the process of starting medical school in one country and finishing in another). On April 14, 1922, the minister of Religious Beliefs and Public Enlightenment, in agreement with the Ministry of Public Health, issued restrictions and instructed the faculty board to evaluate foreign diplomas by scrutinizing the qualifications and determining if they were comparable to the requirements of Polish universities. If the conditions were acceptable, the applicant could apply to have his/her credentials recognized.[56] At the start of the 1930s, the number of students applying to have their foreign diplomas evaluated at Warsaw University increased, probably because many who left to study abroad were returning. During the 1925/1926 academic year, eighteen evaluations took place, four years later there were twenty, and in 1932/1933, there were forty-one cases, of which only nine had successful outcomes.[57]

Thanks to data in my "List of Doctors in the Warsaw-Białystok Medical Chamber" (see appendices to this book) it was possible to calculate that, among the aforementioned 831 Jews registered during 1940–1942, 317 studied abroad, but only 99 (11.9 percent) had their diplomas evaluated before the war. Of this group, 5.12 percent received evaluations from Warsaw University. Among the ninety-nine assessed, three had their credentials evaluated in two countries: Julia Blay, who studied in Zurich, was evaluated in Kazan and Warsaw; of the two who studied in Geneva, Józef Cygielstrejch was evaluated in Moscow and Warsaw, and Helena Gabay, in St. Petersburg and Warsaw.

By the 1920s, the Medical Faculty of Warsaw University understood perfectly why the Jews preferred to have their foreign diplomas evaluated, and so they kept petitioning government officials to forbid the practice. To this end, the faculty board adopted a special resolution, handed to the Ministry of Religious Beliefs and Public Enlightenment on September 23, 1925, and to faculty boards at other universities, before publishing it in the press.[58] The resolution read:

---

56  Więckowska, *Lekarze jako grupa zawodowa*, 134–135.
57  Ibid., 206.
58  Majewski, *Dzieje Uniwersytetu Warszawskiego 1915–1945*, 206.

The matter of medical faculties having to evaluate the credentials of foreign diplomas has become an important social issue, due to the number of applications and the fact that the applicants are alien elements, not desirable in society. . . When deciding to implement the *numerus clausus*, medical faculties at our universities were guided not only by the capacity of their institutes, but also by the capacity of the region and the work security of future graduates. The large number of successful applicants nullifies the calculations on which the medical faculties' *numerus clausus* computations are based. In future, this may lead to a lowering of the standards of doctors' welfare, converting them into the proletariat class among the *intelligentsia*, which is, socially speaking, a very dangerous development. . . . The Faculty of Medicine at Warsaw University believes that the need for doctors in this country is presently fully satisfied, albeit that when compared to culturally more advanced Western countries, their ratio to the population is lower. This can largely be explained by the lower standards of living in Poland, and an inadequate understanding of sanitary needs. . . . It is our conviction that the number of doctors completing medicine in Poland satisfies the demand for doctors in this country, for both the present and the future. The faculty believes that, to prevent an oversaturation of specialists in this field, any further evaluation of diplomas issued by foreign universities should be discontinued, unless the significant scholarly achievement of a foreign candidate can bring the country tangible benefits.[59]

In most cases, applications from Jews were consistently rejected by tacit agreement.[60] Despite difficulties in obtaining a medical qualification in Poland, and (over time) increasingly antisemitic policies at universities, the contribution of Jewish doctors, when calculated in percentage

---

59  Ibid., 206–207. Cited after Warsaw University Archives, RP/WL 3, from the letter by the dean of Medical Faculty dated September 23, 1925. The position of dean in the medical faculty at Warsaw Unversity in the 1926/1927 academic year was held by Prof. Jerzy Modrakowski.

60  Ibid., 206.

points, did not change during this period. In the view of Piotr M. Majewski, this was possibly due to the continuous influx of Jewish doctors who, having been educated abroad, wished to have their qualifications accredited in Poland.[61] Why did the "native Poles" so despise their Jewish colleagues? Here is Majewski's comment:

> The above position [on nostrification], fully supported later by the medical faculty board following discussions with other academic centers, must surely be seen in conjunction with the social and political situation in the country at that time. Even if professors formally used the concept of *numerus clausus* in respect of limiting cases of evaluation, regardless of a candidate's religion, in practice such restrictions affected mostly Jews who were the majority in this group. It is difficult, then, to think that the authors of such a resolution did not share the opinion that there were too many persons of Jewish origin among the medical fraternity, that they did not try to limit their influx to the medical services market—a process facilitated by circumventing their studies in Poland. Moreover, this resolution demonstrates that, in practice, the national interest aligned with the personal interests of the profession, for fear of lowering the material wellbeing of Polish doctors given stiff competition from their Jewish colleagues. The ethical or social aspects of this issue were of little interest to the authors: according to them, the country was lagging in respect of access to medical services, and this was an accepted fact. Although the medical faculty failed to prohibit the evaluation of foreign diplomas on paper, there was no doubt that under this administration, attitudes towards the Jews did not improve. A year before the outbreak of the Second World War, the Medical Faculty Board adopted a resolution to postpone evaluations until 1942.[62]

---

61 Majewski, *Dzieje Uniwersytetu Warszawskiego 1915–1945*, 278.
62 Ibid., 207. Cited here is Majewski's opinion.

## Antisemitism in the Association of Doctors of the Polish State

Among the numerous doctors' associations registered in interwar Poland, the most influential was the Association of Doctors of the Polish State.[63] Thanks to its national scope, it represented almost half of all Polish doctors during the 1930s. According to its charter, adopted on February 16, 1929, the Association aimed to organize doctors and defend their professional interests, in addition to regulating professional ethics. This was the second-most important national professional medical association (the first being the Supreme Council), and only medical doctors were entitled to become members. Its public face was the journal *Medical News*, which began publication in 1927.

From the start, the union was politically connected to nationalist circles.[64] Apart from defending the interests of the medical profession, the union embraced the fight against "Jewification."[65] In the introduction to *Medical Directory of the North-Eastern Lands*, published in Vilnius in 1939, the editorial board wrote: "While consulting the directory, please remember that any concerns for one's health should be guided by one principle: Poles should seek treatment only from Christian doctors." Each page carried slogans like "A Polish doctor will never recommend a Jewish doctor to anyone"; "A Polish doctor will place patients requiring hospitalization in an institution which is maintained and managed by Christian doctors"; "For all kinds of consultations and advice, a Polish doctor will turn to Christian colleagues only"; and "A Polish doctor will call upon Christian nursing personnel to tend to patients."[66] These recommendations were not limited to mutual relations between doctors, but also prescribed a model of cooperation with intermediary and auxiliary personnel while encouraging customers to buy Polish pharmaceutical products.

In the second half of the 1920s, various medical associations employed in *Kasa Chorych* joined the union; the Association of *Kasa*

---

63 Bojczuk, "Wykaz polskich towarzystw," 231–247. She lists 292 organizations, including the Polish Medical Association formed in London.

64 Więckowska, *Lekarze jako grupa zawodowa*, 184.

65 I. Einhorn, *Towarzystwo Ochrony Zdrowia Ludności Żydowskiej w Polsce w latach 1921–1950* (Toruń: Adam Marszałek, 2008), 60.

66 *Informator Lekarski ziem północno-wschodnich* (Vilnius, 1939), edition sponsored by Association of Doctors of the Polish State.

*Chorych* Doctors in Warsaw joined in 1928, and the associations and unions of *Kasa Chorych* doctors in Lviv and Kraków joined in 1932. This led to a consolidation of the interests of doctors employed in insurance companies, who had been treated unfairly by the union. In 1934, activists who supported the decisions of the *Sanacja* government were elected to the union's leadership.[67]

In 1935, the Association of Doctors of the Polish State formed a section for doctors in private practice and, a year later, tried to introduce the Aryan clause. For the first time, representatives proposed a change to the charter on May 17, 1936, during the seventeenth general congress, but the application was rejected. On May 9, 1937, at the request of the General Secretary, Adam Huszcza, the proposal was again subjected to the vote and accepted (140 votes for, 103 against, with four abstentions). Henceforth, only "a doctor, who was a citizen of the Polish Republic and a Christian from birth" could become a member of the Association of Doctors of the Polish State.[68]

The Aryan clause was mainly supported by members in independent practice, as well as members of the hospitals and clinics sections. The chairmen of the Kraków, Lviv, Lublin, Warsaw, Vilnius, and Łódź delegations condemned the discrimination against Jews. The Board of the Association of Doctors in Social Insurance even terminated its agreement with the Association of Doctors of the Polish State, and other associations soon followed suit. At the turn of 1937, doctors who had approved the Aryan clause created a *new* Association of Doctors in the Polish State, which discriminated against Jews.

This split led to a reactivation and revival of antisemitic organizations that previously left the association. Unfortunately, even the Warsaw Association of Doctors in Social Insurance was soon dominated by antisemites. On March 3, 1939, at their insistence, the Aryan clause was pushed through.[69] The withdrawal from the association of those who condemned the clause heralded the dissolution of the organization.

In 1939, doctors affiliated with the Warsaw branch of the Association of Doctors of the Polish State, threatened by their well-educated Jewish colleagues, sent a memorandum to the Medical Chamber signed by

---

67 Więckowska, *Lekarze jako grupa zawodowa*, 192, 194, 201.
68 Ibid., 191.
69 Ibid., 204.

Union President Dr. Roman Sobański, and the secretary, Dr. Janusz Miłaszewski, proposing changes to the electoral law. The document read as follows:

> In recent years the number of Jewish doctors has constantly increased. The situation has reached a point where, in certain medical councils, the number of Jewish doctors exceeds that of Christian doctors. For instance, in the Lviv Medical Chamber, the number of Jewish doctors stands at sixty percent, in Kraków sixty percent, in Łódź fifty-three percent. In other chambers this percentage is lower, but, as stated by the Minister Dr. Piestrzyński, overall Jewish doctors in Poland make up forty-four percent [of the entire cohort]. . . Should the Jewish doctors so desire, they could—in some chambers, including that of Warsaw-Białystok—elect a management team consisting exclusively of Jewish doctors. . . This weakens the import of medical chambers in Polish medical circles, causing constant conflict and misunderstandings, and breeding dissatisfaction with professional life. This is harmful to our country, as the representatives on our medical chambers do not reflect the true face of the Polish medical milieu. . . It is essential that the medical chambers' electoral law be changed so that it formally guarantees that Polish doctors will have the deciding vote in electing the management of regional chambers, and later of the Supreme Medical Council.[70]

However, this memorandum did not reflect the subsequent actions of the medical chamber.[71] In August 1939, the Warsaw-Białystok Medical Chamber called on all doctors to pay attention to the origins of the medicines they prescribed, urging them to give priority to drugs produced locally. It further appealed to doctors to avoid prescribing medicines

---

70 *Lekarskie* 11 (1939): 173–174. Cited after Nasierowski, Świat *lekarski w Polsce*, 61–62. The discussion on the memorandum and the introduction of the Aryan clause in the statute led to violent conflict among the doctors and the disbanding of the Lviv and Kraków branches of the Association of Doctors of the Polish State.

71 R. Zabłotniak, "Zrzeszenie Lekarzy Rzeczpospolitej Polskiej," in *Słownik Polskich Towarzystw Naukowych*, vol. 2, part 2 (Wrocław: Zakład Narodowy im. Ossolińskich, 1990), 366.

produced in Germany, keeping in mind the wellbeing of their patients, and asked they be replaced with non-German remedies, where possible.[72]

## Activities of the Association of Doctors of the Polish Republic

In 1923, the Association of Doctors in the Polish Republic was formed, most likely as a response to the difficulties Jewish doctors experienced when trying to join existing medical organizations.[73] Its mission was to encourage doctors to engage in research, and to facilitate access to libraries and grant bursaries, in addition to organizing conferences and training workshops. The Research Commission, mutual-aid funds, and employment brokers came under its auspices. Membership largely consisted of Jewish doctors. Proceedings were conducted in Polish when no foreign visitors were present. In the years 1923–1939, its members participated in 280 scholarly sessions, and membership increased from 288 to 600. Members maintained close contact with their colleagues in the Polish Society of Social Medicine, established in 1916.[74] The society was linked to the traditions ascribed to the Association of Polish Doctors and considered its main function to be organizing healthcare for the people. Its newsletter was the *Warsaw Medical Journal*, established in 1924. These associations cooperated closely; the *Warsaw Medical Journal* published the proceedings of the Association of Doctors in the Polish Republic and research articles by its members, and several doctors were members of both associations.[75]

---

72  *Wieczór Warszawski* 12, no. 241 (August 1939).

73  Among its founders were the Polish doctor and Esperantist Wilhelm Rubin (Róbin, 1873–1942); the surgeon Henryk Stabholz (1882–1941), the director of the (Jewish Old Order) Czyste Hospital; Teofil Simchowicz (1879–1957), a pioneer of Polish neuropathology and research on dementia and a student of Alois Alzheimer; the surgeon Jan Mutermilch (1889–1940), a member of the tribunal of the Warsaw-Białystok Medical Chamber; the urologist Dawid Szenkier (known as Tadeusz Mazurek after the war, 1886–1963); and the neurologist and social activist Zygmunt Szneur Załmen Bychowski (1865–1934).

74  R. Zabłotniak, "Zrzeszenie Lekarzy Rzeczpospolitej Polskiej," in *Słownik Polskich Towarzystw Naukowych*, vol. 2, part 2 (Wrocław: Zakład Narodowy im. Ossolińskich, 1990), 370.

75  K. Ohry-Kossoy, A. Ohry, "Dedicated Physicians in the Face of Adversity. The Association of Jewish Physicians (ZLRP) and the Jewish Health Organization (TOZ) in Poland, 1921–1942," *Polin: Studies in Polish Jewry* 25 (2012): 456.

Members of the Association of Doctors in the Polish Republic protested against manifestations of antisemitism directed at medical students at Jagiellonian University.[76] Among the members who later became known for their work in the ghetto were doctors Izrael Milejkowski (president of the Jewish Medical Chamber and later, the *Judenrat* Health Department). Another member, Dr. Julian Fliederbaum, who supervised a group dedicated to researching hunger sickness during the ghetto years, was the assistant of Dr. Witold Orłowski, the founder of the Polish School of Internal Medicine.

## Jews in the Warsaw Medical Society

The Warsaw Medical Society was formed in 1820, five years after the Polish Kingdom/Congress Poland was created and became the most prestigious society of its kind. Its establishment was mainly initiated by graduates of German universities and foreign doctors.[77] Its mission was to continually improve knowledge in the field of medicine, and inspire doctors to engage in research and knowledge sharing. The charter of the Warsaw Medical Society was approved on April 10, 1821, by the Kingdom's governor in Warsaw. In accordance with article 4 of the charter, any doctor "residing in Warsaw and legally practicing the art of medicine" could become an active member,[78] whereas any other "doctor residing in the country or abroad" could become a corresponding member.[79] In both cases, the candidate had to accomplish "scientific achievements" known to the society. In 1848, a proviso was added to article 4, stipulating that "each newly accepted member is obliged to write a dissertation on a topic of the member's choice." In 1916, Zygmunt Kramsztyk, a Jewish-Polish ophthalmologist, as well as a journalist and editor, publisher of medical

---

76  Zabłotniak, "Zrzeszenie Lekarzy Rzeczpospolitej Polskiej," 367.
77  R. Zabłotniak, "Towarzystwo Lekarskie Warszawskie," in *Słownik Polskich Towarzystw Naukowych*, vol. 2, part 1 (Wrocław: Zakład Narodowy im. Ossolińskich, 1990), 401.
78  The charter of Warsaw Medical Society, formulated on December 6, 1820, was confirmed by a decree of the Polish kingdom's governor on April 10, 1821. The charter was published by Brothers Hindemith Printing House, on 495 Daniłowiczowska Street, and is now preserved in the society's library. Further amendments to the act and its regulations were introduced in subsequent years of the society's existence, but the article regulating membership of the society remained unchanged.
79  Ibid.

literature and scholar of literature, tried to create an electoral commission to consider the qualifications of colleagues applying for membership of the society.[80]

Members of the Warsaw Medical Society focused on education and promoting practitioners' professional qualifications. During the national uprisings (1830 and 1863) they ran field hospitals for insurgents.[81] Everyone was involved—irrespective of religious orientation, youth, or experience—even titled professors.[82] The contributions of the Warsaw Medical Society to the development of medical thought and the organization of healthcare cannot be overestimated. Its prestige was evident when the Ministry of Health consulted its members to help create medical councils, as it had in 1918.[83]

According to Zofia Podgórska-Klawe, among the first thrty-six doctors to apply for union membership were nine Jews (twenty-five percent of applicants).[84] Joanna Mackiewicz reports Jewish doctors in the Warsaw Medical Society was at five percent in 1820, reaching fifteen percent in the years 1865–1914.

In 1914–1939, no members were listed as Jewish, while ninety-five percent of members were listed as Roman Catholic.[85] Today, it is difficult to establish the true reason for this state of affairs—it is possible that some Jewish doctors changed their religious affiliation to further their

---

80  H. Bojczuk, J. Mackiewicz, M. Paciorek, "Kronika posiedzeń Towarzystwa Lekarskiego Warszawskiego w latach 1916–1939," in *Towarzystwo Lekarskie Warszawskie 1820–2005*, ed. Z. Podgórska-Klawe, part 2 (Warsaw: Zakład Poligraficzny Primum, 2005), 8.

81  Podgórska-Klawe, "Warszawa i jej instytucje," 33.

82  In 1863–1866, Ludwik Natanson (1871–1898) was the president of the Warsaw Medical Society. Natanson was a leader in the Warsaw Jewish community, the founder and editor of *Medical Weekly*, and an advocate of Reform Judaism. Ludwik Maurycy Hirszfeld (from 1875), Dawid Rosenthal (from 1888), Mikołaj Rejchman (from 1914), Henryk Nusbaum (who had been a vice president in 1889–1901, and president from 1928), and Maksymilian Zweigbaum (from 1929) were the society's honorary members.

83  Bojczuk, Mackiewicz, Paciorek, "Kronika posiedzeń," 15.

84  Z. Podgórska-Klawe, "Udział lekarzy Żydów w tworzeniu warszawskiego środowiska lekarskiego," in *Polscy lekarze Żydzi w XIX i XX wieku*, ed. Z. Podgórska-Klawe (Warsaw: n.p., 2010), 61.

85  J. Mackiewicz, "Członkowie Towarzystwa Lekarskiego Warszawskiego," in *Towarzystwo Lekarskie Warszawskie 1820–2005*, ed. Z. Podgórska-Klawe, part 2 (Warsaw: Zakład Poligraficzny Primum, 2005), 323.

professional and academic careers. In Stanisław Konopka's opinion, the decline in membership was caused by new medical societies dedicated to specific fields of medicine—a phenomenon that the society's President, Zdzisław Dmochowski, noted in his 1921 report:[86]

> During the past year, the functioning of the Warsaw Medical Society was weak and lethargic. . . I think that our inaction was a consequence of such factors as the war, difficulties in everyday life, our preoccupation with general issues. . . However, today, having established relatively calm and stable internal relations, and having been given a university with such a degree of organization that didactic and academic work is possible, it seems we are better equipped to look to the future, so hopefully our academic work will be more vigorous next year. Unfortunately, there is reason to suspect that it may not turn out that way, for it appears that reviving the Warsaw Medical Society sessions will not come easily. The cause for my pessimism is the establishment of new specialist medical societies in Warsaw.[87]

As many as five scientific societies, namely the surgical, neurological-psychiatric, pediatrics, ophthalmic, and gynecological societies, which began their existence as parts of the Warsaw Medical Society in 1891, became independent.[88] Dmochowski, who investigated the possible reasons why certain sections opted to break away from the society, found that one of the reasons lay in the desire to follow a foreign example:

> I heard that our society is intolerant and undemocratic, that is why other societies had to be established, which are accessible to

---

86  S. Konopka, "Co dało Towarzystwo Lekarskie Warszawskie medycynie polskiej," paper presented at a conference devoted to the 150th anniversary of the founding of Warsaw Medical Society, April 22, 1972, Warsaw, *Archiwum Historii Medycyny* 35 (1972): 386; H. Bojczuk, "Członkowie TLW w okresie okupacji hitlerowskiej," in *Towarzystwo Lekarskie Warszawskie 1820–2005*, ed. Z. Podgórska-Klawe, part 2 (Warsaw: Zakład Poligraficzny Primum, 2005), 135.

87  *Pamiętnik Towarzystwa Lekarskiego Warszawskiego* 116 (1925): 44. *Memoirs of Warsaw Medical Society* was a yearbook that covered questions of a scholarly nature raised during sessions, as well as organizational issues; it first appeared in 1837. Today its volumes are a valuable source of information on the activities of the society and its members.

88  Ibid., 45.

all. These allegations are not true. People of various convictions belong to our society, as do different religious denominations and nationalities. It is possible that, to a degree, it is exclusive because the society has very high moral expectations, in keeping with its traditions. But, compared with what was the case during the first five decades of the Warsaw Medical Society's existence, we have become much more lenient. Each year, into the ranks of real members (as opposed to corresponding members) we accept young people who have not yet distinguished themselves either in their community or in science. Previously this was not possible: only older people were elected as members, being distinguished and deserving of the absolute trust of the entire membership. . . And this was laudable, because thanks to its seamless selection process, the Warsaw Medical Society has survived an entire century of grave historical catastrophes to which the nation as a whole was subjected. . . For many years, the Warsaw Medical Society was the only place that kept Polish academic endeavor alive. Highlighting the issue of intolerance cannot become the reason why sections are transforming into independent societies.[89]

Members of the new societies lost their membership in the Warsaw Medical Society—which may have contributed to the latter's declining membership. Joanna Mackiewicz writes:

Upon the establishment of the Second Polish Republic, members of the Warsaw Medical Society tried to avoid the ubiquitous politics which dominated many other societies. For example, at the initiative of the Central Agricultural Society to sign a declaration issued by political institutions of the Polish Kingdom, the president of the Warsaw Medical Society commented scathingly: "Our meeting room does not divert to political discussions." This view met with resistance, for there were voices maintaining that even university senates signed a variety of petitions. . .[90] During the interwar period, the society stopped being a meeting place for various cultures.

---

89   Ibid.
90   Mackiewicz, "Członkowie Towarzystwa," 50.

The ranks of the Warsaw Medical Society did not grow, as is evident when paging through the register of new member-doctors of Jewish origin. Although there is no manifestation of systemic antipathy or discriminatory behavior towards them, suspicion of a certain posturing arises when recalling the case of Maksymilian Zweigbaum.[91]

The situation was further aggravated by the economic crisis and laws of exclusion applied to Jews, such as *numerus clausus*, the "bench ghetto" and the Aryan clause. The last time Jewish doctors became members of the Warsaw Medical Society was in 1935, when Marceli Landsberg and Józef Stein joined.[92]

Over the years, many Jewish doctors joined the ranks of the Warsaw Medical Society, many of them graduates of medicine at Warsaw University. Many took an active part in the society, presenting various papers.[93] On numerous occasions they presented lectures, as did distinguished neurologist Henryk Higer, internists Anastazy Landau and Mieczysław Fejgin, world-renowned serologist Ludwik Hirszfeld, and otolaryngologist Zygmunt Srebrny. During the 1925 conference, gynecologist Henryk Altkaufer presented his invention—a transparent antiseptic dressing of stainless mesh covered with the thinnest layer of mica, one of the first so-called active wound dressings.[94] In 1934, neurologist Marek Bornsztajn presented his paper "The Mechanism of Reactive Psychotic Disorders Formation." Internist and infectious diseases specialist Marceli Landsberg explained the mechanism of exudation absorption (1920) and new methods for treating liver disease (1936). In 1937,

91  Ibid., 52. Maksymiliam Zweigbaum (Zwejgbaum, 1855–1943), was member of Warsaw Medical Society since 1887, honorary member since 1929, Chief Librarian in the society's library; after independence he was employed in the Ministry of Public Health. See his personal file at Warsaw-Białystok Medical Chamber, ref. 4413.

92  H. Bojczuk, "Spis członków Towarzystwa Lekarskiego warszawskiego za lata 1820–1951," in *Towarzystwo Lekarskie Warszawskie 1820–2005*, ed. Z. Podgórska-Klawe, part 2 (Warsaw: Zakład Poligraficzny Primum, 2005), 289–319.

93  M. Paciorek, "Referaty wygłoszone na forum TLW w latach 1919–1939," in *Towarzystwo Lekarskie Warszawskie 1820–2005*, ed. Z. Podgórska-Klawe, part 2 (Warsaw: Zakład Poligraficzny Primum, 2005), 325–351. See also appendix 10 in this book.

94  Idem, "Działalność TLW w latach 1915–1939," in *Towarzystwo Lekarskie Warszawskie 1820–2005*, ed. Z. Podgórska-Klawe, part 2 (Warsaw: Zakład Poligraficzny Primum, 2005), 115.

anatomical pathologist (and later director of the ghetto hospital) Józef Stein presented on "The Pathological Anatomy of a Kidney Tumor." Jewish doctors were invited to participate in the society's sessions and present research papers.[95]

From the onset of the occupation, the German invaders suspended the activities of all Polish institutions and scientific societies, including that of the Warsaw Medical Society. According to Halina Bojczuk, at the beginning of 1939, 412 members were registered with the Warsaw Medical Society.[96] From September 1939 to October 1944, membership numbers dropped by 167. Because of the lack of data reflecting the place and date of death of several doctors, it is impossible to calculate the society's membership losses during the Second World War.[97]

Of the twenty-four members of the society who worked in the Warsaw Ghetto, ten people (forty-one pecent) survived, which is relatively high compared to the total survival rate.[98] It is difficult to say why this was the case. Perhaps they had help from prewar friendships with Polish colleagues, or perhaps in some cases the relative material welfare of doctors compared to the others was helpful.

---

95 Among their number were Łucja Frey (1925, 1927), Józef Szper (1927), Seweryn Cytronberg (1931), Leon Blacher (1934), Julian Fliederbaum (1934), Henryk Beck (1934), Emil Apfelbaum (1935), and Natan Mesz (1935). Among the society's corresponding members were Józef Maybaum (from 1910), who administered the first shelter for Jewish children in Łódź and authored *An Outline of Social Childcare*, and hygienist and pulmonologist (phthisiologist) Seweryn Sterling.
96 H. Bojczuk, "Towarzystwo Lekarskie Warszawskie w roku 1939," *Pamiętnik Towarzystwa Lekarskiego Warszawskiego* 153, no. 21 (2017): 233.
97 Ibid., 235. See also idem, "Członkowie TLW w okresie okupacji," 135.
98 According to the aithor's estimates, of the 831 Jewish doctors who were members of the Warsaw-Białystok Medical Chamber, the total survival rate was just under twelve percent (100 individuals)

Chapter 4

# Healthcare during and in the Aftermath of the 1939 Siege of Warsaw

The Second World War began when the German army attacked Poland along their common border on September 1, 1939. After signing the non-aggression Ribbentrop-Molotov Pact between Germany and the USSR, on September 17 Poland was attacked from the East by the USSR and was split between the Soviets and the Germans. Two days before the invasion, Poland mobilized its forces. Along with line infantry, doctors— many serving as reserve officers— nurses, medical staff, and administrators were drafted to establish field hospitals and emergency medical teams.[1]

This caused major shortages of medical personnel in hospitals and clinics around Poland, and particularly in Warsaw, Kraków, and Łódź. During the September Campaign, which lasted until October 6, 1939, approximately 66,000 Polish soldiers and officers were killed by the *Wehrmacht*, 134,000 were wounded and approximately 420,000

---

1  P. Zarzycki, ed., *Plan mobilizacyjny "W." Wykaz od działów mobilizowanych na wypadek wojny* (Pruszków: Ajaks, 1995), 186–187; M. Dutkiewicz, "Wychowankowie i kadra Szkoły Podchorążych sanitarnych wśród ofiar zbrodni katyńskiej (problem badawcze, tło, przebieg i skutki zbrodni)," in *Była taka podchorążówka w Warszawie . . . Wychowankowie szkoły Podchorążych sanitarnych 1922–1939*, ed. Agnieszka Pruszyńska (Warsaw: n.p., 2002), 39.

became prisoners of war, including many medical practitioners.[2] These losses were severely felt in Warsaw as the city came under attack.

On orders of the supreme commander, almost all medical personnel from the Ujazdowski Hospital in Warsaw, which had been transformed into the training center for sanitary personnel, were instructed to leave and assigned to field armies to organize an evacuation zone on Poland's eastern border. Colonel Dr. Bolesław Pawłowski was the first commander of the newly created 104th Field Hospital.[3] When the hospital was about to be evacuated to the East (September 6), he was replaced by Colonel Docent Michał Rosnowski.[4] Ordered to evacuate to Trembowla, the officers were arrested by the Soviets on September 17, 1939, and sent to the camp in Starobielsk, where the majority of them were later shot dead by the People's Commissariat for Internal Affairs (NKVD).[5]

In 1938, Jewish soldiers made up 6.08 percent of the Polish Army.[6] In 1939, almost 100,000 Jewish citizens were drafted, making up roughly 10 percent of the total number of deployed soldiers (approximately 7,000

2   A. Krupa, ed., *Encyklopedia wojskowa: dowódcy i ich armie, historia wojen i bitew, technika wojskowa* (Warsaw: Bellona, 2007), 405–406.

3   Colonel Dr. Bolesław Pawłowski (1892–1946), a surgeon gynecologist, served in the Ujazdowski Training Hospital. See J. B. Gliński, *Słownik biograficzny lekarzy i farmaceutów—ofiar drugiej wojny światowej*, vol. 3 (Wrocław: Urban&Partner, 2003), 343; and Pawłowski's personal file, Warsaw-Białystok Medical Chamber, ref. 2881.

4   Colonel Docent Michał Rosnowski (1897–1940), an army doctor and internist, was the commander of the Paramedics Training Center Hospital, where he worked. Personal file, Warsaw-Białystok Medical Chamber, ref. 3208.

5   H. Odrowąż-Szukiewicz, H. Bojczuk, P. Wiloch, "Szpital Ujazdowski w okresie 1939–1945," in *Jazdów*, ed. Edward Rużyłło (Warsaw: Wojskowy Instytut Medyczny, 2008), 201.

6   T. Gąsowski, "Żydzi w siłach zbrojnych II Rzeczpospolitej: czas pokoju i wojny," in *Udział mniejszości narodowych w różnych formacjach wojskowych w kampanii wrześniowej 1939 r.*, (Warsaw: Wydawnictwo Sejmowe, 2009), 16. A. Felchner states that, according to sources of the Central Military Archives (CAW), healthcare officers of Jewish faith made up only 2.7 percent of the total officers in the Medical Corps. It was not possible to establish what percentage of all medical officers in the Polish Army in 1938 were Jews. See A. Felchner, *Pod znakiem Eskulapa i Marsa. Służba Zdrowia Wojska Polskiego (od jesieni 1918r. do mobilizacji w 1939 r.)* (Oświęcim: Napoleon V, 2016), 236.

were killed).[7] This was about equal to the percentage of Jewish people to the general population in Poland in 1939.[8]

During the war, from 1939–1945, in total 1,700,000 Jews, including thousands of Polish Jews, fought on all fronts.[9] Jews fought in Polish formations in France and the Middle East, they participated in the Battle of Britain, in the battles of the Independent Carpathian Rifle Brigade in North Africa at Tobruk, at El-Gazala and in Cyrenaica.[10] In September, many Polish soldiers and officers escaped to Romania and crossed into France, where detachments were being formed by Poles living in France, Belgium, Holland, and Great Britain. The detachment subsequently became known as the Polish (Sikorski's) Army in France. In 1940, they took part in the second French Campaign.

One who did not survive the war was Dr. Józef Stefan Szper (1883–1942), a surgeon specializing in urology. In 1919–1921 he served as a captain in field hospitals. In 1934 he became the spokesperson for the disciplinary committee of the Warsaw-Białystok Medical Chamber. From 1934 he had worked as head of department of surgery at the Czyste Jewish Hospital. Dr. Szper also participated in the September Campaign

---

7    M. Fuks, *Z dziejów wielkiej katastrofy narodu żydowskiego* (Poznań: Sorus, 1999), 313. Marian Fuks refers to the findings of Szymon Datner and Filip Friedman. Cyryl Chlebowski, "Żydzi w Wojsku Polskim," *Tygodnik Solidarność* 27, July 6, 2001, gives the number of Jews called to arms as 150,000. The article is a review of Benjamin Meirtchak, *Żydzi—Żołnierze Wojsk Polskich polegli na frontach II Wojny* Światowej (Warsaw: Bellona, 2001), where Datner's and Friedman's findings are to be found. However, Jacek E. Wilczur, "Oficerowie-Żydzi w dołach Katyńskich," *Inne Oblicza Historii* 12 (2007): 90–93, refers to Filip Fredman's findings that as many as 32,000 Jewish soldiers died in battles, in camps, or were wounded.

8    It is clear from the incomplete data for 1926–1930 that the professional staff of the Polish Army had only several dozen officers of Jewish origin, mainly physicians, vets, field rabbis, or clerks. For more on the topic, see Gąsowski, "Żydzi w siłach zbrojnych II Rzeczpospolitej."

9    According to Edward Roseman, *The Role of Jews in the Defeat of the Nazis and Axis Powers* (Melbourne: Victorian Association of Jewish Ex-Servicemen and Women, 1992), on all battlefronts of the Second World War, 1,658,000 Jewish soldiers and officers fought—men and women—of whom 50,000 were partisans. For detailed information about the participation of Jews in the Soviet Army and as partisans, see Yitzhak Arad, *In the Shadow of the Red Banner: Soviet Jews in the War against Nazi Germany* (Jerusalem: Yad Vashem, 2010). Cited after Feliks Tych, "Udział zbrojny Żydów w II Wojnie Światowej," http://www.dzieciholocaustu.org.pl/, accessed April 19, 2017.

10  Wilczur, "Oficerowie-Żydzi w dołach Katyńskich," 91.

in Romania, Yugoslavia, and Italy before arriving in France, where he became a medical commander on a sanitary train. After the Germans crossed the frontlines over the Somme and Aisne, he and other wounded soldiers were taken to the training camp at Crawford Castle, in Scotland. He died on January 30, 1942, in Perth, Scotland and is buried in the local cemetery there.[11]

From the start, the *Wehrmacht* violated international law regarding the protection of the wounded and of medical personnel with their bombing of hospitals (even buildings correctly marked as such) and the killing of doctors and sanitation personnel. The 1907 Geneva Convention defines the status of medical personnel who become prisoners of war under "the treatment of the wounded and sick in active armies," according to which "medical personnel involved exclusively in providing care to the wounded and sick, also during their transportation, must not be treated as prisoners of war (POWs). When their help is no longer required, they must be repatriated."[12] Moreover, the Convention provides for repatriated medics to take their personal belongings with them, as well as any medical equipment, weapons and horses that were their private property. Sometimes, in accordance with the Geneva Convention, the Germans released doctors, dentists, chemists and auxiliary personnel. Dr. M.B., captured as a POW near Kamionka Strumiłowa, recalls being treated well. He managed to escape, reaching Pińczów where, as the only surgeon at the hospital, he operated on a few dozen patients in two days. However, there are also stories without a happy ending. Another medic, Dr. Beniamin Oppenheim (1897–1939), worked as a dermatologist at the Social Insurance Company in the Solce. He later served in a field hospital and was wounded when, on September 8, his detachment was attacked by the retreating *Wehrmacht*. He was shot dead by the Germans when exiting a hospital tent bearing the Red Cross.[13]

By the end of September 1939, the Germans captured approximately 20,000 Polish officers and imprisoned them in camps for higher-ranking prisoners, the *Offizierslager* (Officers' Camps). The Germans regularly violated the rights and protection of captives so many Jewish officers (seven percent of prisoners)—fearing persecution—chose not to disclose

---

11 Gliński, *Słownik biograficzny lekarzy*, 357.
12 Dutkiewicz, "Wychowankowie i kadra Szkoły Podchorążych sanitarnych," 52.
13 Gliński, *Słownik biograficzny lekarzy*, 427.

their origins. They were protected in these attempts by their fellow Polish prisoners, even by the antisemites among them.[14]

Dr. M.B. recalls hostilities on the Bzura River:

> They called me to come to a hut in the village of Kamion, to treat wounded soldiers. . . The Germans directed their gunfire at the hut, tossing a grenade inside it. I was shot. In another room, our comrades opened fire. We were completely trapped, and in the end, we raised a white flag and surrendered. We were disarmed and told to stand facing a wall. They took our razors, Swiss army knives, even our matches. When a German officer asked me whether I was a Jew, I pretended not to understand him. We were led to a meeting point, where the doctors were ordered to step forward.
>
> Again, the question: Are you a Jew? I was rescued from this dangerous situation by a doctor, a Pole and well-known antisemite, who replied that I was not. That was on September 19. After that, we were ordered to tend to the wounded.[15]

Some doctors returned to Warsaw relatively quickly. Izrael Rotbalsam, a pediatrician from the Bersohn and Bauman Children's Hospital, came back early in October when his detachment was disbanded on September 23, 1939.[16] Another pediatrician in Kamień Kaszyrski, Jan Przedborski, went to Pińsk until May 1940. In his diary, written while living on the Aryan side in the Soviet-occupied zone, Przedborski wrote he joined a clinic treating the local population. He returned to Warsaw following a prisoner exchange.[17]

An anonymous doctor, D., wrote:

> On March 23, 1939, I was deployed as a doctor-ensign in an infantry regiment stationed in Brześć on Bug. . . In May, as battalion doctor, I went on maneuvers in Tuchola, Pomerania,

---

14  Wilczur, "Oficerowie-Żydzi w dołach Katyńskich," 91.

15  The Ringelblum archives contain three anonymous accounts by Jewish doctors commenting on the events related to September 1939. See "Relacje lekarzy żydowskich chuczestników kampanii wrześniowej 1939 r.," *Biuletyn Żydowskiego Instytutu Historycznego* 2, no. 70 (1969): 109–110. The authors of those accounts were not professional soldiers and were often not precise in describing the course of military operations.

16  An account by Izrael Rotbalsam, YVA O.3/2357.

17  Memoir of Jan (Jonas) Przedborski, Jewish Historical Institute Archives 302/172.

where the regiment provided border protection. . . . The Jews went on a vedette [sentry duty]; they were all great soldiers, disciplined and eager to perform even the toughest of tasks. The colonel's adjutant was a Jew, an advocate, a very intelligent and brave person.[18]

Dr. D. describes his garrison unit's march through Warsaw, from Sochaczew to Siedlce and Żelichowo, where on September 13 the Germans captured him. He subsequently worked as a doctor in a POW hospital in Siedlce until it closed, after which he was released. Dr. Józef Grosglik was a POW in *Oflag* II B in Arnswald (now Choszczno) until May 1940. He was released and returned to Warsaw to resume his private practice.[19]

It is estimated 300 officers held in the officers' camps managed to survive the war.[20] Not all did. In 1943, in one of the camps, a radiologist from the St. Lazarus Hospital, Dr. Henryk Kaltman, died of tuberculosis. Coming back from the eastern borderlands, Dr. Lucjan Chaskielewicz, a gastroenterologist from the Czyste Jewish Hospital, was killed.

Thousands of Polish soldiers were killed or wounded after the Soviet invasion of Eastern Poland, while approximately 250,000 were imprisoned in Soviet camps—including 20,000 Jews.[21] Initially, military medical personnel thought they would be safe, believing the enemy would respect the Geneva Convention. Instead, the Soviet authorities handed sanitary corps officers over to the secret police (NKVD). The majority were sent to POW camps and treated as "a class enemy," an element deemed unsuited for "ideological reeducation."[22]

Some officers managed to escape. Dr. Ludwik Stabholz was sent to a POW camp in Tarnopol where his uncle, Wilhelm Marienstrass (also a doctor and officer in the Polish Army) lived and practiced. Marienstrass

---

18  "Relacje lekarzy żydowskich," 107–108.
19  Several thousands of Jewish soldiers were directed to *Stalags* (camps for rank-and-file POWs *Kriegsgefangenen-Mannschafts-Stammlager*) in Eastern Prussia, and soon afterwards released to return home. See Chlebowski, "Żydzi w Wojsku Polskim."
20  Gąsowski, "Żydzi w siłach zbrojnych II Rzeczpospolitej," 18.
21  Ibid.
22  Dutkiewicz, "Wychowankowie i kadra Szkoły Podchorążych sanitarnych," 53.

delivered a disguise to Stabholz who escaped from a transport and arrived back in Warsaw in early 1940.

Neither the Red Army nor the NKVD were prepared to accommodate 250,000 POWs so most of the prisoners were released. However, the special camps (at Starobielsk, Kozielsk, and Ostaszków) were established to house 15,087 officers who were later shot in the spring of 1940 by the NKVD in Katyn, Kharkiv, and Mednoe.[23]

Among the POWs were Jewish doctors, including Dr. Szymon Lewinson, a urologist from the Czyste Jewish Hospital in Warsaw, who was drafted in September 1939 and ordered to join the auxiliary staff at the First Provincial Hospital. He left Warsaw following an appeal by Roman Umiastowski, head of Propaganda in the Polish Army Headquarters, who, during the nights of September 6–7, 1939, broadcast a call for all able-bodied men to form a new defensive line east of the Vistula River. Dr. Lewinson was a POW in Kozielsk. He was shot in the back of the head by the NKVD in the Katyn forest, sometime between April 3 and May 12, 1940. Also murdered was his brother, Józef Lewinson, a chemical engineer.[24] Dr. Lewinson was survived by his wife Alina (the daughter of the prominent urologist, Aleksander Fryszman), who lived in Warsaw, his thirteen-year-old daughter Janina, and her younger sister, nine-year-old Zosia. From 1942, his wife and daughters hid in Warsaw, and later in nearby towns. They moved often after falling victim to extortionists. After the Warsaw Uprising (August–September 1944) they, together with other Warsaw residents, moved to a village near Kraków, where they remained until April 1945.[25]

---

23 Ibid., 55. Marek Dutkiewicz points out that not all sites of massacre or the names of the massacred are known. He estimates that over 25,000 were killed. Among the 432 survivors were 43 doctors with the rank of officer. Furthermore, as part of the repressions of 1940–1941, hundreds of thousands of Poles were transported to Siberia, the far North, and Central Asia, while many others were subjected to inhumane tyranny. In his opinion, the medical profession was well represented among the prisoners in Kozielsk and Starobielsk. Of the 3,940 prisoners in Starobielsk, 376 were doctors. M. Dutkiewicz, "Personel medyczny ze Wschodnich Kresów II Rzeczypospolitej—ofiary zbrodni katyńskiej," in *Prace naukowe Światowej Rady Badań nad Polonią*, vol. 7, *Przeszłość, teraźniejszości przyszłość Polaków na Wschodzie, Materiały z konferencji naukowej 8–9 maja 2001 r. w Gorzowie Wielkopolskim*, ed. M. Szczerbiński and T. Wolsza (Gorzów Wielkopolski: Światowa Rada Badań nad Polonią, 2001), 189.

24 Ibid., 54.

25 An account by Alina Lewinson, Jewish Historical Institute Archives 301/6816.

The same fate befell Dr. Eli Hirsz Wigdorowicz, an internist and captain-in-reserve. In her diary, his daughter wrote that on September 6 he was in his uniform, hanging blackout shades in front of the dining-room windows ten minutes before he left for war.[26] Done with the curtains, he hugged his wife and cried. In a letter from Kozielsk, he wrote that while all was not well, he did not need much. After two letters and a card printed by the Red Cross, correspondence ceased.

Not all Jewish doctors managed to join army units or reach hospitals or outpatient clinics in time. When the war began, Dr. Anna Szachnerowicz, a pediatrician at the Bersohn and Bauman Children's Hospital, lived in an apartment on 38 Muranowska Street with her husband and daughter. In her postwar memoirs she noted:

> The bombing of Warsaw began. Explosions tore the air. We lowered our heads, thinking the ceiling would come down at any minute. Houses stood in flames. Although it was September, not a drop of rain fell to extinguish the fires. . . Patients [of my husband's] would come down to the basement. "Doctor, please, save us! My husband is in the army, there are four children at home, what can be done about my pregnancy?" Izaak didn't listen to our protestations: "Don't go upstairs, you will be killed by a bomb!"
>
> "I am a doctor, it is my duty to help these poor women," he said. He ran upstairs between raids, kept boiling his instruments. Some women said they had no money. But money was not important now, people needed help. They came and kissed his hands.[27]

After a few days in the basement, the Szachnerowicz family moved into Dr. Szwarc's apartment on Czacki Street. After a few hours, the bombing was so intense that they hid in a shelter. Soon all of Czacki Street was in flames. Between raids, people ran outside to buy a loaf of bread, some butter or sugar. For meat, they cut the flesh off dead horses littering the city streets. One sprinted from one building entrance to another.

---

26 N. Makower, *Miłość w cieniu śmierci. Wspomnienia z getta warszawskiego* (Wrocław: Erechtejon, 1996), 9.

27 A. Meroz, *W murach i poza murami getta. Zapiski lekarki warszawskiej z lat 1939–1945* (Warsaw: Czytelnik, 1988), 8.

The Szachnerowicz family reached the Bersohn and Bauman Children's Hospital on Sienna Street by dashing from doorway to doorway.

During the siege of Warsaw, medical students also rendered medical assistance. Adina Blady-Szwajger, a final-year student at the Warsaw University Medical Faculty and her friend, who was a nurse, organized a makeshift wound-dressing station in the basement of the building where she lived and worked until the capitulation of Warsaw. She wrote:

> I must admit, I had no difficulty in "registering" at the closest healthcare center on Freta Street. We received meager supplies for wound dressing and sterilization of equipment, along with essentials such as scalpels, tweezers, even needles and surgical sutures and forceps. I spent almost three weeks of the siege there, popping upstairs to the apartment from time to time to change or eat something. . . In the shelter I had a baptism by fire, learning how to work under conditions of war. There, in a corner next to the door, I delivered a baby—fortunately it came out by itself. A neighbor's fifteen-year-old son died in my arms, having been hit in the head by shrapnel during the horrendous bombing of the Jewish District on Yom Kippur, September 13, 1939 [sic].[28]

Warsaw capitulated on September 28, 1939. German troops entered the city on October 1 to find the city ravaged by typhoid fever brought on by water shortages and damage to the sewage system. People began to flock to Warsaw—men who, for some reason, had not reached their respective army units, entire families returning after having sought refuge in the east. Henryk Bryskier described three of his friends—an engineer, a doctor and a technician—who, exhausted after a long walk back home, hired a cab:

---

28  A. Blady-Szwajger, *I więcej nic nie pamiętam* (Warsaw: Świat Książki, 2010), 19–20. Dating these events as September 13, Blady-Szwajger might have confused Yom Kippur (Day of Atonement, which in 1939 was September 23) with Rosh Hashanah. According to other sources (such as "Bombardowanie Warszawy (1939)," Wikipedia, https://pl.wikipedia.org/wiki/Bombardowanie_Warszawy_ (1939)), the heaviest bombings in Warsaw were on September 22 and 23, 1939, coinciding with Yom Kippur. The Luftwaffe deliberately concentrated their attack on a suburb inhabited mainly by Jewish families, indiscriminately bombing civilian buildings and synagogues.

The hackney struggled to reach the Kiliński monument [Kiliński led the Warsaw Uprising of 1794, against the Russian garrison]. One of the passengers could see his house in the distance. Its windows were shattered, the frames torn out, the curtains were gone and, the gutters looked like they would break off at the slightest gust of wind. The house had taken a direct hit from a bombing or artillery fire.

The face and eyes of our fellow passenger, a doctor, changed markedly. It was as if he died in that moment. A fear bordering on madness made him pick himself up and set off at a run, which made the horse seem immobile. But the others stopped him, and the cab drew to a halt. They would not let him check for himself if there were survivors. His two friends went to his apartment, leaving him in the care of the other passengers. Judging from the way the apartment looked on the outside, they wanted to spare him the shock of a possible tragedy and planned to remove him by pretending the family was gone. Soon the "emissaries" returned with good news.[29]

Sabina Gurfinkiel-Glocer, a nurse from the Czyste Jewish Hospital, recalled: "The last days of August 1939 were full of anxiety for Czyste. Most of the doctors were called up to the army and left to join their regiments. From our department, that is, the Second Surgical, Doctors Perelman, Fliegel, Lipes, From, and many others went. They left, never to return. . ."[30]

A register published in the *Medical Journal* lists 650 doctors (with the rank of officer) who were murdered by the NKVD and buried in Piatichatki-Kharkov, Katyn, Mednoe, and Kharkov.[31] Fifty-seven of them were members of the Warsaw-Białystok Medical Chamber.[32]

---

29  H. Bryskier, *Żydzi pod swastyką, czyli getto w Warszawie w XX wieku. Pamiętnik* (Warsaw: Aspra, 2006), 14–15.
30  An account by Sabina Gurfinkiel-Glocer, "Szpital na Czystem i ja," YVA O.3/396. She mentions Doctors Mieczysław Perelman, Łazarz Fliegel, Mordechel Lipes, Mieczysław From, and Adam Atlasberg.
31  *Gazeta Lekarska* 9 (2000): 35; and 2 (2001): 28.
32  When the war broke out, of the fifty-seven officers and NCOs, only two, Majors Hipolit Gibiński and Henryk Peche, were deployed as professionals. Jan Władysław Nelken held the rank of colonel (retired). Of the remaining doctors, twenty-six were reservist NCOs, sixteen were reservist lieutenants, nine were reservist captains, and

Dr. Bolesław Ałapin, a neurologist at the Czyste Jewish Hospital, had better luck. After obtaining a medical diploma, he completed three months' training in the school for sanitary ensigns-in-reserve and started working in the communications center in Zegrze. Those six months were equal to a compulsory internship in the field of internal diseases, and after passing his exams, he was employed in Prof. Herman's department at the Czyste Jewish Hospital. On September 6, Ałapin reported to Umiastowski's headquarters and was assigned to Field Hospital 111 in Radom.[33] After September 17 he made it to Lviv, where he volunteered at a university clinic, and post-February 1940, served as head of department at the psychiatric hospital in Kulpartovo. After Lviv fell to the Germans, he returned to Warsaw to the Neurology Department at the Bersohn and Bauman Children's Hospital on Stawki Street.[34]

During the siege and bombardment of Warsaw, hospitals throughout the city were strafed and bombed, among them the Holy Ghost, a branch of the Warsaw district hospital, St. Anthony's and two pavilions of the Infant Jesus Children's Hospital. St. Lazarus lost its administration and urology buildings. The battles claimed the lives of several patients and medical staff at the Holy Ghost and Infant Jesus Hospitals, and destroyed pavilions of the Ujazdowski Hospital, St. Stanisław's Hospital in Wola, the hospital of the Order of Elizabethan Sisters, the Transfiguration of the Lord Hospital in Praga, and a hospital for railroad workers.

It is estimated that during the siege of Warsaw, about 21,000 wounded were treated in hospitals. Approximately 12–15,000 others were outpatients. Among the wounded were civilian casualties and 16,000 soldiers,[35] and many died of their wounds. Unclaimed bodies were buried in the hospital gardens. From October 1939, magisterial officials began issuing lists of the dead, so that they could be buried in cemeteries.

---

three were major reservists. Almost half of the men mentioned in the register were forty to forty-nine years of age. In the thirty-to-thirty-nine-years bracket there were fourteen doctors, while fifteen were aged fifty to fifty-nine. The youngest war fatality was the twenty-nine-year-old Ensign Leon Glikman; the oldest, the sixty-one-year-old Colonel Jan Władysław Nelken.

33  Zarzycki, *Plan mobilizacyjny "W,"* 185.

34  T. Nasierowski, "Bolesław Ałapin (1913–1985)," *Postępy Psychiatrii i Neurologii* 2, no. 4 (1995): 200.

35  A. Wysocki, "Lekarze polscy w czasie II wojny światowej," in *Dzieje medycyny w Polsce*, vol. 2, ed. W. Noszczyk and J. Supady (Warszawa: PZWL Wydawnictwo Lekarskie, 2015), 593.

## The Czyste (Old Order) Hospital for Orthodox Jews

The Czyste (Old Order) Hospital for Orthodox Jews at 17 Dworska Street, founded in 1883, was on the frontlines. Considered the most modern hospital in Warsaw, the first patients were admitted to the hospital in April 1902. For the first time in Poland, a hospital had a central heating system, gas and electricity, a power generating unit, ventilation, sewage and water supply systems, and its own well. On its extensive grounds, each of the eight hospital pavilions housed one or two departments named in the terminology of those times: internal and nervous diseases, surgical, ophthalmic and gynecological, pulmonary, throat and ear diseases, midwifery, skin and venereal diseases, mental and infectious diseases. Pavilions for skin and venereal diseases, along with psychiatric wards, were walled off from the rest of the hospital and had their own gardens. Modern hydrotherapeutic facilities, inhalation chambers, verandas, terraces for resting outdoors and phototherapy equipment were at hand to ensure a speedy convalescence. There also was a morgue, a dissection room, a synagogue and a chapel. The hospital also boasted a pantry, coach house and stables, a disinfection facility, and freezers. There were additional rooms furnished with bookshelves and board games. Meals were delivered from the central kitchen and reheated in special utility rooms, where tea and herbal infusions were also brewed. The bathrooms were equipped with tubs on wheels, showers and toilets. The clinic, its admissions section and the director's office were in the administration building. The maintenance block housed a kitchen, laundry, boiler room, accommodation for service staff, and a nursery for personnel's children, as well as rooms for convalescing patients. The hospital had its own pathology laboratory, radiology section and pharmacy.

The patient observation department (for tuberculosis) was led by a distinguished expert in pulmonary diseases, Dr. Owsiej Bieleńki. He hailed from a poor Jewish family in Eastern Poland (Kresy). After completing his studies at a Russian junior high school, he enrolled at the Faculty of Natural Sciences in St. Petersburg. After four years, he moved to Warsaw where, in 1913, he graduated from the Medical Faculty at Warsaw University and distinguished himself during the rampant Spanish flu epidemic. From 1926 on, he served as head of the Internal Diseases Department at Czyste's Old Order Jewish Hospital working under Prof. Gerszon Lewin.

Not a single Jewish home could be found where Doctor Bieleńki refused to be their doctor or was not asked to be a consultant. In pulmonary disease cases, he was the ultimate authority. His hearing was unparalleled, his experience colossal. It came as no surprise, then, that thanks to his experience, he could detect the outbreak of a disease where others could not.[36]

Tall, slim, with lush black hair and expressive eyes, he had an extraordinary influence on his patients, who worshiped him for his expertise, his quick wit and his good heart. He was well liked by his colleagues, who found him approachable. Bieleńki was chairman of the Charitable Society's Medical Circle.

During the Warsaw blockade, when the power station and water works stopped operating, the foodstuffs and medical supplies that the hospital had hoarded when they realized a war was coming, became invaluable, as did the generator and well that had been dug out on the property.

In the second half of the 1930s, Czyste became the largest closed-circuit medical center in the capital. Before the outbreak of the Second World War, the hospital had 1,500 beds and employed 147 doctors, 119 nurses, and six pharmacists. Architecturally speaking, no other medical institution was better prepared to fulfill the function for which it had been designed.[37]

During the attack on Warsaw, the hospital was understaffed with most of its prewar medical personnel drafted. During sustained German bombings, the surgical pavilions and the operating rooms were destroyed forcing staff to create makeshift facilities. The kitchen was also badly damaged. And yet, by the time the city capitulated to the Germans, the hospital had cared for 5,000 wounded soldiers and civilians.

---

36  An account by Paweł Rajman, YVA O.3/439.

37  The Old Order Jewish hospital in the Czyste suburb consisted of a complex designed by Artur Goebel, an architect and student of Henryk (Enrico) Marconi, in cooperation with Warsaw's chief architect, Czesław Domaniewski. Located at 17 Dworska Street, it functioned from the end of the nineteenth century (now Wolski Hospital on 17 Kasprzak Street). Z. Podgórska-Klawe, *Szpitale warszawskie 1388–1945* (Warsaw: PWN, 1975), 238–240.

Sabina Gurfinkiel-Glocer, a nurse and theater assistant employed at the Czyste Old Order Jewish Hospital, described her experience of September 1, 1939, as follows:

> As I was getting dressed to return home at 4 p.m., there were several loud explosions. We were convinced these were the practice bombings, which had earlier been announced. However, a phone call soon clarified matters. Hospital director Dr. Sztabholc told Dr. Amsterdamski (who had taken the call) that Dr. Orzechowski—the director of the Hospitalization Department, had just informed him that the Germans were bombing Wola–Koło (Warsaw suburbs.) Because it was close to our hospital, all the wounded would be directed to us. The ward became frantic. Everyone immediately thought about their homes, and whether other suburbs would be bombed as well. At the end of my shift I was prevented from leaving and began preparing for operations. There were not many doctors at the hospital—Dr. Amsterdamski, who was the senior assistant, Dr. Kroszczor and Dr. Brewda were assigned to us from gynecology, as was Dr. Brandwajn, who had not yet left for his regiment. He was telephoned and asked to come to the hospital.[38]

The wounded got priority treatment. Shrapnel wounds required surgery, including amputations. There were so many wounded that it was difficult to decide who to operate on first. The doctors and nurses—in fact, all the medical personnel—worked without respite. As Sabina Gurfinkiel-Glocer put it:

> From this day onward, the hospital became hell on earth. Air raids, which lasted the entire day, with brief intervals, produced vast numbers of wounded soldiers and civilians. Later, in bombing the city, the Germans were bent on destroying hospitals, ours included. Bombs fell one after the other, fortunately next to our buildings. One day, some shrapnel hit the isolation ward, rupturing the wall and, with a hiss, landing next to Dr. Amsterdamski's legs. Everyone in the ward congratulated him

---

38   An account by Sabina Gurfinkiel-Glocer, "Szpital na Czystem i ja," YVA O.3/396.

for emerging unscathed from the incident. But it did not take long for the hospital to stop working altogether. A bomb fell on our surgical departments, in one swoop destroying all the [operating] theaters, forcing the three departments to merge into one, with a common [operating] theater, in Dr. Wertheim's department on the ground floor. . . The amount of work in the department was tremendous: thirty or forty operations were performed each day, not to mention the vast number of injured requiring wound dressings.[39]

Each subsequent bombing of the hospital or its vicinity caused panic, forcing people to flee. The nurses could hardly cope with trying to keep patients in their beds. Even amputees scrambled to try and hide. Severe water shortages ensued, making it difficult to sterilize instruments, so the nurses cleaned them in the laundry rooms. Soon the entire hospital became one large surgical department. The first department eliminated was the one for mental health patients. Dr. Stanisław Waller recalled: "After a week, the influx of the wounded was so great that the mental health department, so-called Ward 8, was closed and two surgical departments were created instead. One was assigned to me, the other was led by Dr. Meister-Tempelhofow (who died later in the ghetto)."[40]

Towards the end of September, all the beds were occupied and every available bit of floor space was taken. Managing the hospital was made more difficult by the fact that Dr. Henryk Stabholz, its director and surgeon, had left Warsaw on September 6. He was replaced by Dr. Adam Zamenhof, an ophthalmologist who managed the hospital until his arrest on October 1, 1939.[41] He was replaced by Dr. Julian Rotstadt, a neurologist, head of the Department of Physiotherapy, and a reservist lieutenant. In mid-December he, too, was arrested and later murdered. In the end, the Germans nominated Dr. Józef Stein, from the pathology laboratory in

---

39  Ibid.

40  An account by Stanisław (Shmul) Waller (Walewski), YVA O.3/2358.

41  Dr. Adam Zamenhof was shot dead in Palmiry. His sister, Dr. Zofia Zamenhof, was arrested but later released. During the major deportations in August 1942, Zofia was taken to the *Umschlagplatz* and from there deported to Treblinka where she was murdered.

the Holy Ghost Hospital, as the director of the Czyste Old Order Jewish Hospital—a post he held until the end of the ghetto's existence.[42]

From the start, the Germans were plagued by fear of infectious diseases. Conscious of the immense threat posed by typhus, and the likelihood of a high mortality rate, they did everything possible to isolate themselves from the sources of infection. Isolation was their safest bet as they had no effective vaccinations at their disposal—at least not in the quantities needed to satisfy the demands of officials in the occupied territory. In November 1939, the Germans therefore concluded that the principal aim of any health policy was to prevent the spread of infectious diseases.[43]

## The Bersohn and Bauman Children's Hospital

Another severely affected hospital was the Bersohn and Bauman's Children's Hospital which was founded in 1878. It was housed in two locations, 51 Śliska Street and 222 Sienna Street. After the First World War it fell on hard times and closed in 1923. In 1930, Dr. Anna Braude-Heller organized a takeover of the buildings by the Society of Friends of Children. With funding from the Warsaw Jewish community and the American Jewish Joint Distribution Committee, the hospital was expanded to 150 beds. By the time the Second World War broke out, Bersohn and Bauman had grown to 250 beds and was lucky not to be damaged during the siege.

The hospital admitted children between the ages of three and thirteen, regardless of their religious affiliation.[44] Initially, the property, surrounded by an iron fence, had two buildings: one single-story, and the other a multi-story. A modern kitchen, a staff dining room, and utility

---

42  The accounts of those who participated in the events of 1939 vary as to the sequence and periods in office of the various directors of the Czyste Old Order Jewish Hospital. That uncertainty is resolved thanks to information in Dr. Julian Rotstadt's personal file, which clearly states that he replaced Dr. Zamenhof on October 7, 1939, and was arrested between December 15 and 27 of the same year. Personal files of doctors, members of Warsaw-Białystok Medical Chamber, Old Books Collection, Main Medical Library, Warsaw, ref. 3226.

43  Wysocki, *Lekarze polscy w czasie II wojny światowej*, 598.

44  A. Marek, *Opieka nad chorym dzieckiem w opinii polskiej prasy medycznej Królestwa Polskiego w latach 1801–1908* (Warsaw: Śląski Uniwersytet Medyczny, Instytut Historii Nauki PAN, 2009), 347.

rooms were in the basement. An elevator enabled meals to be delivered to the upper floors, where there was a remarkably well-equipped science laboratory and a conference room with a library. The wings, which once housed a school for pediatric nursing, were now the eye clinic and radiology departments. The hospital also boasted a spacious analytical laboratory.

On the first floor there was a forty-bed surgical department, with well-equipped operating theaters (antiseptic and septic), washrooms, toilets, and an incinerator. On the second floor was a fifty-bed internal diseases department, divided into one for younger children (up to the age of two), and another for older children, as well as a separate room with a washroom and toilet for non-resident breastfeeding mothers. On the third floor was a twenty-seven-bed tuberculosis department, with vast terraces on its southern side. Individual wards were divided by transparent glass partitions, while cots were equipped with loose mattresses to facilitate the raising and lowering of patients.

Each ward had phototherapy equipment. The admissions section was situated in the building adjacent to the main hospital.[45] The L. Dawidson Building, surrounded by gardens, housed an office and outpatient ward on the ground floor, and eye specialists' rooms and nurses' accommodations on the first floor. Before the war, the heads of the departments and clinic were highly respected specialists in their respective disciplines.[46]

At the time, there were two large lumber yards or depots near the hospital. Judyta Braude, Dr. Braude-Heller's sister, recalled how, when the bombing started, they became particularly hazardous for the hospital:

> In the evening, both depots were hit by several incendiary bombs and there was considerable danger that the fire would spread to the hospital buildings at any moment. Tremendous heat

---

45  Subsequent renovations and alterations to the complex were done in 1934, during an epidemic of scarlet fever among the children. During the remodeling, a separate staircase was added to improve access to the first floor.

46  An account by Judyta Braude, YVA O.3/2360. Among them were Dr. Anna Braude-Heller (neonatal ward), Dr. Mieczysław Seidman (pediatric surgery), Dr. Zofia Zylberstein (surgery clinic), Dr. Feliks Sachs (internal diseases department), Dr. Natalia Szpilfogel-Lichtenbaum (internal diseases clinic), Dr. Mieczysław Ganc (infectious diseases), Dr. Teodozja Goliborska (analytical laboratory), and Dr. Beniamin Kryński (radiology).

came off the walls separating the hospital from the depots. . .
Since fires had sprung up across the city and along its streets,
barricading them with rubble from collapsing buildings, the
fire engines could not extinguish the burning warehouses, and
several hours passed before they arrived.[47]

Buildings on Twarda, Pańska, and other streets in the vicinity of the hospital were in ruins or in flames. The priority was to save the children. There were about 100 of them in the hospital, as those on the mend had been sent home. After earnest efforts to find some sort of accommodation close by, Judyta Braude remembered a Christian family living at the corner of Twarda and Pańska Streets—probably the Dąbrowskis—who were the only ones to accept sick children and offered three rooms. "A family offering their apartment was a rare find. As it happened, in the morning their son was supposed to report to the army, at home there was a baby they moved to their neighbors."[48]

During a period of relative quiet, the staff carried sick children to the apartment. Babies' cots were moved using hand-drawn carts, mattresses and bedding were spread on the floor for the older children. Medicines and other indispensable items were also transferred. Children with typhoid fever were placed in a separate room. Although everything around it was still smoldering, the children were moved back to the hospital the next day.

Due to continuous bombings, gas, electricity, and the sewer system were destroyed. As a result, there was no way to prepare meals for the youngest patients. The hospital potter, Mr. Lejbowicz, hastily built a stove from bricks and tiles by dismantling an old fireplace from the former hospital building. Carbide lamps were used to light the wards.

When a shell damaged the water supply, Dr. Anna Braude-Heller shouted in disbelief: "It's not possible! We put up a huge banner with the Red Cross on it! How can we operate without washing our hands? Whoever survives, survives!"[49] Luckily, water was obtained by digging out an old, deep well on the property. Paramedics and patients not seriously injured carried water inside.

---

47  Ibid.
48  Ibid.
49  Meroz, *W murach i poza murami getta*, 13.

Under normal circumstances, food supplies would have lasted for three months. But a few days after the war started, the authorities redirected about a hundred older patients to the Children's Hospital from a makeshift hospital at Warsaw University. Many more civilian casualties were "dumped" over the fence by passersby.

Thieves stole whatever they could, so the situation rapidly deteriorated. There were no adult-sized beds, mattresses lay on the floor in wards and corridors, and even on the landings. Soon there was no free space on the floor. There were attempts to keep the children on the ground floor. "The usually impeccably clean hospital became hell, reeking of congealed blood and pus."[50] Soon the entire building carried the stench of rotting corpses.

The patients lived in fear of air raids. Sometimes, during the bombings, children were moved several times a night to rooms with windows facing away from where the bombs were falling. The walking wounded had to go down to the ground floor. During the worst bombings, Dr. Braude-Heller climbed to the top floor to calm terrified patients too gravely injured to move. Despite such diligent care, some patients remained unhappy about being in a Jewish facility.

> An unpleasant incident involving the nurses happened when, among the injured transferred from the university there were two Jews, both seriously wounded. One was diagnosed with tetanus and given serum, then put in a bed that had just become free. Other wounded patients, lying on the floor, protested, complaining that the man received the bed because he was a Jew, and was laughing at their plight. The unconscious patient indeed had a smirk on his face, which is typical of tetanus sufferers and resembles a smile. Because his condition was critical, he was soon moved to the isolation ward where he died later that evening.[51]

Thankfully, such attitudes were not the norm. Two firefighting officers with less serious injuries expressed their heartfelt gratitude, thanking the

50  An account by Judyta Braude, YVA O.3/2360.
51  Ibid.

doctors, nurses and orderlies, with one of them saying he could never have imagined that such courage and devotion existed.[52]

During the first days of the war, even before the first casualties were brought to the hospital, the facility had no surgeon because Dr. Maurycy Saidman, the surgical specialist, had been assigned to the front. His assistants were called up as well. Dr. Zofia Hurwicz-Zylbersztajn, a consulting doctor in the surgical clinic, was also unavailable.[53] Other specialists were also called up.[54] Eventually, the hospital obtained the services of Dr. Gottesman[55] and his junior colleague, Dr. Bencjan Leneman, a diligent and attentive surgeon. The hospital also welcomed gynecologist Izaak Szachnerowicz and his pediatrician wife, Anna, both from the Czyste Old Order Jewish Hospital. In her book, Dr. Anna Meroz wrote that by then the facility no longer resembled a children's hospital: "Everywhere— in corridors, lecture halls, and laboratories—lay adults who had been dragged out from under the ruins. On seeing a white uniform, they pleaded: "Help me please, I have not had a drop of water to drink in three days!'"[56] Judyta Braude recalled a tragic incident when a patient was left without further surgical help:

> There was a young woman who had recently volunteered to work in our laboratory, the twenty-three-year-old university graduate and analyst, Finkelsztein. . . greatly appreciated for being conscientious and well mannered. Her engineer husband had been in Australia for a while, and made formal arrangements for her to join him, but she did not want to leave her elderly father alone when the war broke out. One night, during the bombing, she arrived at the hospital with her father on a stretcher. One of the bombs had struck their apartment on the second floor in Jerozolimskie Avenue, crashing through the two upper floors and hitting her bedridden father in the legs, as he lay in his anteroom.

---

52  Ibid.
53  Doctors Leopold Rafałowski, Stanisław Hercenberg (both later murdered in Katyń) and Seweryn Wilk.
54  Among them radiologist Dr. Beniamin Kryński (murdered in Kharkov), laryngologist Aleksander Owczarek (murdered in Katyń), and pediatrician Izrael Rotbalsam (who returned to the hospital at the beginning of October).
55  No further information could be found regarding a doctor named Gottesman.
56  Meroz, *W murach i poza murami getta*, 12.

Because there was no surgeon on hand to operate immediately, she had him transferred to another facility. She went to Infant Jesus Hospital on Nowogrodzka Street. That very night a bomb hit the surgical department, even though the hospital had many pavilions. Almost all the patients were killed. Finkelsztein was also killed, while the remains of her father were not found. She was buried in the Warsaw Jewish Cemetery.[57]

The biggest obstacle was a shortage of medical personnel, among them surgeons needed to provide crucial service in the heat of battle. After a week the situation worsened, as more doctors left for the Eastern Front following an appeal by Colonel Umiastowski. The situation in the hospitals improved slightly when several doctors returned as the army began to retreat, as we saw from examples mentioned above.

## The Ujazdowski Hospital

In the first few days of the war, the Ujazdowski Hospital admitted over 5,000 wounded from troop divisions "Poznań," "Pomorze," "Warszawa," "Prusy," "Modlin," and "Łódź."[58] In the first few days of September, they, too, saw a rapid turnover in hospital staff.[59] To cope with the unending stream of wounded, ad hoc hospitals were established in school buildings and private apartments. With the vast number of patients, there were not enough doctors to carry out procedures, and worse, there was limited blood for transfusions. World-renowned immunologist, Prof. Ludwik Hirszfeld, and his coworkers Róża Amzel, Zofia Skórska, and Dr. Olgierd Sokołowski organized blood donation stations. Zofia Mańkowska and Stanisława Adamowicz managed the office, keeping records and

---

57 An account by Judyta Braude, YVA O.3/2360.
58 A. Matuszak, *Ujazdów wojskowy. Wspomnienia* (Warsaw: Aleksy Matuszak, 2014), 35.
59 Until September 15, the hospital's commander was Dr. Józef Konarski. After the military doctors in the "Poznań" division returned to Warsaw, the position of the Ujazdowski Hospital commander was assigned to Colonel Dr. Mieczysław Naramowski. From September 28, 1939, this position was held by Colonel Prof. Dr. T. Kucharski, and Colonel Dr. M. Naramowski served as his deputy. On April 1, 1940, Colonel Dr. Leon Strehl became the new commander of the hospital.

performing administrative tasks, while Irena Nowak served as laboratory nurse and scout Piotr Osiński was their messenger.[60]

In his postwar memoirs, Prof. Hirszfeld wrote:

> The influx of wounded was never-ending. A female doctor from the Ujazdowski Hospital came to the institute [the State Hygiene Institute—M.C.] to say the hospital was being evacuated, that wounded soldiers were left lying without any help, that everything was in short supply. When I asked whether they had organized for blood transfusions, I was told they had not. I immediately donated and then decanted my own blood and that of my assistants into a bottle and reported to the hospital commander. He received the blood with gratitude; after only a few hours it was finished. I proposed organizing a blood transfusion station—a proposal which was enthusiastically accepted. . . The hospital assigned me the bacteriological laboratory to use. I appealed to citizens over the radio and in the newspapers, especially to the women of Warsaw, asking them to donate blood for the wounded. . . In response to my appeal, hundreds of women came forward. After only a few days I had enough supplies to meet the needs of our hospital and hospitals across the entire city. We established a duty roster in the hospitals and handed surgeons the addresses of female donors living in the vicinity. Typically, a trip to the hospital took place under a hail of bombs and bullets, streetcars did not operate. To avoid being hit by bullets, donors had to rush from one entrance to another.[61]

Hospitals with an 800-bed capacity typically accommodated 1,200 wounded, and the branches another 3,000. The conditions under which patients were treated worsened dramatically with each passing hour.

---

60  T. Brzeziński, *Służba Zdrowia w obronie Warszawy we wrześniu 1939 roku* (Łódź: Wojskowa Akademia Medyczna, 1963), 85. Reprint of a thesis in fulfilment of the Doctor of Medicine degree, Military Medical Academy, Łódź, 1963.

61  Hirszfeld, *Historia jednego życia*, 184–186. Ludwik Hirszfeld wrote in his memoirs that, with the outbreak of the war, all the prewar assumptions and preparations proved useless. If blood was needed, doctors donated their own blood, as did the support staff.

Despite its Red Cross markings, the Ujazdowski Hospital came under fire. During one of the air raids, a bomb hit the hospital admissions section, killing seven wounded patients waiting for treatment and injuring many others. "Patients were lying on the floor, there were no medicines, no wound-dressings, no undergarments for them. Everything had to be improvised," Prof. Hirszfeld recalled.[62]

Chief officer of the sanitary detachment, in the "Warszawa" division and the commander of District Hospital no. 1, Colonel Dr. Leon Strehl, began evacuating the wounded. On September 8 and 9, the hospitals in Rudka and Mienia accepted approximately 3,000 convalescing patients, and those with minor injuries from the Ujazdowski Hospital. Several patients were evacuated to Kowle in improvised sanitary trains. During its last days, the Ujazdowski Hospital functioned without water and electricity, anesthetics or bandages. After the capitulation of Warsaw, the next wave of wounded arrived, and the military's sanitary units were disbanded at the hospital. On October 1, 1939, the Ujazdowski Hospital became a POW field hospital.[63]

The first three months of the occupation proved to be very challenging for the Ujazdowski Hospital. Though the *Wehrmacht* was obliged to supply food, medical equipment, medicines, and dressings, they did not. No one received a stipend or salary, since hospital employees had become POWs. According to the Geneva Convention, wounded Polish soldiers with the status of POWs had to be looked after for six months.

Despite this catastrophic situation, the hospital stayed open thanks to the benevolence of Warsaw residents. Owners of workshops and warehouses donated textiles and other necessary items. Private residents also helped. To help the injured, Dr. Eli Lubelczyk, a Jewish radiologist who worked at the Order of Malta Hospital in Warsaw, donated equipment from his own practice.

Although the POW doctors' finances were dire, patients received proper care. Despite a leg wound, Dr. Henryk Fenigsztein worked in the surgical department for the entire year. In an interview years later,

---

62  Ibid., 186.
63  T. Brzeziński, "Ujazdów w dniach obrony Warszawy," in *UJazdów. Materiały sesji naukowej zorganizowanej przez Główną Bibliotekę Lekarską im. Stanisława Konopki oraz Muzeum Historyczne m. st. Warszawy* (Warsaw: Główna Biblioteka Lekarska, Muzeum Historyczne Warszawy, 1992), 40.

he said he shared the ward with four non-Jewish POWs, and all were treated equally: "My roommates and I were comrades in misery. We lived together, shared everything. I was the only one from Warsaw, so they had no families nearby who could supplement the meager diet the Germans provided."[64]

In mid-March 1940, during a briefing of commanders at the POW hospital (attended by representatives from the Polish Red Cross and the Central Welfare Council), Chief Doctor Richter declared that April 1 would end the six-month period when the German army had been obliged to maintain the hospital under the terms of the Hague and Geneva conventions.[65] According to Dr. Fenigstein, convalescing soldiers who did not escape from the hospital earlier were moved to POW camps, while captive officers were released. Doctors, nurses and private individuals helped soldiers and officers escape, despite constant searches by *Wehrmacht* inspectors.

Because of its important role in underground activities, the hospital was called the "Ujazdowska Republic." During the occupation it was instrumental in shaping the patriotic and professional stance of the medical fraternity. The first clandestine lectures for medical students from the ghetto took place there; it also served as a shelter for Jews.[66]

## The Activities of the Jewish Community Organizations

When the war started, the community assisted in defending Warsaw. On September 1, 1939, under the auspices of the Jewish Community, the committee for the defense of the country was established in Warsaw.[67] The committee established five subcommittees—finance, legal, publicity,

---

64 Henry Fenigstein, "Holocaust and I: Memoirs of a Survivor by Dr. Henry Fenigstein as told to Saundra Collis" (unpublished manuscript, undated), 96. Kindly made available by Prof. Claude Romney and Dr. Lawrence Powell.
65 A. J. Chaciński, "Szpital Maltański w okupowanej Warszawie," *Przegląd Lekarski—Oświęcim* 32, bk. 15, no. 1 (1975): 145.
66 Fenigstein, "Holocaust and I," 98.
67 J. Leociak, "Opieka społeczna," in B. Engelking and J. Leociak, *Getto Warszawskie. Przewodnik po nieistniejacym mieście* (Warsaw: IFiS PAN, 2001), 292. Members included Apolinary Hartglas, Maksymilian Friede, Mojżesz Koerner, Leon Lewite, Salomea Lewite, Maurycy Mayzel, Szymon Seideman, Mojżesz Schorr, Rafał Szereszewski, Henryk Szoszkes, Jakub Trockenheim, Samuel Wołkowicz, Abraham Weiss, and Zdzisław Żmigryder-Konopka.

sanitary and social care. On September 13, the Jewish Citizens' Committee received legal status with headquarters in a Jewish Association building. Its members were Abraham Gepner, Mojżesz Koerner, Stanisław Szereszewski, Adam Czerniaków, and Marek Lichtenbaum. Its medical and sanitary care section was headed by Dr. Izrael Milejkowski.[68] On September 14 the Jewish Coordination Committee was established and became a vital link in civilian efforts to defend Warsaw. It became the roots of the future *Judenrat*'s Self-Help organization. The Coordination Committee cooperated with Community Self-Help to help Jews and other victims of wartime hostilities, concentrating in districts predominantly inhabited by Jews.[69]

During the Warsaw blockade, the administrative activities of the Council of the Jewish Community were curtailed, since many of its members left the capital in the first days of the bombardment, including its president, Maurycy Mayzel.[70] Many of the office clerks fled. Because of the bombings, getting to its headquarters was difficult. Yet despite the daily air raids, until the Germans entered the city, four clerks reported for work every day, along with two (and later only one) member of the council.[71] On September 11, Adam Czerniaków, a member of the Community's council and later the head of the *Judenrat*, noted in his diary:

> Management got a fright. I was in my office at 26 Grzybowska Street. At number 27, an explosion killed three people. The wounded were helped on our premises. *He-Khalutz* members were engaged as support staff in forming a Jewish Committee. A meeting was held in Gepner's office, to establish such a committee.[72]

---

68 Czerniaków dates the legalization of the Jewish Citizen's Committee by President Starzyński as September 15. A. Czerniaków, *Adama Czerniakowa dziennik getta warszawskiego*, ed. M. Fuks (Warsaw: PWN, 1983), 47.

69 Leociak, "Opieka społeczna," 292.

70 B. Engelking, "Rada Żydowska," in B. Engelking and J. Leociak, *Getto Warszawskie*, 147–148.

71 *Tak było . . . Sprawozdania z warszawskiego getta 1939–1943 (Wybór)* (Warsaw: ZPPU Zetpress, 1988), 29.

72 Czerniaków, *Adama Czerniakowa dziennik*, 46. He-Khalutz (also he-chaluts, Hebr. החלוץ—pioneer, settler) was a Jewish youth Zionist organization, founded in 1914 in Russia, whose aim was to revive the Zionist movement by conducting preparations for the Jewish population to return to Palestine.

On September 18, without permission and failing to meet conditions for its effective functioning, the Association organized a 100-bed hospital on Zielna Street to treat wounds and dispense medicines.[73] On September 20, Czerniaków approached Warsaw Mayor (also known as the president of Warsaw) Stefan Starzyński, and requested formal authorization to dispense medical care. On September 22 Starzyński nominated him to replace Maurycy Mayzel as the president of the Jewish Community.[74]

Self-help activities among the Jews in the besieged capital were also undertaken by Jewish political parties and organizations that had been active before the war. Along with the work of the Jewish Community, community institutions provided care for ailing Jews. Initially known as the Coordination Committee of Jewish Social Organizations, in January 1940 it was renamed the Jewish Self-Help Society and in October 1940, the name was changed again to the Jewish Society for Community Welfare.[75]

Later, the *Judenrat* Self-Help absorbed all social, charitable, and cultural associations.[76] The Community Self-Help Warsaw branch became the Jewish Welfare Society and assumed control over Jewish community and charitable organizations. These included the Towarzystwo Ochrony Zdrowia Ludności Żydowskiej (Society for Safeguarding the Health of the Jewish Population; referred to as TOZ) established in Warsaw in 1921;[77] the Society for Abandoned and Orphaned Children (CENTOS); Włodzimierz Medem's sanatorium in Miedzeszyn;[78] the Bikur Cholim

---

73 Ibid., 48.
74 During the hostilities of September 1939, the work of the Jewish Community's various committees was disrupted because its chairperson left, and most of its council's members stopped carrying out their duties except for funeral services.
75 For more on Jewish Self-Help structural changes, see chapter "Instytucje i urzędy," in B. Engelking and J. Leociak, *Getto Warszawskie*.
76 A regulation dissolving all community, charitable, and cultural organizations was issued on August 1, 1940, in *Dziennik Rozporządzeń Generalnego Gubernatorstwa* ("Journal of General Government Regulations"). See Einhorn, *Towarzystwo Ochrony Zdrowia*, 106.
77 The Towarzystwo Ochrony Zdrowia Ludności Żydowskiej (Society for Safeguarding the Health of the Jewish Population; TOZ) was established in Warsaw in 1921, when the Polish branch of the Saint Petersburg-based Obshchestvo Zdravookhraneniia Evreev (Society for the Protection of Jewish Health, OZE, later, Oeuvre de Secour aux Enfants; OSE) became a specific national organization.
78 CENTOS's principal doctor was Zofia Rosenblum. Miedzeszyn sanatorium boasted the Włodzimierz Medem Therapy and Education Institute. The management office of

society (a group that helps the sick) providing care for the indigent; the Society for the Care of Indigent Patients (Linas Hatzedek); Brijus (Health), the Jewish Tuberculosis Prevention Society, and its sanatorium in Otwock; the Society for Mentally Ill Jews and its Zofiówka hospital; and maternity facilities such as the Institute for Assisting Destitute Mothers and the Institute of the Society for the Care of Jewish Infants. All these institutions, which had existed before the war, had a direct (or an indirect) influence on the development of community medicine and healthcare for infants and children. TOZ, funded by memberships, donations, and foreign Jewish philanthropies, looked after the welfare and wellbeing of Jewish citizens in independent Poland, promoting their health and the health of their children. It was most influential in the area of preventative medicine, concentrating on mitigating and treating tuberculosis and trachoma by establishing clinics and sanatoria.[79] TOZ's Warsaw branch was one of a few therapeutic pneumothorax clinics in Poland, with a special tuberculosis prevention clinic at 43 Gęsia Street, directed by Dr. Gerszon Lewin.[80]

The clinic was equipped with a radiology laboratory and examined children periodically to prevent infection. It had an analytical laboratory, physiotherapy units, a phototherapy unit, and a dispensary for basic medicines and cod-liver oil.[81] There were ringworm prevention clinics and dermatology clinics that treated crusted ringworm infections with X-rays. The TOZ sanatorium for children and youths at Otwock accepted

---

Wł. Medem's Child Sanatorium Society (Stowarzyszenia Sanatorium Dziecka im. Wł. *Medema*) was located on 2 Leszno Street in Warsaw. The sanatorium, under principal doctor Natalia Szpilfogel-Lichtenbaumowa, was closed by the Germans on August 20, 1942.

79  For the genesis and establishment of TOZ and accounts of its work in Poland between 1921 and 1950, see Einhorn, *Towarzystwo Ochrony Zdrowia*. The TOZ chairman was Dr. Marek Koenigstein.

80  Gerszon Gabriel Lewin von Hersz (1867–1939), a doctor, pulmonologist and phthisiatrist (a TB specialist), community activist and author writing in Hebrew and Yiddish, died in Warsaw on October 24, 1939.

81  The phototherapy unit was headed by doctors Regina Judt and Jakub Gelbfisz, assisted by Maria Sucharczuk. The TOZ mother-and-child unit was managed by Dr. Emma Mościsker, the infant care unit by Dr. Hanna Hirszfeld. The TOZ surgical institute on 34 Pańska Street was served by doctors Dawid Amsterdamski, Michał Eljasberg, and Julian Ajzner, and obstetrics on 11 Elektoralna Street was headed by Dr. Nikodem Szenkier. From the first days of war, organizing dispensary services represented a marked challenge for clinic employees.

sick and recovering patients free of other infectious diseases or psychiatric illness. Treatments cost between three and four zlotys per day.[82]

When the war started, the activities of Warsaw TOZ was centralized. Its manager, Dr. Jakub Rozenblum, an energetic and resourceful man, had a disability affecting his mobility. To expedite TOZ's work and assist him, Drs. Menachem Mendel Schwalbe (former chair of the Łódź TOZ branch) and Icchok Chain came to work with him.[83]

Following the bombardment and siege, the first multiple cases of typhoid fever appeared in Warsaw. TOZ organized transportation for the sick, making use of hand-drawn carts to take patients to the Czyste Jewish Hospital. The winter of 1939/1940 brought an increase in the number of typhus cases, which led to the Bersohn and Bauman Children's Hospital becoming a facility for infectious diseases. At the same time, it was deprived of income from private patients. When the German authorities forced the Social Insurance Company and the City Council to stop paying into its account, the hospital was forced to rely on TOZ.[84] In January 1940, together with the American Jewish Distribution Committee (JDC), TOZ took over all patients' expenses at the Zofiówka psychiatric facility in Otwock.[85]

In his postwar memoir, Mojżesz Mieczysław Tursz recalled how TOZ helped Jews living in Warsaw that September:

> In their despair, the Jewish people . . . could turn to one address only: the TOZ building on 43 Gęsia Street . . . the largest sanitary and medical center which arose almost spontaneously in a northern suburb of Warsaw. There were two qualified nurses (sisters Reinfeld and Kopel), long-time employees in TOZ's tuberculosis prevention clinic. There

---

82  H. Kroszczor and R. Zabłotniak, "Towarzystwo Ochrony Zdrowia Ludności Żydowskiej w latach II Rzeczypospolitej," *Biuletyn Żydowskiego Instytutu Historycznego* 1, no. 105 (1978): 65.

83  An account by Icchok Chain (Józef Gołębiowski), YVA O.3/2355.

84  *Gazeta Żydowska* 13 (1940): 2.

85  The Zofiówka facility was situated on 2 Kochanowski Street in Otwock. Dr. Stefan Miller was its director, Dr. Jan Przedborski its curator. Zofiówka's office was on 6 Elektoralna Street in Warsaw. During the liquidation of the Otwock Ghetto, Dr. Maks Maślanka committed suicide on the sanatorium grounds. The director and his wife, Dr. Irena Themerson-Miller, also a psychiatrist, both committed suicide two days later in Mińsk Mazowiecki.

was also a doctor living in the vicinity of TOZ, but at the heart of the action was the old faithful stoker and janitor, F. Wroński. He could be everywhere at once, he would extinguish an incendiary bomb on the roof and a moment later lug a heavy crate with wound dressings from the cellar, and immediately after that rush out onto the street to help a badly injured person inside. As long as we had a telephone connection, the TOZ sanitary team received moral support and encouragement from Dr. Jakób Rozenblum, a member of the TOZ Warsaw branch management, an institution deeply concerned with the fate of the Jewish population from the very beginning. Unfortunately, because he lived in the center of the city and walked on a prosthesis, it was impossible for him to get to Gęsia Street. . . Luckily, the TOZ building was not bombed. Several bullets scarred the third-floor walls, depriving the building of windows while a few incendiary bombs were disarmed with sand, just in time. In the second half of September, Warsaw was in ruins, turned to ash. Only with the passing of time did it become obvious that ruins could still be turned into more ruins, that ashes could cover an even larger area, when for the Jews, death became an almost common occurrence.[86]

Before the war, TOZ had been involved in various health promotion activities but was not involved in healthcare as such. When the war started, the number of people turning for help to TOZ on Gęsia grew with each passing day. Initially, only those with minor injuries came, but later also the seriously ill arrived—people who had been hiding in cellars, hungry and in constant fear. Hundreds turned up to have their dressings changed. Slowly, bandages and medications ran out, and there were not enough personnel to handle the patients.

Fortunately, Dr. Jakub Rozenblum reached the TOZ office and with the approval of the JDC directors and the TOZ chairperson, was appointed general secretary of its Warsaw branch.[87] Under his direction,

---

86  An account by Mojżesz Mieczysław Tursz (Thursz), "Jak kształtował się sanitariat w ghetcie warszawskim," YVA O.3/438.

87  Ibid.

TOZ arranged a cooperation agreement with the Brijus Sanatorium for Tuberculosis Sufferers in Otwock.[88] According to Mieczysław Tursz, the JDC financed facilities like the Bersohn and Bauman Children's Hospital, the Brijus Sanatorium, the Zofiówka Psychiatric Institute, and the Society for the Friends of Children through TOZ agencies—right up to the moment the United States joined the war against the Nazis, when all American contact was blocked.[89] From its founding, TOZ leased a small office building on 11 Leszno Street and oversaw a number of institutions dispersed across the city.

Care centers served as counseling and advisory clinics where pediatricians attended to sick children and implemented prevention programs (vaccinations), in addition to teaching mothers the basic principles of hygiene. Financially, the centers depended on the Society for Abandoned and Orphaned Children (CENTOS). Medical supervision was in the hands of TOZ. Doctors were assisted by nurses who had previously worked in the Bersohn and Bauman Children's Hospital. Judyta Braude, whose sister revived the hospital before the war, acted as secretary for all three mother-and-child centers until the end of 1939.

In October of that year, Society of the Friends of Children opened a Mother-and-Childcare Center on Elektoralna Street; it was the third such center for children of four to fourteen years of age. Every day the children received breakfast and lunch in a common room. The center offered a feeding program for almost all its charges by distributing rations (flour, cereal, honey, sugar, tins of condensed and fresh milk) received from CENTOS. Medications were also distributed.

As Mieczysław Tursz noted:

---

88 The Brijus Jewish Tuberculosis Prevention Society ran a sanatorium with the same profile on 55 Reymont Street in Otwock, with Dr. Mieczysław Levi as its director. For more on this facility, see Jewish Historical Institute Archives, ref. 311/15, 17, 18 (bequest of Henryk Kroszczor).

89 Tursz, "Jak kształtował się sanitariat w ghetcie warszawskim." The Friends of Children society emerged in 1919 on the initiative of Stefania Sempołowska, a renowned community activist, educator, journalist, and writer, who offered Polish socialists an opportunity to include in their program the struggle to improve the lives of workers' children.

Extremely poor people kept coming, jobless and without any means to survive. Before the war, the tuberculosis prevention clinic had dispensed basic medicines in the form of tablets, along with other remedies, to the sick. Now this action resumed without the necessary authorization. At so-called medicine distribution points, hundreds of people received basic and essential medicines.[90]

The International Red Cross sent TOZ parcels from Geneva containing medicines, wound dressings, malt, vitamins and anti-typhus vaccines, but the Germans looted these, appropriating everything they considered useful.[91] Together with CENTOS, TOZ organized feeding programs to help young patients and destitute children. Doctors visited schools (with the permission of the Department of Education) and vaccinated children against typhoid fever and dysentery.[92] Two to three times a week, eleven doctors and fifteen nurses visited more than twenty kitchens and ten hubs to examine the children and staff (keeping a health record for each child). At the end of every month, a doctor would prepare a report on each kitchen. A medical doctor and a principal hygienist would also inspect the kitchens on behalf of TOZ. The section which oversaw kitchens serving adult employees employed four doctors, each taking care of approximately fifteen to eighteen kitchens, which were inspected once a week.[93] The Central Sanitary Unit organized courses for home caregivers and paramedic training.[94]

In October 1940, by order of the German Social Insurance Commissioner, TOZ had taken over the medical services of Jews who had been insured. According to their oral agreement, the Social Insurance Company undertook to pay TOZ 10,000 zlotys a month, allowing the insured to seek medical help from the Department of Medical Assistance, paying twenty to thirty groszes for a consultation. But regular payments were not made into a TOZ account. Most of the funds went into the coffers of German insurance companies.

---

90  Tursz, "Jak kształtował się sanitariat w ghetcie warszawskim."
91  Ibid.
92  *Gazeta Żydowska* 13 (1940): 2; 73 (1941): 3, 39 (1942): 2.
93  "Sprawozdanie z kontroli w Towarzystwie Ochrony Zdrowia 'TOZ,'" Jewish Historical Institute Archives, Ringelblum archives, Ring. II/ 92, 1–49.
94  The lecturers were: Akiwa Uryson, Jakub Rozenblum, Izaak Lejpuner, Hipolit Boczko, Menachem Schwalbe, Mojżesz Tursz, Rudolf Kirszblum, Icchok Chain, Henryk Makower, Bernard Szeps, Ilia Janowski, and J. Mitz.

Chapter 5

# Healthcare Prior to the Creation of the Ghetto

After the invasion in September 1939, the German authorities issued discriminatory regulations targeting Jews in particular with their properties confiscated and their civil rights denied. Marked by armbands featuring the blue Star of David, they were beaten and humiliated on the streets and forced to do senseless tasks. In addition to being stripped of their property, Jews were forced out from their homes and, later, locked behind the walls of the ghetto. Noemi Makower wrote that "being rounded up for the so-called labor camps . . . and being shot at near the ghetto gate by passing motorcyclists became a daily occurrence."[1]

Marek Edelman wrote:

As early as November 1939, the first "exterminating" decrees were made public: the establishment of "educational" camps for the Jewish population as a whole and the expropriation of all Jewish assets in excess of 2,000 zloty per family. Later, one after another, a multitude of prohibitive rules and ordinances appeared. Jews were forbidden to work in key industries, in government institutions, to bake bread, to earn more than 500 zloty a month (and the price of bread rose, at times, to as high as 40 zloty a pound), to buy from or sell to "Aryans," to seek comfort at "Aryan" doctors' offices, to doctor "Aryan" sick, to ride on trains and trolley-cars, to leave the city limits without

---

1    Makower, *Miłość w cieniu śmierci*, 61.

special permits, to possess gold or jewelry, etc. After November 12, 1939, every Jew twelve years of age or older was compelled to wear on their right arm a white armband with the blue Star of David printed on it (in certain cities, e.g. Łódź and Wloclawek, yellow signs on the back and chest).[2]

These armbands made the wearers instantly recognizable and subjected them to abuse by the Germans and their collaborators. Initial acts of violence were limited to beatings or to cutting off the beards and sidelocks of visibly Orthodox Jews.

Soon German officers, soldiers, and *Volksdeutsche* began to invade private apartments, raiding them for money, valuables, and personal items. In time, as Judyta Braude put it, this "looting of apartments and businesses assumed an organized, systematic character." Works of art, jewelry, and, in the case of doctors, medical equipment they kept at home became prized booty. Many of these items were officially confiscated or obtained through blackmail and extortion.[3] While the official requisitioning of property was done on the order of the Office of the Governor of the Warsaw District, many Germans participated of their own volition.

> Soldiers came to Docent Brookman to steal. They were surprised that he owned very few shirts. . . A young medical officer came to the meritorious senior otologist [ear doctor] Dr. Srebrny, and without ceremony removed his library. Doctor Srebrny had published valuable research, among others, in German. A book in German was lying on his desk. The following conversation ensued between the two: "Is this your work?" asked the German doctor. "Yes, I wrote it at the time when Germans still respected science." "Times have changed," responded the German. "Didn't you hear that Archimedes was killed by a Roman soldier?" To this, Doctor Srebrny offered an answer which should make every German burn with shame: "True, but I know, you know, and everyone else knows the name of Archimedes, while nobody remembers the name of that Roman soldier."[4]

---

2    Marek Edelman, "The Ghetto Fights," in *The Warsaw Ghetto: The 45th Anniversary of the Uprising* (Warsaw: Interpress Publishers, n.d.), 17–39.
3    An account by Judyta Braude, YVA O.3/2360.
4    Ibid., 196.

Wealthy Jews were arrested preemptively to prevent them from hiding their possessions or transferring their property abroad.[5] To protect their possessions, some doctors placed notices on their doors, stating: "In service of combating the epidemic." Soon after that, they were called to Blank's Palace, where Oskar Dengel, the Nazi-commissioned mayor, told them that such notices could only be posted with permission of the authorities.[6]

During the spring and summer of 1940, Jews began to accept the inevitability of being forcibly moved to the ghetto, which was "justifiably" created as a result of a typhus epidemic. Many tried to trade their apartments outside the ghetto with Poles inside the area in advance, while others moved their assets to summer houses or to homes of friends living outside of Warsaw. One of the ironies of creating the ghetto around Warsaw's Jewish Quarter meant that many poorer Jews had the advantage of staying in their own homes. Then Jews from outlying areas were brought to the ghetto, and apartments that barely managed to house one family housed as many as five, as food and medical supplies dwindled.

Doctors were, comparatively speaking, in a better position than other Jews, because many had friends who could help them hide their valuables. For instance, the doctors at the Bersohn and Bauman Children's Hospital were helped by Dr. Wacław Skonieczny, the commission-appointed administrator of the hospital.[7]

The authorities forbade anyone from assisting Jews and the City Council's Department of Healthcare was ordered to dismiss all Jewish employees.[8] Jews lost their right to healthcare and medical assistance, and Jewish patients were evicted from hospitals. Jewish medical personnel were ordered to leave non-Jewish institutions immediately.[9] All efforts to stabilize healthcare provisions (and especially hospitalization) made by the Warsaw Department of Healthcare, the Jewish Association and other community organizations were for naught after Jewish patients

---

5 J. Grabowski, *Ja tego Żyda znam. Szantażowanie Żydów w Warszawie 1939–1943* (Warsaw: Centrum Badań nad Zagładą Żydów, 2004), 19.
6 An account by Icchok Chain (Józef Gołębiowski), YVA O.3/2355.
7 An account by Izrael Rotbalsam, YVA O.3/2357.
8 Leociak, "Opieka społeczna," 292.
9 *Dzieje medycyny w Polsce. Opracowania i szkice*, vol. 2, W. Noszczyk, J. Supady (eds), Warsaw 2015, p. 587.

were removed from the insurance system and funds and supplies were cut off.

## The Polish Medical System under Occupation

After the outbreak of the Second World War, the German authorities retained Polish laws enacted prior to 1939, provided they did not endanger military security and were aligned with German military interests. General Friedrich von Cochenhausen, Kommandierender General des Stellvertretenden Generalkommandos des XIII Armee-Korps, became the military commander of Warsaw in charge of a civilian administration. At its helm was SS-Standartenführer Harry von Craushaar. Helmut Otto was the Reich commissioned mayor of Warsaw. Before the war, he was mayor of Düsseldorf. Dr. Oskar Dengel, the former mayor of Würzburg, served as his deputy.[10] The commander and his offices were housed in Blank's Palace.

Given the urgent need for doctors in 1939, medical university graduates were permitted to work in hospitals, without being on the published list from the Ministry of Social Care, dated July 17, 1940.

## Creation of the Judenrat

On October 7, 1939, the Germans appointed Adam Czerniaków, deputy president of the Jewish Community in Warsaw, as chairperson of the Council of Elders, which became the *Judenrat*.[11] Lothar Beutel, chief of the Operational Brigade, who also commanded Task Force IV, the SS-Brigadeführer and commander of Einsatzgruppe IV (a mobile squad),

---

10 Helmut Otto was the first Nazi Reich commissioned mayor (president) of Warsaw (October 1, 1939–November 4, 1939), the second was Oskar Rudolf Dengel (November 4, 1939–March 1940).

11 The first task the Germans gave the *Judenrat* was to conduct a census of Jews. Statistics show that in October 1939, almost 360,000 Jews were living in Warsaw. When on October 30, 1939, Reichsführer-SS Heinrich Himmler ordered the resettlement of Poles and Jews from Polish territories under German occupation to areas controlled by the *Generalgouvernement*, that number increased considerably. Between November 1939 and October 1940, approximately 90,000 displaced Jews flowed into Warsaw. See B. Engelking and J. Leociak, "Kalendarium," in their *Getto Warszawskie*, 54.

ordered Czerniaków to select twenty-four councilors from the prewar members of the board of the Jewish Community (Dr. Josef Meisinger signed the order by plenipotentiary). They were confirmed on October 15, 1939, and were headquartered at 26/28 Grzybowska Street.[12] By the time the first meeting was set on November 4, 1939, the council faced debts of approximately a million zlotys.[13] Neither its clerks nor its suppliers had been paid for two months yet the German authorities imposed further financial obligations on the council and exacted financial contributions from it.

The mission of the health departments created by the *Judenrat* included:

1. Maintaining the health of the Jewish population, which included providing prophylactics and preventative services (establishing and maintaining bathhouses, laundries, delousing chambers and immunization centers) as well as medical care (support for hospitals, outpatient clinics, pharmacies);
2. Establishing and maintaining contact with the health authorities;
3. Coordinating the work of the health departments in the *Judenrat*;
4. Extending assistance to small towns where no Jewish doctors were present;
5. Regulating relationships between Jewish doctors in the community;
6. Maintaining contact with charities, TOZ, and the JDC.[14]

## The Functioning of the Medical Chambers

With the ceasefire, the medical chambers resumed their operations.[15] On November 18, 1939, Jost Walbaum, director and health superintendent of the *Generalgouvernement* Health Department, and Werner Kroll, the spokesman in the Governor-General's Office for Health Affairs, issued a decree defining regional doctors' duties as representatives of the medical

---

12  *Tak było*, 30.
13  Ibid., 33.
14  *Gazeta Żydowska* 29 (1940): 6.
15  Z. Wiśniewski, *Lekarze i izby lekarskie w Drugiej Rzeczypospolitej. Naczelna izba lekarska* (Warsaw: Naczelna Izba Lekarska, 2007), 376.

chamber. Walbaum had been responsible with others for allowing euthanasia to be performed on patients in psychiatric hospitals in the occupied Polish territories (in Chełm Lubelski, Kobierzyn, Kulpartów, Tworki, and Otwock).[16]

Polish medical chambers were supposed to continue functioning as before but under German administrators. These regulations, which also covered the pharmaceutical chambers operating under the medical chambers, went into effect in May 1940. Regional doctors had to prepare lists of active doctors and keep them up to date. The lists had to state names, surnames, addresses and the nationality of each doctor. They also issued regulations encompassing the range of activities of medical chambers inside the borders of the *Generalgouvernement* (the Kraków, Lublin, and Warsaw-Białystok chambers). A compulsory annual membership fee of twenty-one zlotys was instituted, and Jewish doctors had to "evacuate" their apartments and practices. Unemployed Aryan Polish doctors were permitted to take over deserted practices and abandoned apartments.[17]

Before the German occupation, Colonel Dr. Adam Julian Huszcza was president of the Warsaw-Białystok Medical Chamber. On January 26, 1940, Johann Kaminski, a district doctor, ordered the National Medical Chamber in Warsaw to close.[18] By order of Governor Hans Frank, on February 28, 1940, the National Medical Chamber was established in the *Generalgouvernement*, headquartered in Kraków. Walbaum was chamber president and Kroll was his deputy.[19]

As Marian Cieckiewicz recalled:

> On a designated day, in the company of the city's chief medical officer, Dr. Owsiński and three German officials reported

---

16 Dr. Jost Walbaum (1889–1969), a doctor and member of the NSDAP (National Socialist German Workers Party) and the SA (abbreviation from *Sturmabteilung*, Assault Division), with the rank of colonel, was a director in the Health Department (*Abteilung Gesundheitswesen*) of the *Generalgouvernement* until December 1942. P. Strekowicz, "Dr. Jost Walbaum, kierownik wydziału zdrowia w tzw. Rządzie Generalnego Gubernatorstwa," *Przegląd Lekarski—Oświęcim* 46, bk. 29, no. 1 (1989): 136–140.

17 Zespół Izba Zdrowia w Generalnym Gubernatorstwie (*Gesundheitskammerim Generalgouvernement*), Jewish Historical Institute Archives, ref. 251/1, Zarządzenia i okólniki. It was impossible to establish whether this really happened.

18 Kordel, *Geneza, struktura*, 36.

19 *Zdrowie i życie* 2 (1940): 16.

to the Medical Council in Kraków. One of them introduced himself as Dr. Walbaum, who became minister of Health in the *Generalgouvernement*. The conversation with these gentlemen was merely informative, and at that stage we didn't know what the Germans were planning regarding the transfer of the Supreme Medical Council. A few days later, having already been nominated as president of the Medical Chamber, Dr. Kroll arrived, along with the later-infamous Von Würzen as his secretary.[20]

In October 1940, district health chambers were established for Kraków, Lublin, Radom, and Warsaw.[21] The manager of the Warsaw District Health Chamber was a Dr. Lambrecht. The medical manager was Tadeusz Alkiewicz, who as a member of the Polish resistance, was instructed to take up this position by the High Command of the Union of the Armed Struggle. In January 1944, Alkiewicz was arrested and imprisoned in Pawiak, but was later released thanks to the efforts of the Central Welfare Council.[22]

The first order of business of the German occupation, was to separate and remove Jewish doctors from society. Jewish doctors' bulletin boards were marked with a six-pointed blue Jewish star affixed in the top left corner. Walbaum ordered doctors' stamps and prescriptions to feature the Star of David. A few months later, when all doctors, as members of medical chambers, were obliged to complete questionnaires, there, too, the Star of David was used to identify Jews.

In March 1940, Jews were ordered to stop treating Aryan patients, with a subsequent addendum on May 7, 1940, that allowed Jews to treat Aryans in situations when an Aryan doctor was not available. Each time, permission for such treatment was issued by regional doctor, for a period

---

20  M. Ciećkiewicz, "Izba lekarska w dobie okupacji niemieckiej i na przełomie," *Dziennik urzędowy izby lekarskiej w Krakowie* 1 (June 1945), http://izbalekarska.pl/izba-lekarska-w-dobie-okupacji-niemieckiej-i-na-przelomie/, accessed August 23, 2016.
21  *Zdrowie i życie* 7 (1940): 51–54; and 8 (1941): 57–60.
22  P. Bayer, *Służba zdrowia Warszawy w walce z okupantem* (Warsaw: Wydawnictwo Ministerstwa Obrony Narodowej, 1985), 49.

not exceeding four weeks.[23] From that moment on, Jewish medical personnel could only officially practice in Jewish hospitals and organizations (such as TOZ), or in private rooms where only Jewish patients were to be treated. This made it impossible for hundreds of Jewish medical professionals, who had for years worked in city hospitals or done well in private practice, to earn a living.

Governor Frank divided doctors into two nationality groups. This was possible because they had to state their nationality in writing when filling out "questionnaires for the initial declaration of medical professions." According to the racial policies adopted by the Reichstag on September 15, 1935, including the laws on citizenship rights, a Jew was anyone who had three or more grandparents who were racially, fully Jewish. A descendant of two Jewish grandparents was considered a "crossbreed [*Mischling*] of the first degree," and someone with only one set of Jewish grandparents was deemed a "crossbreed of the second degree." A person's religious denomination did not count. This was also the case with anyone who, prior to September 1, was a member of the Jewish community or was married to a Jew. To reflect this in the questionnaire, individuals were categorized accordingly. A doctor had to demonstrate his or her pure Aryan blood by listing the nationalities of his/her grandparents. If a doctor was considered Jewish, the questionnaire's first page was annotated with the word *Jude.*

The so-called group of doctors of Jewish nationality was called the Jewish Medical Chamber and housed at 11 Tłomackie Street, a building that bore the coat of arms of the Polish government, a white eagle. Towards the end of December 1940, the chamber moved to 3 Leszno Street, and Dr. Izrael Milejkowski became its president.

A "List of non-Aryan Doctors" is in the archives of the Jewish Historical Institute dated May 1, 1940.[24] Above the title is an annotation: Warsaw-Białystok Medical Chamber, Warsaw, 37 Koszykowa Street, which suggests the list was prepared for the newly established Jewish Medical Council. The list is typewritten, in alphabetical order, with the

---

23  *Gazeta Żydowska*, October 1, 1940, reports that the regulation forbidding Jews from treating Aryans was implemented on March 6, 1940. *Gazeta Żydowska* 21 (1940): 6. See also *Tak było*, 13.

24  It is possible that the reference 806/I/94 on the document belongs to another archive. No information is available on the source of this copy.

last eight names added later.[25] The list contains the names, surnames, and addresses of 737 doctors,[26] including people who, when the list was being prepared, could not fill out their registration questionnaires. This was the case with Dr. Benno Aron, who was imprisoned and later killed by the Soviets, or Dr. Abraham Rakower, Dr. Karol Rozensztrauch, and Dr. Izaak Szachnerowicz, who were arrested in January 1940 and executed soon thereafter. The list was prepared prior to their arrest, or their names were added because there was no news of their demise.[27]

Membership in the Jewish Medical Chamber did not automatically guarantee the right to practice medicine. Each Jewish doctor had to reapply for a permit to practice in Jewish residential districts. To register, a doctor had to complete three forms, supply three copies of his or her medical diploma, a certificate of previous employment, a certificate confirming their right to practice medicine, and four photographs. Copies had to be certified in the chamber's main office by Dr. Izrael Milejkowski, and there was a registration fee of five zlotys.

Doctors living and working in Warsaw before the war usually had no problem renewing their permits, but those living outside Warsaw, or doctors completing their post-diploma internships, faced serious obstacles. Dr. Henryk Fenigsztein, who graduated in June 1938 and completed an eleven-month internship at the Holy Ghost and at the Czyste Hospital before being called up for military service, was refused a permit after being discharged from the Ujazdowski Hospital in March 1940, where he had been a POW patient.

Although his application for a private practice permit was submitted at the beginning of April, and he was turned down by State Doctor Joachim Kaminski, he continued to work at the Czyste Jewish Hospital

---

25  It has not been established at whose request the list was prepared. Among these last-minute additions are Dr. Benno Aron (who died in Kharkov), Dr. Pejsach Berendt (held in a POW camp until February 24, 1940), Dr. Tobias Gitler (held in a POW camp until May 8, 1940), and Dr. Jan Przedborski (who remained in Kamień Koszyrski until May 10, 1940).

26  There are 737 surnames, but the name of Malwina Biro features twice, whereas the name of her husband, Maksymilian Biro, does not appear.

27  There are no names of some doctors known for their work in the ghetto, or of interns. Next to the names of Michał Eliasberg, Anna Jokisz Grynbergowa, and Albert Mazur there is a note: "Attention Mr. Taflowicz—as far as I know Dr. . . . left Łódź for Warsaw when the war started; in 1942 he was brought back to the Łódź Ghetto with forty other doctors." Please see appendix 4.

but was not allowed to practice privately or earn additional income. The hospital director, Dr. Józef Stein, initially employed Dr. Fenigsztein in one of the laboratories and in June assigned him to the pathological anatomy department because there were no posts in the surgical ward where Dr. Fenigsztein dreamed of working. At the end of August, Dr. Fenigsztein married Sala Gniazdo, a pharmacy student, and they lived in one of the hospital rooms. Due to his war injuries not being fully healed, Fenigsztein walked with the aid of a cane. In December 1940, the director wrote a petition to Adam Czerniaków asking the Jewish Association to support the young doctor because he was the only assistant in pathological anatomy and his work was vital. They agreed to help. Fenigsztein was finally registered as a doctor and received permission to practice privately in the ghetto.[28]

On February 28, 1940, Governor Frank had issued a directive ordering all those registered with the Medical Chamber to fill out a "questionnaire regarding once-off contributions paid by all medical professionals to the relevant medical chamber," an additional two-page declaration of total income earned in 1938 and in each month of 1940. Based on the income declared, doctors had to pay a fee to the relevant medical chamber. In Warsaw, this was administered by Kamiński, the state doctor. In addition to fees and donations, each doctor was compelled to subscribe to *Life* magazine, a journal issued by the Kraków Medical Chamber, which published decrees regarding the medical professions. These payments exceeded a hundred zlotys and had to be paid monthly.[29] Many doctors managed to pay the required amount by selling their rations of spirits or kerosene on the black market, and at great expense to their family budgets.

Affiliation with a medical chamber granted doctors membership cards with a "safeguard clause," protecting them against having their apartments and property requisitioned. In truth, that did not protect anyone from being looted but it saved them from having lodgers housed in their medical rooms.[30] Some doctors had passes entitling them to be outside the ghetto and on the streets at night. Such a pass allowed Marek Edelman, a hospital courier and a Polish political and social activist—and

---

28  Fenigstein, "Holocaust and I," 100.
29  Bryskier, *Żydzi pod swastyką*, 156.
30  Ibid., 157.

later, the last leader of the Warsaw Ghetto Uprising—to go outside the ghetto to deliver samples for testing to the National Institute of Hygiene. Dr. Henryk Makower and Prof. Hirszfeld were issued long-term passes.[31]

To deal with outbreaks of infectious diseases such as typhus and tuberculosis, venereal diseases, scabies, hunger, and infant mortality, the Jewish Medical Chamber created the Health Commission with Dr. Anna Braude-Heller as chairperson and Dr. Makower as secretary. Doctors Akiwa Uryson and Aleksander Wertheim who was soon replaced by Dr. Anna Margolis, served as members. Its weekly meetings were held in the Medical Council office at 3 Leszno Street. Frustrated by a serious shortage of medications, Dr. Makower summed it up succinctly: "We were fighting against windmills."[32]

The Germans forced the Medical Chamber to choose doctors to work in the camps. But the chamber also helped people find employment outside Warsaw. According to Dr. Józef Bergson's documents, he was transferred from Warsaw to Staszów with permission of the regional office in Sandomierz. In a letter dated June 1941, the regional doctor wrote to the Medical Chamber in Kraków: "Please let me know if I can grant permission to Józef Bergson, a Jewish doctor who currently works in the Warsaw Ghetto, to settle and practice in Staszów. This person works in the field of gynecological surgery and obstetrics and agrees to practice exclusively among the Jewish population. I support Dr. Bergson's request."[33] Permission was granted by the chief sanitary inspector, Dr. Werner Kroll.[34]

The chamber also corresponded with doctors in the Warsaw region as some lived in the capital but worked on the outskirts. Dr. Alicja Holländer, a psychiatrist at the Czyste Jewish Hospital, moved to Otwock and later to Biała Rawska. In the regional doctor's letter to the District Medical Chamber requesting her documents, he added a note: "Not required, because Otwock Ghetto has closed down." Dr. Holländer escaped the Otwock Ghetto before its liquidation in August 1942 and

---

31  Engelking, "Rada Żydowska," 159.
32  H. Makower, *Pamiętnik z getta warszawskiego. Październik 1940–styczeń 1943* (Wrocław: Ossolineum, 1987), 105.
33  Zespół Izba Zdrowia w Generalnym Gubernatorstwie, Zarządzenia i okólniki.
34  Staszów Jews were enclosed in the small ghetto in mid-1941. It was liquidated on November 7 and 8, 1942.

survived the war thanks to Aryan documents issued in the name of Stefania Jasińska.

## The Fight against Epidemics

Prof. Dr. Anton Richter, the medical chief of staff in the commander's office, was responsible for maintaining sanitary conditions and providing general medical care. Before the war he had been a professor of venereal and skin diseases at the university in Królewiec (now Kaliningrad, Russia).[35] In charge of controlling the typhoid epidemic caused by devastatingly unsanitary conditions in Warsaw after the bombardment and siege, he established a committee of Polish and Jewish practitioners to cooperate with city authorities.[36] Their collaboration included intensifying sanitary controls and enforcing compulsory immunizations against typhoid fever, which succeeded in eliminating most of the disease by January 1940.[37]

In November 1939, Richter appointed Kurt Schrempf the official head doctor of Warsaw.[38] His office was in the Brühl Palace on Wierzbowa Street, which also housed the Department of Healthcare. Prof. Ludwik Hirszfeld, who survived the war and wrote his memoirs in the 1960s, characterized Schrempf as a man of vigor and brutality:

> He treated doctors as if they were orderlies; he addressed them as he would grooms in a stable, on many occasions threatening them with his revolver. . . He would dispose of the most meritorious hospital directors, sending some of them to death camps, and replaced them with rather young and inexperienced ones.[39]

---

35 J. Starczewski, "Uwagi o służbie Zdrowia w okupowanej Warszawie," *Przegląd Lekarski–Oświęcim* 33, bk. 16, no. 1 (1976): 106.

36 An account by Icchok Chain (Józef Gołębiowski), YVA O.3/2355.

37 L. Fischer, *Warschau unter deutscher Herrschaft* (Kraków: Burgverlag Krakau, 1942), 238–239.

38 Starczewski, "Uwagi o służbie Zdrowia w okupowanej Warszawie," 107. The official German head doctors were Kurt Schrempf, Hans Vieweg, Wilhelm Hagen, and Fritz Janik.

39 Hirszfeld, *Historia jednego życia*, 198.

Julian Kulski, mayor commissioner of the city, described Schrempf as a "hyena who preyed on the misfortune of others."[40] He likened Schrempf's mentality to that of the German doctors in the death camps.[41]

Schrempf ordered the community's Health Department to combat the epidemic, but did not provide resources to achieve it.[42] Despite imposing "sanitation checks" where all doctors had to make daily rounds in assigned residential areas, searching the apartments for people infected with typhus, only a few cases were reported. As Dr. Ebin recalled, the German authorities . . . were furious that they did not receive reports of typhus in the ghetto, whereas on the Aryan side of Warsaw it was spreading. They were furious because their conception of the ghetto (it was called the infectious zone) was explained by the need to protect Aryan citizens from typhus, since only Jews were its carriers. Meanwhile, in the entire ghetto only two cases were reported.[43] This happened even though failure to report a case of typhus infection was punishable by death.[44]

The next major outbreak of typhus in Warsaw was reported in February 1940, with sixty dead among the Jewish population, along with five non-Jews.[45] During the first months of the German occupation, all Jewish hospitals were closed, ostensibly to prevent the spread of typhoid. Personnel were not permitted to leave the hospitals, and police cordoned off buildings.

In April 1940, the Germans required the *Judenrat* to erect a wall around Muranow, Warsaw's Jewish district, and demarcate it with bulletin boards announcing it was a plague-infected area. Fearing a typhus epidemic, during the first days of April, a three-week sanitary blockade was created on Krochmalna Street, leaving 18,000 people without any

---

40  J. Kulski, *Z minionych lat życia 1892–1945* (Warsaw: Państwowy Instytut Wydawniczy, 1982), 286.

41  Idem, *Zarząd Miejski Warszawy 1939–1944* (Warsaw: PWN, 1964), 86.

42  R. Zabłotniak, "Epidemia duru plamistego wśród ludności *żydowskiej w Warszawie w latach II wojny światowej,*" *Biuletyn Żydowskiego Instytutu Historycznego* 4, no. 80 (1970): 4.

43  An account by Leopold Ebina, YVA O.3/440.

44  Z. Szymańska, *Byłam tylko lekarzem* (Warsaw: PAX, 1979), 143; Makower, *Miłość w cieniu śmierci,* 63; Makower, *Pamiętnik z getta warszawskiego,* 106.

45  P. Kłodziński, "Sytuacja sanitarna okupowanej Warszawy w sprawozdaniu Wilhelma Hagena," *Przegląd Lekarski—Oświęcim* 32, bk. 15, no. 1 (1975): 140.

means of survival because they were not permitted beyond the cordon.[46] The street was closed off for three-week periods during May and August, each time disinfections were conducted with chaos and violence.[47]

A year and a half later, another large-scale sanitary action was conducted on Krochmalna Street, but even the orders of the cruelest Germans, such as Kałusz, Keller, or Franz, proved ineffective.[48] People hid linens, fought with disinfection officials and even with Jewish police officers. Abject poverty and squalor reigned, the area was littered with corpses of people who starved to death, prompting disinfection units to consider setting fire to entire streets. Twelve disinfection units, consisting of doctors from the Jewish Health Department, Polish doctors, a hundred Jewish Police officers, German gendarmerie and the Polish Blue Police (Polish auxiliary police) carried out the action.[49] Residents were ordered to leave their apartments and assemble in the main market square. Several thousand terrified men, women and children expected the worst. Unlocked and unsecured apartments became easy targets for thieves, who accessed the buildings on Krochmalna by traversing the roofs. Where doors were locked, the police hacked them open with axes until, in the afternoon, locksmiths were ordered to open them. Chaos ensued. Hundreds of people were sent to disinfection pools. That night it rained heavily, but there was no shelter for those waiting to be disinfected. Some people returned to their apartments after midnight, while others arrived home the next day.[50] Dead bodies were removed and those with typhus were taken to hospitals.

---

46  Ibid., 102.
47  Leociak, "Służba zdrowia," 284.
48  The names of the persons listed here could not be established.
49  The Polish Police in the *Generalgouvernement* (*Polnische Polizei im Generalgouvernement*), better known as the Blue Police (*Blaue Polizei*), a community policing organization, was financed by Polish self-governing bodies, under the supervision of the German civil administration and subordinated to the commanding officers of local German Order Police (*Ordnungspolizei*). M. Getter, "Policja Polska w Generalnym Gubernatorstwie 1939–1945," *Przegląd Policyjny* 1–2 (1996): 74.
50  Two anonymous accounts exist: "Akcja sanitarna na ulicy Krochmalnej [in September 1941]," Jewish Historical Institute Archives, Ringelblum archives, Ring. I/93, Mf. ŻIH–776.

## The Activities of TOZ

In February 1940, in the face of growing numbers of typhus cases, TOZ created the Division for Combating Epidemics.[51] Led by Dr. Sara Syrkin-Binsztejn, its efforts were directed at promoting the hygiene of ghetto residents, providing them with disinfectants, soap, and, if possible, undergarments. The Division organized wide-ranging information and prevention interventions emphasizing the importance of community participation. They organised makeshift beds in refugee shelters and regulated health standards in community kitchens. In 1940, Warsaw had seventy-one soup kitchens serving some 30,000 regulars.[52]

District sanitary managers and officials from the Division for Combating Epidemics trained sanitary delegates from house committees. Through them, disinfectants, soap, bleaching agents, brushes, and instruction leaflets in Polish and Yiddish were distributed to the population. TOZ and CENTOS presented public talks to different groups in Polish and Yiddish.[53] Liaison agents who did not know Yiddish attended special courses to learn basic communication.[54]

Rabbis and well-known community activists attended some of these meetings. With difficulty, a "hygiene week" was organized, with nurses from the Division for Combating Epidemics, sent to visit basement and attic dwellings to help residents to clean rooms, scrub floors, windows and tables. A laundry was opened to service hostels and night shelters. People from the house committees distributed free tokens to the poorest residents, allowing them to wash their clothes. The *Jewish Gazette* regularly placed announcements notifying the public when free washes were available.

## The Czyste Jewish Hospital

Initially, the authorities decided the hospital would serve only civilians. All wounded soldiers were removed, and Polish and Jewish civilian patients were moved in. But before the new arrivals could be registered,

---

51 *Gazeta Żydowska* 13 (1940): 2.
52 *Gazeta Żydowska* 4 (1941): 3.
53 *Gazeta Żydowska* 47 (1940): 3.
54 Ibid.

the Germans changed their minds and declared it an army hospital. This decision was then retracted, and the hospital was allocated to Jewish patients. The Czyste Old Order Jewish Hospital was then renamed the Czyste Jewish Hospital for Infectious Diseases.

On December 15, 1939, the *Judenrat* was forced to take over the Czyste Jewish Hospital. The *Judenrat* health commission recruited doctors and nurses to work in the Czyste Jewish Hospital and in two isolation hospitals (on 86 Żelazna and 109/111 Leszno Streets), which were opened at a cost of almost 200,000 zlotys.[55] Responding to Czerniaków's appeal, house committees began collecting linens and undergarments for hospital use. Because approximately 250,000 zlotys were needed to cover the monthly cost of hospital care, the *Judenrat* began compulsory collections.

In line with its policy of persecuting the Jewish population, the Germans forbade the Warsaw City Council from continuing to finance the hospital. Sabina Gurfinkiel-Glocer, a nurse and operating assistant, wrote:

> And thus began the isolation of the Jewish hospital from other hospitals and the Hospitalization Department. . . The nursing staff, with Head Nurse Fryd at the helm, worked under very difficult conditions. Everything was in short supply, there were no undergarments because there was no laundry room, there was no food because the kitchen was inadequate, there was no money to pay wages. All we heard was "no." Although there were many sick Jews requiring our care, other patients were brought to us—Jews who had been beaten up or injured by the Germans.[56]

Dr. Heinrich Sikorski, from Poznań, was nominated as superintendent for Czyste. Dr. Fenigsztein (Henry Fenigstein) recalls Sikorski "was constantly drunk and had little to do with the actual administration of the hospital," while engineer Ignacy Stabholz, the administrative director,

---

55  *Tak było*, 36.

56  S. Gurfinkiel-Glocer, "Szpital Żydowski w Warszawie (na Czystem) w czasie okupacji (1939–1943). Fragmenty pamiętnika (skrót)," *Biuletyn Żydowskiego Instytutu Historycznego* 1, no. 41 (1962): 101.

assumed responsibility for everything.[57] Sabina Gurfinkiel-Glocer notes that his attitude towards the Jewish doctors and personnel was good.[58]

Dr. Bieleńki, as head of the Internal Diseases Department, continued his work at the Czyste Jewish Hospital, and cooperated with Prof. Hirszfeld during disinfection actions in the ghetto. In his book, Prof. Hirszfeld wrote:

> I witnessed the faces of maltreated people becoming more cheerful when they saw him. "If Dr. Bieleńki participates [in the disinfection]," they would say, "then no harm will come our way." I learned that he took part in the defense of Warsaw and led a sanitary unit in the most dangerous sections. He had always shown initiative. During the epidemic, he served as hospital director. He responded to the call during the typhus epidemic. He was one of those soft-hearted people who were hard, but only on themselves. When he entered the hospital, he was surrounded by a swarm of children begging for money. "They will be dead in a month, but I cannot stop trying to help," he said. As is the case with many Jews, he loved learning. I frequently tried to invite him to give a lecture, because I detected a zeal and a heart in him, although he was not a talented orator. He was the kind of doctor who not only cures, but also heals the soul.[59]

The persecution of Jewish doctors was not limited to physical abuse and the plundering of their possessions. The first arrests took place in mid-December 1939, during the typhus epidemic, when Schrempf visited the Czyste Hospital. He was furious when he learned the disinfection equipment was not yet functional. The doctors were fired a few days later, but the week after that, Schrempf threatened further arrests if there were delays in getting the delousing chamber in working order.[60]

---

57  Henry Fenigstein, "The History of 'Czyste.' The Jewish Hospital in Warsaw from 1939 to 1943 during Nazi Regime" (Toronto, 1990, unpublished), xiii–xiv. The manuscript was kindly made available by Prof. Claude Romney and Dr. Lawrence Powell.
58  The account of Sabina Gurfinkiel-Glocer, "Szpital na Czystem i ja," YVA O.3/396.
59  Hirszfeld, *Historia jednego życia*, 217–218.
60  Fenigstein, "The History of 'Czyste,'" xi.

In January 1940, Andrzej Kott, a member of PLAN, a resistance organization, was captured but escaped from the Gestapo. The resulting mass arrests had an impact on the Warsaw population.[61] Among 255 Jews arrested was a gynecologist, Dr. Izaak Szachnerowicz, taken hostage at the Czyste Old Order Jewish Hospital. When the Gestapo came for him, he was performing a medical procedure. The Gestapo said they weren't barbarians and let him finish.[62] Szachnerowicz's wife, Anna Meroz, wrote that ten doctors were arrested at the hospital that day. Please refer to the list of doctors in appendix 1. Unfortunately, despite the efforts of Czerniaków, the hostages were executed (most probably in Palmiry or in Saski Park).[63] Dr. Antoni Wortman, the director of the Hospitalization Department of the *Judenrat*, was the only one released.[64]

The complex, having suffered through the initial German bombardment, was in a lamentable state: The majority of its pavilions had no windows, wards had no beds or linens, the dispensary had no medicines, and the laundry had no caldrons for boiling the linens. As the number of typhoid fever cases in the city grew, patients could not be admitted because of the catastrophic state of the facilities, yet they needed to be quarantined. The hospital itself suffered through a six-week quarantine. The hospital perimeter was not, however, impermeable: one of the nurses recalled how a colleague crawled through a small window at the Czyste Old Order Jewish Hospital to visit her baby daughter, while others jumped over the fence next to the dissecting room.[65]

---

61  A. Rutkowski, "Sprawa Kotta w środowisku żydowskim w Warszawie. (Styczeń 1940 r.)," *Biuletyn Żydowskiego Instytutu Historycznego* 2, no. 62 (1967): 66. A group of activists from the Polish People's Action for Independence (*Polska Ludowa Akcja Niepodległościowa PLAN*) was arrested on January 14, 1940, based on a report by the provocateur Stanisław Izdebski.

62  Meroz, *W murach i poza murami getta*, 18.

63  Rutkowski, "Sprawa Kotta," 67.

64  In Ringelblum's archives there are two lists of hostages who were arrested; these were delivered to the *Judenrat* in August 1940. On the first there are 165 surnames with "deceased" noted in pencil, on the second there are 90 surnames with annotations reading: "alive." Please see appendix 1 for more details.

65  Gurfinkiel-Glocer, "Szpital Żydowski w Warszawie," 101.

## The Bersohn and Bauman Children's Hospital

During the first weeks of the German occupation, the hospital lost its subsidy, which it had previously received from the Warsaw city budget and the Social Insurance Company. The funding needed to maintain the hospital thus came mainly from the JDC, which functioned legally until the moment the United States joined the Allies against the Axis. Both formally and financially, Bersohn and Bauman Children's Hospital was assigned to TOZ, as were the Brijus Sanatorium and Zofiówka Institution in Otwock.[66]

Like the Czyste Jewish Hospital, the Bersohn and Bauman Children's Hospital was placed under quarantine in early 1940. The entire staff was locked in with the patients, and "blue" policeman (*granatowy policjant*) stood guard at the gates.[67] Staff slept in the large library hall on the ground floor, with the portraits of the hospital's founders looming over them. The dinners they ate in the canteen consisted of watery porridge, and they used a makeshift washroom set up in what was once the admissions hall. Judyta Braude recalled:

In the Children's Hospital the quarantine was also enforced out of the blue. One day, the announcement came that no hospital employee would be allowed to leave for six weeks. Those wishing to leave were subjected to a two-week quarantine. Polish police were stationed in front of the hospital to stop anyone from leaving the premises. Some doctors, nurses and maintenance staff left because of their families and for personal reasons, prior to the Jewish Police directing them to compulsory quarantine facilities at the end of Leszno and Wolska Streets.[68]

---

66 An account by Mojżesz Mieczysław Tursz (Thursz), "Jak kształtował się sanitariat w ghetcie warszawskim," YVA O.3/438.
67 *Granatowa policja*, lit. The Blue Police (*Blau Polizei*) was a common name for the Polish police during the Second World War, established by the German regime in occupied Poland (the *Generalgouvernement*). The entity's official German name was *Polnische Polizeiim Generalgouvernement* (Polish Police of the General Government, subordinate to Order Police (*Ordnungspolizei*). The adjective "blue" originates from the dark blue uniforms worn by its functionaries. See: https://en.wikipedia.org/wiki/Blue_Police (transl.)
68 An account by Judyta Braude, YVA O.3/2360.

Difficult working conditions and the enforced stay brought about unexpected results. "The German authorities' nightmarish move of locking people up in quarantine, separate from their families and homes, and condemning them to starvation and inconvenience, made the personnel unite—a bond nothing could ever break."

## Pharmacies

According to the "official register of doctors, dentists, pharmacists, medics, nurses, certified midwives, and independent dental technicians" in the Ministry of Social Care, in January 1939, 797 pharmacists were registered and employed in 140 Warsaw pharmacies.[69] The pharmaceutical industry was represented by the Polish Pharmaceutical Society[70] and the industry's workers had their own trade union. Pharmaceutical chambers had been established shortly before the war.[71] As early as October 1939, the Germans forbade Jewish pharmacists from managing their own pharmacies,[72] and ordered them to dismiss all non-Aryan personnel. Jewish pharmacies were placed under receivership and their former owners promised a monthly allowance.[73]

## Emergency Services

In September and October of 1939, the Emergency Services of the Warsaw Society for Emergency Medical Aid functioned with little interference from the Germans. In December 1939, the Germans established a commission for emergency services, headed by a German named Kleiman, who immediately disbanded its Polish management.[74] When the ghetto was created, ambulances were dispatched to both Aryan and Jewish patients, while staff and their families lived at 58 Leszno Street.

---

69  *Urzędowy spis lekarzy*, 18.
70  *Urzędowy spis lekarzy*, part 3: *Farmaceuci.*
71  Ustawa o Izbach Aptekarskich, Dz. U. RP. no. 55, pos. 346, June 26, 1939.
72  Bryskier, *Żydzi pod swastyką*, 139.
73  Ch. A. Kaplan, *Scroll of Agony: The Warsaw Diary of Chaim A. Kaplan*, ed. A. I. Katsh (London: Macmillan, 1999), 53.
74  H. Bojczuk, *Warszawskie Pogotowie Ratunkowe 1897–1945. Od Okólnika do Poznańskiej*, part 1 (Warsaw: Wojewódzka Stacja Pogotowia ratunkowego i Transportu Meditrans, 2010), 78.

## The Threat of Labor Camps

In February 1940, the Germans imposed obligatory work duties on all male Jews between fourteen and sixty years of age, and *Judenrat* doctors in the Health Commission on Solna Street were forced to assess their fitness for work.[75] The cost of registration and examination was borne by the *Judenrat*. Each examinee had to pay five zlotys, the equivalent of a doctor's pay for one hour of work. After the assessment, a candidate could receive a deferment of up to six months, or a total exemption for a monthly fee of between 15 and 100 zlotys.[76] The association determined each sum on a sliding scale, and later a committee to determine fees was established. Persons unfit to work received an official sick card exempting them from being transported to a labor camp. These cards were issued by the Labor Department on 2 Walicόw Street. Complaints were addressed to officials at 6 Twarda Street.[77]

When people were sent to the labor camps, doctors were needed to care for them on site. In spring 1940, the Germans demanded that three doctors be chosen to work in the newly established Bełżec labor camp, and the Jewish Medical Chamber had to choose them.[78] At the time, Bełżec housed Roma and Jews. The only doctor permanently on duty there was Dr. Fejgels, who had been assigned by the Lublin *Judenrat*.[79]

Seventy unmarried doctors who worked at Czyste participated in a raffle, and Doctors Ludwik Stabholz and Jankiel Piekarski were chosen. They were promised they would be recalled after a month when replacements would be sent. Living and working conditions in the camp were terrible. People suffered from hunger; they were beaten, humiliated, and prone to frequent accidents, and the doctors did not have enough medication or bandages to do their jobs.

Despite the camp officials' promises, the prisoners' conditions systematically worsened, and the expected relief teams of doctors never materialized. Since doctors were not surveilled in the way prisoners

---

75 Jewish Historical Institute Archives Central Committee of Polish Jews (AŻIH CKŻP) 101/303.
76 Bryskier, *Żydzi pod swastyką*, 45.
77 *Gazeta Żydowska* 42 (1941): 2. Among them were Jakub Korman, Henryk Landau, Boruch Lando, Henryk Makower, Ignacy Rejder, and Salomon Uzdański.
78 Doctors Owsiej Bieleńki and Ichaskil Wohl were members of this commission.
79 *Gazeta Żydowska* 13 (1940): 2.

were, Stabholz and his colleague managed to escape. They left the camp at night, arrived in Warsaw, and complained to hospital management about the delay in sending their replacements. The next two doctors sent to Bełżec never returned.[80]

One of the few to volunteer to go to Bełżec was Dr. Leopold Ebin, who was paid 500 zlotys to take a colleague's place. He sent the money to his wife, who was hiding on the Aryan side with their two children and who had sold what was left of their belongings when she moved to Warsaw from Łódź.

Recruitment drives for work in the camps made it sound tempting, because they promised easier work, army rations and the protection of the Jewish Police. Dr. Ebin was sent to work in the Krychów labor camp located in a swamp the Jews were draining by digging trenches. Daily food rations consisted of a soup made of worm-infested broad beans, and meat was provided only when German supplies were putrefied. The camp commander was exceptionally "good" because he did not kill inmates for escaping but allowed prisoners to be severely beaten.

After seven weeks of working in Krychów, Ebin moved to a private practice in Lublin to replace a Dr. Bromberg, who was murdered in Auschwitz in 1940 (the camp started taking prisoners on June 14, 1940).[81] After the head of the SS, Heinrich Himmler, visited Lublin, working conditions in Krychów deteriorated and Ebin returned to Warsaw, but not to the ghetto.[82]

## Treatment of Jewish Converts

Many Jewish doctors in Poland converted to Christianity—most for social reasons—to give them the ability to get important positions in medicine, the sciences or other academic and important posts. Others converted for reasons of faith. But in the end, all these conversions failed to save them from the onslaught.

Jewish patients, depending on their degree of observance, either respected converted doctors and used them for their own healthcare, or avoided them altogether—preferring rabbis. Those Jews who converted

---

80  An account by Ludwik Stabholz, YVA O.3/861; *Gazeta Żydowska* 19 (1940): 3.
81  Name not established.
82  An account by Leopold Ebin, YVA O.3/440.

for faith reasons were regarded as traitors to the religion—*meshumadim*—and were less likely to be called upon by the Orthodox.

Jews who had earlier converted, or hailed from the families of converts, hoped to retain their property and get treated better than Jews who were still Jews. When the decision was taken to create the ghetto, the converts tried to obtain permission to remain outside the ghetto and hoped the Germans would establish a separate ghetto for them. There were rumors circulating of a Christian enclave for Jewish converts being created in the suburb of Żoliborz.[83]

In response to a request from the German authorities, the president of the Central Welfare Council, Adam Roniker, handed over a list of converts from Judaism.[84] The German police used the list to move everyone named on it to the Warsaw Ghetto. Prof. Ludwik Hirszfeld and Dr. Aleksander Wertheim, both converts, were among those who were forced to move with few or none of their possessions. As Prof. Hirszfeld wrote, they took everything from him: "position, property, house, furniture, paintings, and books."[85] In the end, a nameless soldier (with his superior's permission) appropriated even his undergarments and the little food he had for the road.

---

83  E. Ringelblum, *Kronika getta warszawskiego*, ed. and introd. Artur Eisenbach (Warsaw: Czytelnik, 1988), 327.

84  The Central Welfare Council (also translated as the Main Social Services Council) functioned with the permission of the occupying authorities, receiving financial assistance and other material benefits from both the occupying authorities and from abroad (mainly the United States government), clandestine donations from the Polish Government in Exile, and the generosity of the community. The council functioned as a charitable institution, organizing feeding programs, medical care, assistance to orphanages and the homeless, as well as professional courses and artisans' workshops.

85  Hirszfeld, *Historia jednego życia*, 204.

# Chapter 6

# Healthcare after the Sealing of the Warsaw Ghetto

On September 3, 1940, the manager in the Department of Health in the Office of the District Chief, Arnold Lambrecht, informed Governor Frank of the growing number of typhus cases in Warsaw and proposed closing off the ghetto for health reasons.[1] After several days, Frank summoned Walbaum, director of the Health Department in the *Generalgouvernement,* who approved the proposal. On September 12, Frank also approved the plan, and the order to create a Jewish residential district in Warsaw was issued by the governor of Warsaw, Ludwig Fischer, on October 2, 1940, thus establishing the ghetto.

The Germans announced the creation of the Warsaw Ghetto on October 12, 1940. Every Jew in Warsaw was required to move to Muranow, the Jewish quarter designated as the ghetto. The walls, built by the *Judenrat,* were ten feet high and topped with barbed wire, with German Battalion 61 (a mobile squad known as an *Einzatsgruppe*) serving as sentries. Hundreds of thousands of Jews from Warsaw and the surrounding suburbs were packed into a space of 1.3 square miles. For those who already lived in the quarter, it was difficult. It was even more difficult for those who had to adjust to living in cramped quarters.[2] According to

---

1   Ch. R. Browning, *The Path to Genocide: Essays on Launching the Final Solution* (Cambridge: Cambridge University Press, 1992), 151. Browning refers to Dr. Lambrecht's Report of September 3, 1940, YVA, ref. JM 814.

2   "Warsaw," USHMM Holocaust Encyclopedia, https://encyclopedia.ushmm.org/content/en/article/warsaw, accessed March 6, 2020.

Ruta Sakowska's estimate, on average, six to seven people lived in one room in a typical ghetto apartment.[3] It was terrible even when epidemics were not ravaging the population. Starvation and deprivation ruled. It was a living nightmare even for those older residents who had stayed in their own apartments, now packed with relatives or strangers.

The ghetto gates were closed on November 16, 1940. Approximately 450,000 Jews were locked behind the walls. On April 3, 1941, Fischer listed the political, economic and sanitary reasons used to justify sealing off the ghetto. He explained it was necessary to isolate the Jewish population to effectively combat the epidemic. In his view, if Jews were permitted to move around freely, there would be a constant threat of a typhus epidemic.[4] Crowded into the former Northern District, and deprived of all rights, the Jews became an easy target for rank-and-file German soldiers, officers and functionaries.[5] The Gestapo entered Jewish apartments at night, taking away one person (or even entire groups of people), sometimes to Pawiak prison. They killed Jews in front of their homes.[6]

The situation became worse with each passing day. Edelman's vivid eyewitness testimony is devastating. He describes streets filled with humans deformed by malnutrition, covered with open wounds, wrapped in dirty rags, "beggars, the aged, the young and the children, in the streets and courtyards."[7] Everywhere he looked, children were begging, inside and outside the ghetto walls. Six-year-olds were used to smuggle foods into the ghetto by scrambling under the barbed wire and snatching packages from the hands of passersby on the Aryan side. People were literally dying of hunger in the streets. Every day, before dawn, funeral carts would gather the corpses, some of them dumped in the gutter after their families had stripped them of their clothing. And into this living nightmare, the Germans again packed the ghetto with more Jews brought in from other regions, and the streets and courtyards filled with penniless, hungry and sick refugees.[8]

---

3    R. Sakowska, *Ludzie z dzielnicy zamkniętej* (Warsaw: PWN, 1993), 29–30.
4    A. Eisenbach, *Hitlerowska polityka zagłady Żydów* (Warsaw: Książka i wiedza, 1961), 214–215.
5    Makower, *Pamiętnik z getta warszawskiego*, 51.
6    "Pamiętnik Sabiny Gurfinkiel-Glocer. Szpital Żydowski w Warszawie (na Czystem) w czasie okupacji (1939–1943)," Jewish Historical Institute Archives, ref. 302/160.
7    Edelman, "The Ghetto Fights," 17–39.
8    Ibid.

Well before deportations began, 100,000 ghetto residents (almost twenty-five percent) died of starvation and/or disease.

## The Doctors in the Ghetto

Over 700,[9] and perhaps almost 1,000 doctors worked in the ghetto—with the consent of the occupying authorities—between November 1940 and April 1943. This is confirmed in the personal documents of several doctors, recovered and supplemented with additional information from my "List of Non-Aryan Doctors" (reproduced here as appendix 2) and "List of Jewish Doctors Working and Living in Warsaw in 1940–1942" (reproduced as appendix 3). Some of the photographs in appendix 7 are obtained from these registration questionnaires. The combined lists contain 948 names, which falls within the range provided by other sources.[10]

Before the war, these doctors had worked in twenty-three hospitals or institutes, the clinics of Warsaw University, in health centers and out-patient city clinics, in emergency medical services and in private practice, usually located in a home office or in private clinics. When the ghetto was sealed off, many of those clinics were located on the Aryan side. Doctors in private practice posted change-of-address notices in the November/December 1940 issues of the *Jewish Gazette*. After being locked in, they could work only in hospitals and clinics managed by the *Judenrat* or other Jewish community and charitable organizations.

Some doctors chose to remain hidden on the Aryan side. Dr. Leopold Ebin decided to move to the ghetto, even though his wife urged him to stay with her in their rented apartment on the Aryan side but he wanted to be "freer, to practice and earn his living instead of living in constant

---

9   Leociak, "Służba zdrowia," 237. Leociak estimates that it was 750 to 1,000 doctors. According to *Urzędowy spis lekarzy*, 2,815 doctors were registered in Warsaw. According to the personal documents in the Warsaw-Białystok Medical Chamber, in 1940–1942, 831 Jewish doctors completed registration questionnaires. Please see appendix 3. Considering that it was not a fixed number, but represented all the collected questionnaires, 750 seems the most probable number for 1940. Emanuel Ringelblum also gives this number in his diary (entries of December 7–10, 1940). It is possible that retired doctors remained in the ghetto and applied for permission to practice. A list of Jewish doctors dated May 1, 1940, in the Jewish Historical Archives features 737 names. Please see appendix 2.

10   Leociak, "Służba zdrowia," 237.

fear on the Aryan side of Warsaw."[11] Initially, he worked as a sector physician, responsible for sanitary care in several buildings on Leszno Street, but his main duty was to report typhus cases and oversee immunization efforts.

## Activities of the *Judenrat*'s Health Department

The Health Department on Leszno Street supervised several branches tasked with caring for orphans and the elderly, underprivileged patients, refugees, POWs, and a branch devoted to individual patients. The department also oversaw two outpatient clinics on 6 Twarda and 6 Nowiniarska Streets (the latter was outside the ghetto walls), an orphanage on 28 Jagiellońska Street, a shelter for those unfit to work (in Broszków), and a home for POWs and displaced people at 34 Świętojerska Street.[12]

Given the rapidly growing needs of those in the ghetto, and the frequent outbreaks of infectious diseases, a commissioner, Dr. Tadeusz Ganc, was appointed to combat epidemics and the Central Health Council was created in the summer of 1941. It was affiliated with the Health Department. The *Jewish Gazette* of August 18 reported the *Judenrat*'s Health Department established a special council to combat infectious diseases and consolidate everyone's efforts to improve health conditions in the ghetto.[13] The Health Council formed separate sections to deal with the spread of information on the need for sanitary conditions, financial information, bathing protocols and notices about buildings where cases of infection had been recorded. There were representatives from the district health councils at the health centers and representatives from Jewish institutions; from the Council for Aid to Jews, and hospital custodians.[14] Three deputies were elected during its first meeting: Jan Koral, Adolf Lewiński, and Izaak Filskraut. No chairman was elected. When Prof. Hirszfeld offered his help, Dr. Makower brought his offer directly to the director of the *Judenrat*'s Health Department, Dr. Milejkowski, of whom he had this to say:

---

11  An account by Leopold Ebin, YVA O.3/440.
12  *Gazeta Żydowska* 24 (1940): 2.
13  *Gazeta Żydowska* 60 (1941): 5.
14  H. Kroszczor, "Szpital dla Dzieci im. Bersohnówi Baumanów 1939–1942," *Biuletyn Żydowskiego Instytutu Historycznego* 73, no 1 (1970): 39–40.

This small man with the rather pretty, intelligent and pleasant face, was a distinguished community activist. As a dermatologist, he enjoyed general esteem, but despite dedication to community service, his practice came first. He was courageous and knew how to talk to the Germans. He expressed a lot of goodwill and knew how to work methodically and fairly. At the same time, he was conceited, and woe to those who tried to tease him: he fought tooth and nail any effort to limit his influence which, under the circumstances, was considerable because President Czerniaków trusted him a great deal.[15]

The portrait Dr. Makower paints of the "totalitarian, sanguine" Dr. Milejkowski is somewhat different from the remembrances of his colleagues. Mieczysław Tursz wrote that Dr. Milejkowski was completely devoted to and loving toward the tormented Jewish humanity, bravely assuming full responsibility for them. Dr. Milejkowski wrote a memo about combating typhus in the ghetto and handed it to the Germans, fully expecting serious consequences for blaming them for failing to stem the epidemic.[16] Dr. Abram Icchok Chain also had good things to say about Dr. Milejkowski, noting that he was an "unimpeachable man with untarnished hands."[17] Zofia Rosenblum wrote that when he was praised for eradicating the typhus epidemic, Dr. Milejkowski responded with great dignity and unheard of bravery by saying it was not the doctors who achieved this feat, because they were never given a chance to provide effective treatment.[18] Dr. Milejkowski eventually accepted Hirszfeld's offer of help; Czerniaków may have intervened on Hirszfeld's behalf. On June 27, 1941, his diary noted, "[Auserwald] ordered to take Milejkowski in hand. I had trouble convincing him that Milejkowski should have a

---

15  Makower, *Pamiętnik z getta warszawskiego*, 107–108.
16  An account by Mojżesz Mieczysław Tursz (Thursz), "Jak kształtował się sanitariat w ghetcie warszawskim," YVA O.3/438; "Memoriał Komisji Zdrowia Grupy Narodowościowej Lekarzy Żydowskich w Warszawie w sprawie zagrożenia epidemicznego w getcie warszawskim (28.06.1941 Warszawa)," Jewish Historical Institute Archives, Ringelblum Archives, Ring. I/214. Mf. ŻIH–280.
17  An account by Icchok Chain (Józef Gołębiowski), YVA O.3/2355.
18  Szymańska, *Byłam tylko lekarzem*, 144.

dictator to deal with epidemics."[19] Prof. Hirszfeld became this "dictator" towards the end of August and the beginning of September.

The Ghetto was divided into six zones with administrative, policing and sanitary divisions.[20] Each zone had a health center under the Health Department, responsible for disease prevention and treatment. Each zone had a medical unit charged with overseeing clinics and doctors in private practice. The doctors treated a certain number of the poor, either at their practices or by making house calls (free of charge or at reduced rate); 150 doctors declared that they had consulted 2,500 times and completed 690 house calls, in addition to the 4,800 free (or reduced-fee) treatments and additional house calls.[21]

New divisions were formed: Healthcare, Inspection, Infectious Diseases, Pharmacies and Refugee Care. The department also oversaw the sanitation repository and disinfection units.[22] To meet the needs of *Judenrat* employees, a polyclinic was opened on 6 Twarda Street.[23] It had its own pharmacy, a laboratory, and radiology and phototherapy departments.[24] Vouchers issued by the Department of Healthcare to the Community's employees and other privileged persons[25] enabled them to receive free treatments and house calls.[26]

Much-needed financial resources, essential to keeping the hospitals running, were collected by the billing department, under Councilor Edward Kobryner. On Czerniaków's instruction, the Jewish Police collected payments and compulsory donations to the hospitals (linens, mattresses, pillows, duvets). After the *Judenrat*'s reorganization of the

---

19  Czerniaków, *Adama Czerniakowa dziennik*, 196.
20  Ibid.
21  *Gazeta Żydowska* 4 (1941): 4.
22  Leociak, "Opieka Społeczna," 292.
23  Makower, *Pamiętnik z getta warszawskiego*, 8.
24  *Gazeta Żydowska* 40 (1941): 2. Doctors Stefan Ałapin, Henryk Grynberg, Szymon Gladsztern, Henryk Makower and Jan Przedborski worked in the clinic, with Dr. Zygmunt Fajncyn serving as chief doctor.
25  Engelking, "Rada Żydowska," 192.
26  The number of consultations appeared in the *Jewish Gazette*. For instance, *Gazeta Żydowska* (35 [1942]: 2) stated that in February 874 patients had consultations at the clinic at a reduced rate, and 712 were treated for free; there were 3,664 fully paid medical procedures, 366 procedures were performed free of charge; there were 1,976 fully paid house-calls, fifty-four at a reduced rate, eighty-five for free; there were 857 fully paid dental consultations, while 170 were performed free of charge.

twenty-six departments in May 1941, an independent Health Department was created by merging the Hospitalization Commission with the billing department.

Hospital supervision was in the hands of the Hospitalization Department (also called the Hospitalization Commission) led by Dr. Milejkowski. It consisted of two branches—one tasked with administration and management, and the other with medical care. The Czyste Jewish Hospital, the quarantine station on 109/111 Leszno Street and the quarantine and disinfecting pool in the corner building at 86 Żelazna Street/80 Leszno Street were subordinated to the Hospitalization Department. The quarantine station and disinfecting pools were referred to as quarantine hospitals. The Hospitalization Department oversaw administrative and medical matters, including renovations, purchasing supplies, bookkeeping, recruitment drives, and contact with city management officials.[27]

On February 10, 1941, Dr. Wilhelm Hagen replaced the much-hated Kurt Schrempf as official doctor of Warsaw and held the job until February 29, 1943. In his report, Hagen noted the manager of the Jewish Health Services, Dr. Izrael Milejkowski and Dr. Józef Stein, the director of the Czyste Jewish Hospital, turned to him for help every day, but the Germans did nothing to improve the provision of medicines and food, since they were only concerned with the needs of the *Wehrmacht*.[28] Dr. P. Waller described Hagen in his notes:

> I first met Dr. Hagen, the German public health officer in Warsaw, in 1941, in the Warsaw Ghetto. He was about forty, medium height, with reddish-blond hair. He visited the hospital frequently, since it was one of the medical facilities under his supervision. Thus, I had a better chance to learn more about his manner.
>
> His attitude to Jewish doctors was not particularly brutal. He was even considered a "friend" of the ghetto hospital director, Józef Stein. However, he was also a hypocrite... being considered Stein's friend, he never hinted that he knew of the threat hanging over Jewish doctors. And yet, as we now know,

---

27  *Gazeta Żydowska* 24 (1940): 2.

28  M. Ciesielska, *Tyfus—groźny zabójca i cichy sprzymierzeniec* (Warsaw: Stowarzyszenie EKOSAN, 2015), 45.

they deluded themselves at the beginning, hoping that they and their families would escape total annihilation. Not once did Dr. Hagen hint at anything which would make the Jewish doctors vigilant, or perhaps cause them to take steps to avoid being killed.[29]

Judyta Braude also recalled Hagen as a decent man who treated Jewish doctors well. Shortly before the *Grossaktion*, he apparently told Stein to save himself, but refused to reveal anything more. Likewise, Dr. Heller formed a good impression of him, because unlike Schrempf, he treated her kindly.[30]

In November 1941, the *Judenrat* established the Committee for Refugee Care (later the Jewish Society for Community Care), responsible for the medical care in all refugee facilities in twenty-two districts, each served by one doctor and a nurse. At the time, twenty-six doctors and twenty-seven nurses were employed.[31]

Work on the formal charter continued until July 1942. Despite difficulties in reaching agreement on the wording of the charter, the Council continued to take a number of actions: supplying hospitals with food; appointing engineer Aleksander Szniolis from the State Hygiene Institute as a disinfection expert; launching a project to combat TB and venereal diseases; organizing vaccination actions (smallpox, typhus, dysentery), and presenting an exhibition on ways to combat typhus.[32] Hirszfeld admitted the meetings were usually too long, because each member felt obliged to express a view on every issue, and personal animosities presented obstacles.

Dr. Icchok Chain, representing TOZ, wrote that the Council was established to develop scientific theses for combating disease and examining common ghetto illnesses.[33] It is difficult to determine the tangible outcomes of the Council's impact, because they had few means to fight the epidemic. As Mojżesz Tursz noted:

---

29  An account by Stanisław (Shmul) Waller (Walewski), YVA O.3/2358.
30  An account by Judyta Braude, YVA O.3/2360.
31  "Sprawozdanie z kontroli w Towarzystwie Ochrony Zdrowia 'TOZ,'" Jewish Historical Institute Archives, Ringelblum Archives, Ring. II/ 92, 1–49.
32  *Gazeta Żydowska* 33 (1942): 2.
33  An account by Icchok Chain (Józef Gołębiowski), YVA O.3/2355.

The Council did not do much to bring health to the tormented. In the Warsaw Ghetto, typhus ran its course, in keeping with the principal biological laws of any epidemic: after a period of great intensity, came a gradual decline in the number of cases. Some sufferers acquired active immunity, others—having been vaccinated—had passive immunity or contracted a milder form.[34]

Hirszfeld had a similar attitude to this "success," which he claimed was due to the reversal of regulations that had previously made things worse rather than any actions that they carried out which did not receive the necessary resources to be effective.

Operating against all odds, the *Judenrat* Health Department, as well as community organizations offering medical care, concluded their work in September 1942, when the *Grossaktion* was over.

## The Fight against Epidemics

Health centers supervised immunizations and issued proof of vaccination—required to obtain food ration booklets. Their duties also included systematically cleaning buildings and apartments during the "hygiene week," as ordered by the *Judenrat*. Committees from the *Judenrat*, the Health Department, Self-Help, sector doctors, and the Jewish Police inspected apartments, buildings and the surrounding terrain. The names and addresses of people who failed to comply with the order were submitted to a health center for sanction (fines and mandatory sanitizing baths).[35]

In 1941, the doctors discovered that using the same tactics they used in 1939 failed to stop another typhus epidemic. Moreover, despite threats, doctors did not report all outbreaks of the disease, often because they were aware of the tragic consequences of enforced block quarantines and the appalling conditions in the hospitals. Others failed to report cases because they saw them as an additional source of income. Dr. Noemi Makower described the work of a block doctor as having "a

---

34  An account by Mojżesz Mieczysław Tursz (Thursz), "Jak kształtował się sanitariat w ghetcie warszawskim," YVA O.3/438.
35  *Gazeta Żydowska* 7 (1940): 2.

policing as well as a medical component." She admitted to reporting only cases, which, in her opinion, were warranted by epidemiological or social reasons. She recalled days when, in the three blocks under her care on Nowolipki Street, the number of cases exceeded 170.[36]

The families of patients stricken with the disease, even the poorest of the poor, would hide their sick rather than send them to the hospital. Some padlocked their apartments and refused to let her in, while others attempted to bribe her, because certain doctors expected to be paid handsomely for their silence and agreed to treat patients even under adverse conditions.[37] As Noemi Makower wrote:

> On many occasions, however, I would send infected families for delousing, and order the premises to be disinfected. The poor were crowded in basements and attics. In a tiny room there would often be three or four families, and several children. Dressed in rags, grey, gaunt, with stick-like limbs, they all looked old, and they all looked alike. Children differed only in size from their parents and in their will to live.[38]

Efforts to combat lice infestations were hopeless because of the lack of soap, water, and clean clothing. Enforced delousing actions were led by units of Jewish disinfection officials, overseen by a *Judenrat* doctor, the Jewish Police, and Polish doctors. These actions did not deliver the expected results—instead, they added to the torment of the ghetto residents. Emanuel Ringelblum noted:

> Sanitary detachments extorted money from the rich in exchange for exempting their lodgings from disinfection. In doing so, they colluded with doctors. For a bribe, the disinfection baths issued certificates, which explains why those who should have bathed did not do so. The sulfur used for disinfection was weak, so it did not kill the lice. In truth, the entire action aimed at preventing an epidemic was a huge con, led by the doctors and sanitary detachments.[39]

---

36  Makower, *Miłość w cieniu śmierci*, 63.
37  Makower, *Pamiętnik z getta warszawskiego*, 106.
38  Makower, *Miłość w cieniu śmierci*, 64.
39  Einhorn, *Towarzystwo Ochrony Zdrowia*, 117.

Following the intervention of Doctors Milejkowski and Hirszfeld, eventually only Jews were employed at disinfection stations. Paradoxically, in Hirszfeld's opinion, were it not for the corruption, the situation in the ghetto would have been much worse. He believed that the best place to treat the sick, given the circumstances, was in their own homes, under the care of their families.[40] Dr. Hagen, the German Health Services manager in Warsaw, ordered specially appointed commissions to decide whether an apartment "was fit to house the sick" (meaning it had to have a bathtub and toilet). In the summer of 1941, less stringent penalties were imposed, and typhus patients could be treated at home.[41] Despite this move, every case of infection still had to be reported.

Disinfection baths became obligatory for all residents of a building, as did the superficial and ineffective sanitizing of their living quarters. This led to possessions being damaged and to the spread of lice.

> If a building had two or three thousand residents—and there were such conglomerations (e.g. 19, 23 and 37 Nalewki Street, 58 Miła Street)—then the building was sealed off by the police until the torture of being subjected to the baths was completed. In the meantime, people were locked up and deprived of even the watery soup, which usually came from a communal kitchen. Upon returning home, they found remnants of their "disinfected" (read: charred) possessions, or more likely they found nothing because they had been robbed blind. After fourteen days at most, the procedure would be repeated, because someone among the "disinfected" had fallen ill.[42]

Somewhat better results were achieved when steam-sulfur fumigation was conducted on clothing, together with mandatory sanitizing baths at the five bath centers in the ghetto. Every month 17,000 people went through these baths, which were barely sufficient for the ever-increasing number of displaced. The baths were located on 4 Solna and 43 Gęsia (TOZ), 21 Stawki, 20 Niska, and Waliców Streets.[43] Baths outside

---

40  Hirszfeld, *Historia jednego życia*, 234.
41  Makower, *Pamiętnik z getta warszawskiego*, 106.
42  An account by Mojżesz Mieczysław Tursz (Thursz), "Jak kształtował się sanitariat w ghetcie warszawskim," YVA O.3/438.
43  Leociak, "Służba zdrowia," 281.

the ghetto were well frequented, among them those on 93 Leszno, 109 Leszno and 15 Spokojna Streets, to which newly displaced people arriving in Warsaw were directed.[44]

At a bath station, possessions were taken away for disinfection and people were directed to the baths. Meanwhile, their luggage was ransacked for any valuable items. Identifying markers were removed in the ghetto storehouses to create chaos and disorder when people reclaimed their possessions.[45] People were left standing out in the cold for hours, waiting to claim their property. Often, people went away infested with lice.[46]

## TOZ Activities after the Sealing of the Warsaw Ghetto

When the ghetto was sealed off in November 1940, the well-equipped TOZ facilities and its head office were on the wrong side of the wall along with the Society of the Friends of Children. As a result, TOZ was forced to close two recently opened surgeries and an obstetrics unit.[47] In mid-November, to meet the enormous demand for medical consultations, TOZ turned hostels at 43 Gęsia Street into a clinic. Displaced people and burn victims were moved elsewhere; some were given financial assistance and sent home.[48] The tuberculosis prevention clinic became a multi-specialization polyclinic,[49] employing thirty-five doctors from various specializations, and ten nurses.[50]

---

44 On June 29, 1941, Czerniaków notes in his diary: "We received another bath for 1,000 people per day on Prosta Street." Czerniaków, *Adama Czerniakowa dziennik*, 196.

45 Bryskier, *Żydzi pod swastyką*, 67–68.

46 An account by Mojżesz Mieczysław Tursz (Thursz), "Jak kształtował się sanitariat w ghetcie warszawskim," YVA O.3/438.

47 *Gazeta Żydowska* 41 (1940): 2. Before the war, the center on 34 Chmielna was the property of Dr. Orko Sołowiejczyk, and the one on 23 Hoża, that of Dr. Eliasz Miszurski.

48 *Gazeta Żydowska* 13 (1940): 2.

49 Leociak, "Służba zdrowia," 243.

50 Information obtained from the files of doctors who, as members of the Warsaw-Białystok Medical Chamber, had filled out personal questionnaires between 1940 and 1942. The files list entries identifying their workplace during a given period. Of the eighty persons listed, as many as twenty (twenty-five percent) indicated the institution on 43 Gęsia as their place of employment. There were only three at the facility on 34 Chmielna, two on 17 Ceglana, and one on 23 Hoża Street. Eight people indicated that they were employed elsewhere, under the TOZ umbrella: they manned refugee shelters, working in a ringworm station or at a radiology department.

TOZ was also involved in providing medical personnel for quarantine stations. These stations and staging points for the displaced failed to combat the epidemic, which was branded "a dreadful ghetto disease."[51] Hirszfeld wrote:

> People on bunks or on the floor, positively starving. Toilets unfit to be used, so they relieve themselves on the floor. Totally louse-ridden. Because how can anyone delouse these multitudes? And what is quarantine, but economic ruin for the family—the final blow.[52]

Tursz also commented on the catastrophic conditions at TOZ staging points for the displaced:

> Every day there were new points. I am at a loss for words to describe them accurately . . . dreadful hunger and cold, almost everyone has bloody diarrhea. The only lavatory at the point is under constant siege. Frequently, people cannot even reach it. They dispose of their bodily wastes where they stand or lie.[53]

Often shelters were sealed off for weeks as new typhus infections were registered. Begging in the streets became impossible. To improve the sanitary and medical care at over ninety staging points, the TOZ assigned a nurse and a doctor to each.[54] Depending on the number of persons at a given point, each doctor had two or three layover points to take care of. Over forty doctors were employed in this way. TOZ supplied medicines, soap and disinfectants. Dr. Sara Syrkin-Binsztejn served as their principal doctor. As Tursz noted, she was not a *homo novus* in the field of social work. She had already worked as a JDC doctor in Poland after the First World War. Later, she retired from active work in Jewish sanitary

---

51  Makower, *Pamiętnik z getta warszawskiego*, 106.
52  Hirszfeld, *Historia jednego życia*, 234.
53  An account by Mojżesz Mieczysław Tursz (Thursz), "Jak kształtował się sanitariat w ghetcie warszawskim," YVA O.3/438.
54  Mieczysław Tursz (YVA O.3/438) gives the number of points resorting under the TOZ as 92. Leociak, "Opieka Społeczna," 311, notes that in January 1940, 6,000 refugees were living in the 108 hostels, and by April 1941, as many as 17,000, when there were 165 shelters.

institutions, but her energy and organizational talents continued to be acknowledged.[55]

Despite the efforts of many, the work at the refugee shelters seemed hopeless. Dr. Naftuli Trachtenherc complained that his "point was simply a death house" and a source from where "typhus spread."[56] In 1941, in quarantine on 86 Żelazna, 77 Leszno, 109–111 Leszno and 20 Niska Streets there were over 9,000 convalescents and suspected typhus cases.[57] In the first half of September 1941, all quarantine sites were liquidated; only those for the resettled remained.[58]

At the turn of 1941/1942, there was a sharp increase in the number of tuberculosis cases in the ghetto, and the progression of the disease was devastatingly rapid. Dr. Milejkowski called a meeting with representatives from the Health Council, the Health Department, TOZ, CENTOS and hospital directors, the JDC directors and leading ghetto community activists. They established the Tuberculosis Prevention League with an office in the TOZ building, four tuberculosis prevention clinics and two hospital departments. They agreed that food rations for the sick and those susceptible to tuberculosis had to be increased, whatever the cost; they presented a wide range of informative seminars and took preventive action.[59] Not much came of those plans.

At TOZ's initiative, during the deportations, a rescue and "First Aid" station run by nurse Ala Gołąb-Grynberg was created on the *Umschlagplatz*, where people were taken and put on the trains to Treblinka and Auschwitz.[60] When the deportations ended, of 580 TOZ personnel only ten survived.[61]

The outpatient clinic was revived after Yom Kippur 1942. Dr. Mendel Szwalbe was formally its director, under supervision of the *Judenrat*. On January 18, 1943, the TOZ head, Dr. Jakub Rozenblum was deported,

---

55  An account by Mojżesz Mieczysław Tursz (Thursz), "Jak kształtował się sanitariat w ghetcie warszawskim," YVA O.3/438.
56  Makower, *Pamiętnik z getta warszawskiego*, 26–27. Makower mistakenly gives the name as Trachntenberg.
57  *Tak było*, 57.
58  Leociak, "Opieka społeczna," 310.
59  An account by Mojżesz Mieczysław Tursz (Thursz), "Jak kształtował się sanitariat w ghetcie warszawskim," YVA O.3/438.
60  Ibid.
61  Ibid.

possibly in the same transport as Doctors Syrkin-Binsztejn and Izrael Milejkowski.[62]

## Emergency Services

Once the ghetto was sealed off, the staff of the Emergency Services moved to a building on Sienna Street, and the ambulance station was handed over to the *Judenrat*. Between November 1940 and May 1941, the Assistance to the Destitute Sick Society on Nowolipki Street was the only emergency service functioning in the ghetto. The *Judenrat* took over the Society in 1941, using it to maintain the pharmacy and outpatient clinic, and to offer medical assistance at night.[63] The night medical emergency station active in the ghetto was most likely a satellite reporting to TOZ.[64]

In May 1941, Jewish Emergency Services (JES), also called the "Red Police," was organized and housed at 13 Leszno Street. The founders were people from the Office for Combating Usury and Speculation, the so-called "Thirteens." Officers in the JES, the "Red Service," wore blue armbands and blue caps with a red rim and the Star of David.[65] At the opening ceremony on May 15, 1941, "hardened social activists from the ghetto, headed by the editor, Mr. Gancwajch," were present.[66] Juliusz Sirota was the manager, Salomon Mejłachowicz was chief doctor. At the time, the *Jewish Gazette* described it as a beneficial institution, whose purpose was to extend ad hoc help to the poorest residents of the ghetto.[67]

The JES headquarters was supposed to have two ambulances to transport patients free of charge, and stations for polyclinical consultations. The plan was to open an infirmary with 150–200 beds as a small observation hospital. A dispensary was planned, where medicines and consultations would be made available either free of charge or for a

---

62  Ibid.
63  Its chief doctor was Paweł Berlis. Also employed by the society were, among others, doctors Feliks Fiszel, Feliks Majnemer and Salomon Świeca.
64  Meroz, *W murach i poza murami getta*, 25.
65  Bryskier, *Żydzi pod swastyką*, 123. Under the cover of providing emergency assistance, the "Red Emergency Service" was involved in smuggling, and had little to do with saving people.
66  *Gazeta Żydowska* 40 (1941): 2.
67  *Gazeta Żydowska* 38 (1941): 2.

minimal fee to the poorest of the poor.[68] The *Jewish Gazette* reported that the JES had two fully equipped ambulances for ad hoc emergencies.[69] In honor of Abraham Gancwajch's wife, one of them was named "Miriam." Henryk Bryskier sarcastically noted that, immediately after the blessing ceremony, "the ambulance headed out into the city to collect its ready and plentiful quarry."[70] Jonas Turkow described the same ambulance:

> The poor horse was bent down pulling it, as it was laden with goods and contraband, while the brothers Sirota (one of them being the manager of the ambulance service) would spend the contents of their bulging pockets on Leszno Street, where every second building housed a café, restaurant, or exclusive shop and, in the evenings, they would attend cabaret performances.[71]

The JES was organized with the sector doctor or paramedic subordinate to a ward delegate (who oversaw about 40 buildings) who, in turn, was subordinate to an area delegate (overseeing 400 buildings). Building, sector and area delegates were charged with maintaining sanitary conditions in the residential buildings assigned to them, especially among the poor. Depending on their condition, the sick had to be referred to a clinic or hospital. The assistance the JES offered relied on the goodwill of the population and doctors who were prepared to work for free. Contributions were collected by designated collectors supervised by a regional manager. About 20,000 members paid monthly premiums of between fifty groszes and one zloty. Some contributions were made in kind, in the form of medicines or wound dressing materials, or surplus from requisitions.[72]

Not much came of the ambitious plans for the emergency services, except for the distribution of bread and sweetened tea to the poorest at regional stations.[73] Mounted sanitary patrols appeared on the streets, equipped with first-aid portable sets containing reviving tonics, bandages, slices of bread and flasks of tea. Those who needed help were

68  Ibid.
69  *Gazeta Żydowska* 39 (1942): 3.
70  Bryskier, *Żydzi pod swastyką*, 124.
71  J. Turkow, *C'était ainsi, 1939–1943. La vie dans le Ghetto de Varsovie* [fragment in Polish translation], http://warszawa.getto.pl/index.php?mod=view_record&rid=2007199812335200012&tid=zdarzenia, accessed February 18, 2017.
72  Leociak, "Służba zdrowia," 245.
73  Bryskier, *Żydzi pod swastyką*, 123.

taken to the hospital in a rickshaw. JES ambulances were kept busy transporting contraband, while the area offices did not even have telephones. Charitable organizations were, for the most part, propaganda machines, with their activities having been reduced to distributing food parcels. In August 1941, the *Jewish Gazette* noted that no one in the ghetto knew anyone who had ever been "rescued" by this service, nor could they give a date for when such an event had occurred.[74] In July 1941, the JES was formally incorporated into the Jewish Police.

By 1941/1942, the *Judenrat* Self-Help established the Doctors' Emergency Services (DES) in a building at 58 Leszno Street with Albert Gotlib as its principal doctor. DES was mainly staffed by surgeons.[75] The ground floor had a waiting room, a registration desk and a twenty-four-hour polyclinic. There was also a blood donation station, although it did not operate smoothly.[76] The staff rendered assistance free of charge, but patients were welcome to donate to pay for bandages. Only transportation had to be paid for. Doctors and sanitary personnel were not paid but received food in exchange.[77]

To distinguish themselves from the JES "Red Service," DES doctors called their service "Blue Emergency"—a name inspired by their dark blue caps with the lighter blue-and-white rim and an international red cross. When the Warsaw Emergency Services withdrew from the ghetto, they left behind several vehicles, all of them in bad states of repair, while supervision of the remaining equipment was left in the care of a paramedic authorized to have access to the ghetto.[78] They transported the sick to hospitals in rickshaws equipped with stretchers. A tandem rickshaw was pulled by two paramedics.[79] If transport was not required, a doctor made house calls in an ordinary rickshaw. DES had only one ambulance, an old yellow Citroën, which took patients to the sanatorium in Otwock.

---

74 *Gazeta Żydowska* 77 (1941): 2.

75 An account by Jerzy Ros (Rosenberg), YVA O.3/3440. Among the doctors were surgeons Jakub Korman, Stefan Jerzy Rotmil, Joel Liebfeld, and Kazimierz Pollak, laryngologist Dr. Józef Frank, and internist Aron Gotlib.

76 Ludwik Hirszfeld established a blood donation facility, requesting assistance from the Jewish Police, but its staff refused to donate. Students of the underground medical school eagerly agreed to donate their own blood.

77 An account by Jerzy Ros (Rosenberg), YVA O.3/3440.

78 Bojczuk, *Warszawskie Pogotowie Ratunkowe*, 80.

79 Bryskier, *Żydzi pod swastyką*, 124.

Dr. Alina Brewda reported spending a few days there. In an interview, she said:

> I had not been feeling well since my mother died. I noticed that half of my face was paralyzed. I could not see out of one eye, nor could I eat, because my mouth was numb, I couldn't move it. I decided to ask permission to go to Otwock, a small town in a pine forest, some 30 km from Warsaw. There was a pre-war sanatorium for poor Jews, with two or three pavilions for tuberculosis sufferers and one or two for the mentally ill. . . It had previously been managed by a charitable society, but the Germans changed it into a convalescent home, and the stay there was payable. Some rich Jews, despite being in good health, spent time there in relative comfort, thanks to the bribes they paid. I received permission for a ten-day stay and was driven to Otwock in an ambulance.[80]

Helena Szereszewska recalled that her grandson, Maciuś, contracted pleurisy in the ghetto. After two months of treatment, Dr. Henryk Brokman recommended a stay in Otwock, and a Dr. Wacław Skonieczny issued the necessary permit. The boy was sent to the Zofiówka sanatorium for the mentally ill in Otwock, where they opened a center for convalescing patients. Szereszewska recalled that the ambulance was white and marked with the blue Star of David.

Doctors and paramedics in the DES also helped people who were dying of hunger on the streets of the ghetto. Such assistance was illusory, because it was frequently limited to offering the dying companionship during the last moments of their lives. As Jerzy Ros (Rosenberg), a driver and paramedic in the DES emphasized, personnel opted not to transport the dying to hospitals, knowing they would not be admitted. The only solution would be to give them adequate nutrition, which ghetto hospitals did not have.

---

80  R. J. Minney, *I Shall Fear No Evil—The Story of Dr. Alina Brewda* (London: William Kimber, 1966), 51–52. Similar sentiments are expressed in Bryskier, *Żydzi pod swastyką*, 125.

## The Czyste Jewish Hospital

The sealing of the ghetto left the hospital on the Aryan side and some doctors received passes allowing them to leave the ghetto to work. Sabina Gurfinkiel-Glocer recalls that most employees did not receive passes so those wishing to work were forced to live in the hospital. According to Henryk Fenigsztein, in December 1940, the Czyste Jewish Hospital employed 200 doctors, and only seventy-five had passes on which the *Judenrat* levied a five zlotys tax per pass. Each morning, the doctors with passes gathered near a *Judenrat* outpatient clinic at 6 Twarda Street and from there were led in a column to the hospital.[81] Often gangs of juveniles threw stones at them. Sometimes the security police on duty at a ghetto gate would confiscate a pass without explanation and order the victim to perform humiliating squats. Soon beatings started.[82] Fortunately, such harassment was not directed at the sick who were transported to the hospital in horse-drawn carts.

When the Germans took control, they put the hospital under the auspices of the city magistrate, who handed it off to the leaders of the city's Jewish community. Then, by German decree, Czyste, which until that point was serving patients from all walks of life, became a solely Jewish facility. All non-Jewish patients and staffers were forced to leave and Jews were brought to Czyste from other hospitals in the city. The facility was massively overcrowded with patients in hallways, in overcrowded wards, in the attics and on the floors. Then in the fall of 1939, when the typhus epidemic broke out, Czyste was quarantined for six weeks with devastating results.

In December 1940, the Germans ordered Czyste to move into the ghetto.[83] Ringelblum noted in his diary that before it was moved, the hospital administration had to restore and renovate the building, including the laundry and bakery destroyed during the siege in September 1939.[84] Finally, at the end of January 1941, the staff moved patients and pieces of

---

81 Fenigstein, "The History of 'Czyste,'" xv–xvii.
82 Gurfinkiel-Glocer, "Szpital Żydowski w Warszawie," 102.
83 In J. Leociak's view, the beginning of evacuations from the Czyste Jewish Hospital took place on December 13, 1940. See J. Leociak, "Przebieg i zmiany granic getta warszawskiego," in B. Engelking and J. Leociak, *Ghetto Warszawskie*, 90.
84 Ringelblum, *Kronika getta warszawskiego*, 214.

hospital equipment to different buildings in the ghetto.[85] The move from Czyste took place in winter, during the fiercest cold. At night, patients were transported by ambulance, without suitable clothing. In line with the directive of the occupying authorities, only the most crucial items could be taken. The newly created hospital had no medical equipment whatsoever, and nurses decided to take along as many items as possible. During its move, the surgery department transported priceless surgical instruments in their patients' makeshift pillows. When the German gendarmerie conducted a search, the nurses forced their patients to keep their heads inclined on those hard pillows, which were stuffed with linens and medical instruments instead of feathers, telling the Germans that their patients had a high fever, which usually proved to be an effective deterrent.[86]

With the move into the ghetto, the hospital was renamed the Czyste Jewish Hospital for Infectious Diseases. In February 1941, about three months after the Warsaw Ghetto was created, the by-then-deserted premises of the Old Order Czyste Jewish Hospital were given to the Holy Ghost Hospital and the Treasury Hospital.[87] After the attack on the Soviet Union in June 1941, Germans evicted Poles from the Holy Spirit Hospital and set up a military hospital for their troops in these buildings.

When the Czyste Jewish Hospital moved to the ghetto, its three surgical (300 beds in total), laryngology and radiology departments were relocated to 1 Leszno Street which had been the Treasury Hospital. The internal and infectious diseases departments and the analytical and pathological laboratories were moved to the city's old archive building and the adjacent elementary school at 6/8 Stawki Street. Internal Diseases and the bacteriological laboratory were moved to 21 Stawki Street/20 Niska Street. A building at 21 Stawki Street housed several hospital departments (apart from infectious diseases), including cardiology and gastric diseases. In one of them, Dr. Emil Apfelbaum conducted research into hunger disease, one of the leading causes of death in the Warsaw Ghetto. Gynecology and Ophthalmology moved to one of the

---

85 Fenigstein, "The History of 'Czyste,'" xv.
86 Gurfinkiel-Glocer, "Szpital Żydowski w Warszawie," 102.
87 When preparations for war with the Soviet Union started, these facilities were moved to the grounds of the Ujazdowski Hospital, while the Czyste Jewish Hospital became a backup facility for German soldiers injured on the Eastern Front.

Leonardi tenement buildings on Tłomackie Street which used to house Dr. Fryszman's Urology Institute.[88] The hospital pharmacy, sterilization unit and library were moved to what had been the Holy Ghost Hospital on Elektoralna Street. The surgical, laryngology and radiology departments were managed by Doctors Aleksander Wertheim (First Surgical), Dawid Amsterdamski (Second Surgical), Ignacy Borkowski (Third Surgical), and Józef Jabłoński (laryngology).

Surgeon Dr. Stanisław Waller had this to say about the head of his department:

> Before the war, Dr. Wertheim, presently the head of department in the ghetto hospital, headed up surgery in a military hospital on Ujazdowski Alley. But before that he was an assistant to Doctors Krajewski and Sawicki. After Sawicki's death, he was ideally placed to assume the position of head of department at the Infant Jesus Hospital, but the magistrate remained reluctant to consider the candidacy of a man who, although converted, was nevertheless a Jew. Thus, it was announced that there would be competition for the position, and Dr. Wertheim was rejected. Eventually, in 1938, when the then head died, he became head of department at Czyste. This happened against the wishes of a Jewish nationalist group, who believed the position should go to Dr. Grynberg. Dr. Wertheim was happy to be considered Polish, and proudly reported that his grandfather had been "a banker of the January Uprising" in 1863—he had financed the activities of the insurgents. Wertheim was not popular with Jewish patients who, when he entered a ward, did not receive him kindly. "Luckily for me, I am not in the hands of a *meshumad* [derogatory term for a convert]," a happy patient would say if Wertheim was not his or her doctor.[89]

When the hospital was moved to the ghetto, no one minded Dr. Wertheim being an Evangelist. What mattered were his vast knowledge and experience. The department boasted six permanent assistants, many medical

---

88 This part of the street was excluded from the ghetto on March 20, 1942, and staff began working in the building at 1 Leszno Street.

89 An account by Stanisław (Shmul) Waller (Walewski), YVA O.3/2358.

students, and graduates from the dental academy.[90] "Each morning this entire white troupe," as Dr. Noemi Makower called herself and her colleagues, followed the chief from his rooms to participate in a ward round. Beds were placed very closely, with only a tiny nightstand separating them. The number of people seeking treatment increased daily and soon patients were being left on stretchers. Cases of severe frostbite, abscesses and gunshot wounds were most prevalent. Many patients needed urgent amputations.

Nearly all required additional nourishment but the hospital's food rations only offered lumpy bread and watery soup. Starvation caused nearly all patients to suffer from diarrhea. There were no linens as they were being stolen on their way to the hospital laundry. In some cases, hospital sheets were for sale at the Kiercelak market. Nurses, especially the head nurse, Altszul, and the wound-dressing nurse Finkiel, always had their hands full, yet they remained patient. Sometimes mere words of consolation had to suffice. In the end, even a single bed became a luxury.

A similar situation prevailed at 1 Leszno Street: the hospital became a mirror image of the ghetto, with grime, starvation, epidemics, gunshot wounds and, as Noemi Makower stated, "murders committed in clear daylight, in the name of the law," the order of the day.[91] Despite it all, the hospital became an asylum where the Germans did not interfere, which is why some beds went to "recommended" patients—the fathers and mothers of deserving nurses, and later those of influential councilors from the *Judenrat*, eager to save their family members from death.[92] There were instances of doctors breaking limbs of family members, just to admit him or her to the hospital, as was the case with Dr. Brandwajn, who temporarily saved his mother-in-law from deportation.[93]

The Department of Internal and Infectious Diseases on Stawki Street housed between 1,000 and 1,400 patients—often two to a bed.[94] Many were in grievous or critical condition, making the work of nurses and support staff remarkably difficult and strenuous. With the continued

---

90  Makower, *Miłość w cieniu śmierci*, 26.
91  Ibid., 44.
92  An account by Stanisław (Shmul) Waller (Walewski), YVA O.3/2358.
93  An account by Adolf Polisiuk, "Pamiętnik w kolekcji Abrahama Adolfa Bermana" (see "Czworobok"), Ghetto Fighters' House Museum, ref. 3182.
94  Fenigstein, "The History of 'Czyste,'" xix.

shortage of medical personnel, students assisted doctors, and support staff helped the nurses. For nourishment, patients received a bowl of watery soup once a day. The supply of medicines and wound dressings at their disposal proved entirely inadequate. When the typhus epidemic was at its most severe, these units, combined, housed as many as 3,000 patients.[95]

Dr. Józef Stein had been chief of the anatomopathological laboratory in the former Czyste Old Order Jewish Hospital since November 1940.[96] When Stein later became the hospital director, he was accused of securing a promotion because he was an Evangelical Augsburg who surrounded himself with "converted" Jews. His nomination was received with skepticism, mainly because he replaced the well-liked and much-valued Dr. Adam Zamenhof, who was executed in Palmiry soon after his arrest in 1939. As Dr. Stanisław Waller observed:

> Dr. Józef Stein was a Jew by birth, but he converted. . . When the hospital moved from Czyste to Leszno Street, from the very beginning Dr. Stein surrounded himself with a retinue of doctors who were converts. At that time, work in the Jewish hospital was highly valued and sought after, because of the mistaken conviction that it would safeguard doctors and nurses from annihilation. That is why Dr. Stein selected, from the many candidates eager for the hospital job those he could relate to, who like him, were converted Jews, yet still had been forcefully moved to the ghetto. But truth to be told, I must add that those converted Jews (usually highly qualified specialists and well educated), even the administrative staff, were generally honest people who did not steal and abided by ethical principles.[97]

---

95  Recollections by Stanisław (Shmul) Waller (Walewski), YVA O. 3/2358.

96  Dr. Józef Stein was a graduate of the Medical Department at Warsaw University and an acknowledged pathologist at the Holy Ghost Hospital. Before the war he devoted himself to cancer research, thanks to a bursary from Count Jakub Potocki. Stein published scientific papers in medical journals, and popularized science in his radio talks. Personal Files of Doctors, Members of the Warsaw-Białystok Medical Chamber, in the Old Books Collection, Medical Library, Warsaw. Personal file of Józef Stein. ref. 3580.

97  An account by Stanisław (Shmul) Waller (Walewski), YVA O.3/2358.

Dr. Waller wrote that Dr. Stein owed his directorship to the patronage of the former caretaker at the Holy Ghost Hospital, the *Volksdeutsch* Piątkowski. This might not be the case, but allegations against Dr. Stein did not end there. Dr. Waller believed the director was guided by personal sympathies and ignored the opinions of other doctors serving as heads of departments, and appeared to favor students who, in the evenings, gathered in his home, sharing inside information about what was happening in the various departments.

Toward the end of 1941, the head of one of the infectious diseases departments, Dr. Jakób Munwes, objected to the meetings and started a campaign against the "supremacy" of "converts" at the hospital. The campaign aimed to dismiss the current management and institute new managers, with candidates being proposed by the *Judenrat* Health Department. Munwes' initiative was rejected by his coworkers: his younger colleagues believed such a move would not alter what was a universally dire situation and defended the "converts" as honest people.[98]

Despite dissatisfaction with his promotion and the way he managed the hospital, Dr. Stein was valued as an excellent anatomical pathologist. Many of the specimens he prepared could be found in German museums.[99] Deep down, he was a scientist and too gentle to deal with the daily demands of managing a hospital. His wife, Anna Welk-Stein, an ambitious and energetic woman, helped him with administrative tasks and more.

Director Stein managed the hospital through all phases of its ghetto existence, participating in the underground medical courses while researching hunger disease. Dr. Makower summarized Dr. Stein's work and conduct in the ghetto as dignified and decent, especially considering that he frequently sneaked out to the Aryan side, where his young daughter was in hiding. Although he could have stayed outside, he kept returning.[100] His legacy is based on the results of postmortems and histopathological examinations he conducted with two assistants, Doctors

---

98  Ibid.
99  Hirszfeld, *Historia jednego życia*, 297.
100  T. Stabholz, *Siedem piekieł* (Kraków: AGAT-PRINT, 1992), 89. Dr. Stein had a daughter, Ludwika, born in 1937, who lived with her mother, Anna Welk-Stein, on the Aryan side.

Henryk Fenigstein and Siegfried Gilde. The team performed over 3,000 autopsies, with 500 pertaining to research on hunger disease.[101]

Since the Jewish faith demands human bodies be buried intact, the number of autopsies performed is hugely impressive. This may have been because Warsaw's official German doctor, the tyrannical Kurt Schrempf, ordered compulsory postmortems for all hospital deaths. Although Dr. Fenigstein had two unqualified assistants to help him, he was sometimes under pressure not to perform an autopsy, and sometimes was offered bribes not to. One way or another, postmortems were performed soon after a death occurred, usually less than twelve hours after death and occasionally within four to five hours. Most corpses did not exude unpleasant odors because putrefaction had not yet set in. The deceased were also emaciated to such a degree, there was little left to decay. Students of the ghetto underground medical courses observed the dissections, but according to Fenigstein, the sight of gaunt corpses often caused emotional trauma.[102]

Even though Fenigstein was Stein's second-in-command in the prosectorium, a crucial contribution was that of Siegfried Gilde, the second doctor, who hailed from Germany. Despite his apparent kindness, he was not liked by the students; they considered him an autocrat and were angry because he was offended when someone called him a Jew.[103]

Renowned specialists such as Mojżesz Gosblat, Henryk Jakób Landau, Jakób Munwes, Jeszaja Bejles, and Ichaskil Wohl, served as heads of departments with Dr. Stanisław Markusfeld in charge of dermatology and venereal diseases units. Physiotherapy was in the hands of Dr. Ida Asz. Dr. David Wdowiński was the psychiatric consultant, and his wife, Antonina Wdowińska, worked as stomatology consultant—a specialist on diseases of the mouth. The department of mental and nervous disorders was run by Dr. Eufemiusz Herman, an eminent specialist in neurology, and a student and associate of Prof. Edward Flatau. From October 1, 1941, when Dr. Bolesław Ałapin returned from Lviv with his

---

101 E. Apfelbaum, ed., *Choroba głodowa. Badania kliniczne nad głodem wykonane w getcie warszawskim w 1942 roku* (Warsaw: American Joint Distribution Committee, 1946), 32.

102 Fenigstein, "Holocaust and I," 129–130.

103 Ibid., 136.

wife, Dr. Stanisława Ałapin, he became one of the assistant doctors. His wife worked there, too. She wrote:

> I worked in the ghetto in Prof. E. Herman's department, which, at the time, dealt with neurological complications arising from typhus. There were many cases of encephalitis and meningitis. We had no medicines, and treated patients by giving intramuscular injections of their own cerebrospinal fluid and through autohemotherapy (aka self-blood therapy). These so-called "Herman methods" probably did not harm anybody. But the death rate was extremely high, there was a mass epidemic, conditions were inhuman. The sick lay two to a bed, they had no undergarments, there was no food or medicine. Bolesław became infected with typhus and was terribly ill, but fortunately he rallied while others died by the hundreds.[104]

From Dr. Ałapin's account we may infer that the mentally ill people were not hospitalized in the Department of Mental and Nervous Disorders, except for those with psychiatric complications resulting from typhus.

The Fifth Department, for typhus patients, was led by Dr. Jakub Penson and a staff of twenty doctors and several students from advanced medical courses.[105] After the war, Dr. Jerzy Szapiro, a staff doctor, remembered Dr. Penson as an excellent clinician and teacher.

In addition to a five-room laboratory, a lecture hall was built at 6/8 Stawki Street, with diagrams and charts hanging on the walls. Vital equipment like microscopes were donated by doctors. The head of provisioning, Abraham Gepner, helped them buy another microscope. An incubator was given to Prof. Hirszfeld by engineer Kurowski, who lived on the outside. When underground medical courses were given, the lecture hall and laboratory served as classroom space for the more advanced students.[106]

---

104  Quoted in T. Nasierowski, "Bolesław Ałapin (1913–1885)," *Postępy Psychiatrii Neurologii* 2, no. 4 (1995): 193.

105  M. Małecka, *Prof. Dr. med. Jakub Penson (1899–1971). Życie, działalnośći i dokonania* (study supervised by Dr. Zbigniew Machliński, Medical Academy in Gdańsk, Institute of History and Philosophy of Medical Sciences, Gdańsk, 2008), 178.

106  Hirszfeld, *Historia jednego życia*, 225. The analytical laboratory in the Bersohn and Bauman's Children's Hospital was led by Dr. Teodozja Goliborska-Gołąbowa, and

## The Bersohn and Bauman Children's Hospital

When the Ghetto was sealed off on November 15, 1940, the hospital became part of the "small ghetto," with Dr. Braude-Heller remaining as director. On the first floor was Dr. Sewryn Wilk's surgery, on the second was Dr. Natalia Szpilfogel-Lichtenbaum's internal diseases department and on the third, Dr. Regina Elbinger's contagious diseases department. The tuberculosis sub-department was headed up by Dr. Anna Margolis, the laryngological consultant was Dr. Kazimierz Lewin, and the hospital laboratory was in the hands of Dr. Teodozja Goliborska.[107]

Initially functioning without being subjected to harassment, the situation deteriorated very quickly. Among its young patients, a number had to be treated for scabies, lice, fungal infections, starvation, and tuberculosis.[108] On May 12, 1942, Czerniaków, head of the *Judenrat*, noted in his diary: "A delegation came from the hospitals to see me, led by (Commissioner) Skonieczny. They explained that Dr. Hagen could not help them, that there was no food. I dictated a memorandum, addressed to the authorities, which I promised to deliver in person."[109]

In the spring of 1941, at the height of the typhus epidemic, children were placed two, sometimes three, to a bed. Despite the Germans' order to hospitalize every case, the hospital could not accept more patients. According to Henryk Makower, Henryk Kroszczor, Judyta Braude and Adina Blady-Szwajger, in October 1941 it became possible, thanks to Dr. Braude-Heller, to open a branch of the Bersohn and Bauman Children's Hospital[110] on the corner of 86/88 Żelazna Street and 80–82 Leszno where they accommodated 400 children.[111] "It was a grim, three-floor building next to a gate in the ghetto wall."[112]

---

on Stawki, Dr. Maria Temkin.
107  An account by Izrael Rotbalsam, YVA O.3/2357.
108  Blady-Szwajger, *I więcej nic nie pamiętam*, 51.
109  Czerniaków, *Adama Czerniakowa dziennik*, 179.
110  Ibid.
111  Stanisław Waller states that, in the winter of 1941, the building of the elementary school on the corner of Leszno and Żelazna Streets was appropriated for use by the hospital. The head of this branch was Dr. Paweł Lipsztat. In my [MC] opinion Waller could have confused a Czyste Jewish Hospital department with the Quarantine and Refugee Center which functioned there until August 1941. See Stanisław (Shmul) Waller (Walewski), YVA O.3/2358.
112  Blady-Szwajger, *I więcej nic nie pamiętam*, 68.

As Edelman wrote:

> All hospitals, by now handling contagious diseases exclusively, were overcrowded. Daily 150 sick were being admitted to a single ward and placed two or three in a bed, or on the floors. The dying were viewed impatiently—let them vacate quicker for the next one! Physicians simply could not keep up with it. There had not been enough of them in the first place. Hundreds were dying at a given instance. The gravediggers were unable to dig fast enough. Although hundreds of corpses were being put into every grave, hundreds more had to lie around for several days, filling the graveyard with a sickening, sweetish odor. The epidemic kept growing. It could not be controlled. Typhus was everywhere, and from everywhere it threatened. It shared mastery over the ghetto with the overpowering hunger. The monthly mortality rate reached 6,000 (over two percent of the population).[113]

Previously, the larger rooms (most likely, classrooms) had been used for quarantining patients. There were doctors' duty offices and rooms for the nursing personnel. A long table with desk-type drawers was placed in the hall, where doctors could take down patients' medical histories. Admissions, the kitchens, and the disinfection chamber were accessible from the backyard.[114] Dr. Adina Blady-Szwajger, who worked in the branch on Leszno Street, left the most poignant description of this place:

> There, in those halls, on wooden bunks and paper mattresses without linens, lay children covered by the same kind of paper mattresses. In every corner there were tin buckets because there were no bedpans, no chamber pots, and children who suffered from hunger disease could not reach the toilets in time. Thus, in the morning, upon entering the ward, there were overflowing buckets, spilling their contents onto the floor; the stench of blood, pus and feces was unbearable. On the bunks lay skeletal children, or huge swollen lumps. Only their eyes were alive. Anyone who saw those eyes, those faces of the famished

---

113  Edelman, "The Ghetto Fights," 17–39.
114  Ibid., 70–71.

children with their open mouths resembling black hollows, their wrinkled, parched skins, knew what life could become.

But we wore white coats, our bodies were not swollen because, after all, we had received purified alcohol, so it is possible that those eyes observed us with hatred. Yet, we were there not to face the horrors, but to help them die in peace. But, most of all, to save them, because even if things were very bad, the worst, we refused to believe there was no point, trusting that if we endured, we would save those children, that they would live. So, we saved them with crumbs of food, a bit of medicine, some injections. Some children did survive. And when their health improved, when from those swollen lumps emerged little skeletons, we sometimes thought we saw something resembling a smile.[115]

Dr. Braude-Heller and her family lived in a building belonging to the hospital. From there, for a couple of hours each day, she went to the hospital on Śliska Street, to work with Dr. Anna Margolis, a temp from Łódź. The running of the hospital remained in the hands of Henryk Kroszczor. The infant-care section on Żelazna Street was led by Dr. Hanna Hirszfeld, infectious diseases by Dr. Henryk Makower, and internal diseases by Dr. Helena Keilson. Dr. Braude-Heller, in charge of disinfections, deployed an intern, Adina Blady-Szwajger, to the newly opened branch.

By winter 1941/1942 the hospital was in a lamentable condition because there was no space for patients to die in peace. The wards were icy, and young patients developed pneumonia. In the spring, meals secured from the JDC and the *Judenrat* Health Department were so calorie-deficient, personnel turned to the community for help, since there still were a considerable number of rich people in the ghetto. Czerniaków's wife established a group of women to organize collections for the benefit of hospitalized children. With their help, the children's nutrition improved, as did their health.[116] Bunks in the wards were replaced with beds and normal mattresses; linens, blankets, bedpans, and chamber pots, cups and bowls also appeared.[117]

---

115  Ibid., 72–73.
116  An account by Izrael Rotbalsam, YVA O.3/2357.
117  Blady-Szwajger, *I więcej nic nie pamiętam*, 74.

The newly opened branch was right next to a security gate guarded by Polish and Jewish gendarmes. The neighborhood proved to be dangerous: shots were fired at passersby on the ghetto side from the direction of Leszno or Żelazna Street, seemingly for fun and games. The worst culprit was nicknamed Frankenstein, because he shot children smuggling goods:[118]

> He would wait until four or five "targets" had gathered before shooting, sorting them all out with a single shot. If any of them still whimpered, we would bring the child to hospital and Dr. Wilk would come. Sometimes it was still possible to move such a child to the surgery on Śliska, but usually there was no point.[119]

The building on Żelazna Street, although modern, was not suitable for a hospital. Working there was monstrously difficult. The number of young patients soon reached 400, with the number of doctors continually decreasing as some moved to the Aryan side. With each passing day, the nursing and auxiliary personnel, too, decreased in number. By contrast, the number of adult patients in the hospital steadily grew as staff sought refuge for relatives. Dr. Henryk Makower, who sheltered his mother in this way, wrote that during her entire stay she felt the nurses' animosity "because she was the mother of a doctor who tried to save her, while their families could at best hide in a cellar. Anyhow, such opinions were not concealed."[120]

## The Hospital at 109 Leszno Street

The quarantine station on 109–111 Leszno Street deserves mentioning because in some memoirs it is referred to as the "hospital on the other side" or a "hospital branch."[121] It served as a quarantine station for the Department of Hospitalization.[122] In December 1939, Czerniaków, in his

---

118  SS-Rottenführer Josef Blösche was called Frankenstein.
119  Blady-Szwajger, *I więcej nic nie pamiętam*, 84.
120  Makower, *Pamiętnik z getta warszawskiego*, 71–72.
121  For instance, Henry Fenigstein calls this place a "hospital branch," adding that it was transformed into a *Dulag*, an internment camp for Jews awaiting deportation to the labor camps. See Fenigstein, "The History of 'Czyste,'" xxx.
122  *Gazeta Żydowska* 1940, no. 24, p. 2.

diary, lists two quarantine stations funded by the *Judenrat* and designated for suspected cases of typhus and recovering patients.[123] The stations were located in buildings at the corner of 86 Żelazna and 77 Leszno Streets, and at 109–111 Leszno Street. Almost from the very beginning of the German occupation, the latter building housed quarantine facilities and disinfection baths for refugees and the displaced, as reported by Henryk Bryskier and Samuel Puterman.[124]

By April 1942, the number of deportees from Germany had skyrocketed. Upon arrival they were transferred from a side-track on the *Umschlagplatz* to the quarantine facility at 109 Leszno, then to shelters in the Main Judaic Library building and the Great Synagogue on Tłomackie Street.[125] Henry Fenigstein's notes make mention of the Infectious Diseases Hospital branch on 109 Leszno Street,[126] with Dr. Pawel Lipsztad as director.[127] A note by Rozenfelt, preserved in the Ringelblum archives, says it was established on December 15, 1941.[128]

The hospital had 216 beds for patients with infectious diseases. The patients were brought in by ambulance after being referred by the center on Stawki Street. The hospital's financial administration was in the hands of Halber, a Jew from Pomerania, whose wife was a *Volksdeutsche*. Using his position, Halber kept pigs and geese on the premises, feeding them cereal and potatoes intended for the patients. His wife had a canteen and a grocery store with two workers who were remunerated by the *Judenrat*. Because groceries were considerably cheaper on the Aryan side than in the ghetto, hospital personnel eagerly purchased small quantities of products to bring to the ghetto.

From December 1941, to safeguard his profits, Halber conducted personal searches at the entrance, confiscating any items that had not

---

123 Czerniaków, *Adama Czerniakowa dziennik*, 72.
124 Bryskier, *Żydzi pod swastyką*, 67–68; Memoir of Samuel Puterman, Jewish Historical Institute Archives, ref. 302/27.
125 Leociak, "Opieka społeczna," 309.
126 Fenigstein, "The History of 'Czyste,'" xxx.
127 Stanisław Waller, however, in his account (YVA O.3/2358), mentions Dr. Wajnbaum (no name stated).
128 B. Rozenfeld, "Szpital po tamtej stronie," series: "Hospitals," Jewish Historical Institute Archives, Ringelblum archives, Ring. I, no. 581/2, published in M. Tarnowska, *Artyści żydowscy w Warszawie 1939–1945. Katalog* (Warsaw: Żydowski Instytut Historyczny, Polski Instytut Studiów nad Sztuką Świata 2015).

been bought from his wife's store. He suspended anyone who was ill-disposed towards him, accusing them of fabricated offences. Office clerk L. Paryżer, for instance, was accused of corrupting and demoralizing Halber's Aryan children. Products destined for feeding the patients found their way to his wife's store. The Jewish authorities tolerated this because they were afraid of Halber's threats to use his Aryan wife's influence.[129]

Towards the end of July 1942, the hospital-quarantine facility at 109 Leszno became a *Dulag* (internment camp) for Jews waiting for deportation to labor camps after being "selected" on the *Umschlagplatz*.[130] In his memoir, Marek Stok describes a German commission carrying out perfunctory inspections on Jews about to be deported to the labor camps.[131] The *Dulag* also quarantined people returning from the camps.

## Pharmacies

When the ghetto was sealed off, there were about twenty pharmacies in the ghetto area with the majority in private hands. Apart from pharmacies, there were also dispensaries belonging to Jewish charitable societies such as "Medical Assistance," "Brotherly Help," and the Old Order Jewish Community (which dispensed some medicines for free), the Social Insurance Company, and the pharmacy in the Holy Ghost Hospital (which was bombed in September 1939 and the hospital did not operate in the ghetto). Chaim Kapłan wrote that when the ghetto was created, there were twenty-one drugstores within its walls with seven of them belonging to Jews, while Leonia Grynberg-Donat (who managed one of the drugstores) remembered twelve or thirteen pharmacies in the ghetto.[132] When the ghetto was established, pharmacies within its walls continued to operate and initially supplied medicines as they had before. Aryan staff employed in those outlets had passes authorizing them to enter the district and work in Jewish-owned pharmacies.[133] As Emanuel

129  Ibid.
130  Fenigstein, "The History of 'Czyste,'" xxx.
131  Memoir of Marek Stok, Jewish Historical Institute Archives, ref. 302/144.
132  L. Grynberg-Donat, "Apteki w getcie warszawskim," Jewish Historical Institute Archives, ref. 333–575 (bequest of Bernard Mark), 1. Leonia Grynberg-Donat (Łaja Grynberg, neé Liberman), born in 1904, held a Master's degree in pharmacy (1929) and lived in Warsaw at 5 Orla Street. See *Urzędowy spis lekarzy*, part 4: *Felczerzy*, 25.
133  Kaplan, *Scroll of Agony*, 203.

Ringelblum noted in his chronicles on October 20, 1940, "long lines of people stood in front of the pharmacies, waiting to buy up almost anything."[134] Helena Szereszewska described such a site: "Pharmacy at the corner, next to it a beggar, just one step over a high threshold, and you were in a clean, bright interior with two cheerful shop windows."[135]

Eventually, the Aryan owners received orders to move their pharmacies to designated locations outside the ghetto walls, with some of the ghetto outlets being acquired by the *Judenrat*'s Department of Pharmacies which had been established at the beginning of 1941 to organize and supervise the functioning of these outlets. The pharmacies were overseen by two pharmaceutical inspectors.[136] The Pharmaceutical Inspectorate was managed by the respected pharmacist, Salomon Sander. The *Judenrat* ended up leasing between twelve and fourteen facilities[137] and nine dispensaries. Despite its tight budget, the *Judenrat* was expected to fund the required equipment. Before August 1941, the *Judenrat* opened an additional six pharmacies and dispensaries to meet the needs of the ghetto population (please see appendix 5). Despite the growing number of pharmacies, the customers waited a long time for their medications to be prepared and dispensed.[138] There were also other facilities in the ghetto, such as Wholesale Pharmaceuticals, owned by Henryk Fuks, who made ampules of the most-needed medicines, and had a sanitary repository, which supplied mostly disinfectants.[139] There was also a private workshop, which produced tablets; one that made sulfur candles for disinfection, and a facility producing mineral water sold through pharmacies. Although it was against the law, some multi-purpose suppliers (cosmetics and chemicals) also manufactured tablets. In August 1941, during a council session, Henryk Gliksberg reported that additional pharmacies would be opening, bringing the total number of working outlets to nineteen, which he considered sufficient to meet the needs in the ghetto.[140]

---

134  Ringelblum, *Kronika getta warszawskiego*, 174.
135  H. Szereszewska, *Krzyż i mezuza* (Warsaw: Czytelnik, 1993), 60.
136  *Gazeta Żydowska* 35 (1941): 2.
137  *Gazeta Żydowska* 28 (1941): 3.
138  Leociak, "Służba zdrowia," 241.
139  Bryskier, *Żydzi pod swastyką*,140.
140  *Gazeta Żydowska* 70 (1941): 3.

Most Aryan pharmacy owners stripped them of everything when they left the ghetto, leaving behind empty (not always undamaged) walls. Pharmacies had to be rebuilt from scratch: new shelves, cabinets, scales, restocking medicines and apparatus. Thus, not all pharmacies were ready in time, but their neat and tidy interiors contrasted sharply with the scruffy appearance of the ghetto.[141]

Helena Szereszewska, at that time a nursing student, remembered a pharmacy manager, Henryk Gliksberg (Glücksberg).[142] Before the war, the Gliksbergs lived on Polna Street, and in the Ghetto at 6 Lubecki Street. Their apartment in the ghetto was filled with antiques, paintings, furniture, and carpets, which the Germans used as a set for the filming of a propaganda movie to demonstrate how wealthy Jews lived in the ghetto.[143] Others representing the *Judenrat* were Hurwicz and Filskraut, co-owners of a pharmaceutical wholesale business; the brothers Szternberg, who were pharmaceutical merchants, and pharmaceuticals vendor and apothecary Abram Rudnicki.

Some pharmacies were open at night. Issues of the *Jewish Gazette* published between April 1941 and April 1942 reported that some chemists kept their stores open at night, mostly in the northern part of the district. In the southern part, some pharmacies, possibly seven, traded at night too, as did the one on Grzybowski Square.[144]

Henryk Bryskier wrote that though the *Judenrat* formally owned the pharmacies and dispensaries, they actually belonged to the group of shareholders financing them.[145] All facilities brought their daily revenues to the Department of Pharmacies, and the *Judenrat* deducted a forty-percent interest from the sale of medicines.[146] The department established drug prices and personnel wages. Former pharmacy owners generally became managers, with their salaries set at 1,000 zlotys per month. Bernard Mark, a departmental employee, wrote that "nonprofessional

---

141 L. Grynberg-Donat, "Apteki w getcie warszawskim," Jewish Historical Institute Archives, ref. 333–575 (bequest of Bernard Mark), 1.

142 Henryk Gliksberg (Glücksberg), engineer and doctor of chemistry, councilor in the *Judenrat*, disappeared with his wife Stefania and two sons, Tadeusz and Stefan, from the ghetto during the January deportations.

143 Szereszewska, *Krzyż i mezuza*, 112.

144 *Gazeta Żydowska* 53 (1941): 2; 56 (1941): 2; 70 (1941): 3; 39 (1942): 3.

145 Bryskier, *Żydzi pod swastyką*, 139.

146 Ibid., 139.

staff (working at the tills or as pharmacy assistants) were employed under the same conditions as other institutions—on the basis of favoritism and bribes."[147] The lowest salary, 150 zlotys per month, was paid to the pharmacies' runners.[148] During the spring of 1941, 150 pharmacists were employed in the ghetto, with approximately 120 auxiliary personnel.[149]

In 1941, the *Judenrat*'s Health Department organized a nine-month pharmaceutical course, run by Prof. Hirszfeld and, according to announcements in the *Jewish Gazette*, scheduled to start in November.[150]

According to the *Jewish Gazette*, different patent medicines were sold in the ghetto: mixtures for getting rid of lice, various remedies, local and foreign herbs, ointments to combat frostbite, among other miscellaneous items.[151] Repositories offered local and foreign remedies, candles and fresh leeches. However, cotton wool and Vaseline could be obtained only by prescription, and later, soap was as well. Additional soap and washing powder were given to doctors, veterinarians, pharmacists, dentists, midwives and other professionals caring for the sick and for infants. They received a bar of soap and 250 grams of washing powder. Doctors collected soap and washing powder vouchers from the Medical Council and purchased the required products at a pharmacy.[152]

The pharmacists were also involved in the battle against the never-ending typhus epidemic, which was the biggest challenge to the doctors, medics and nurses working in the ghetto. The main problem was not being able to get enough glucose ampules, physiological salts and pyramidon tablets to reduce fevers. The department's management blamed the Pharmaceutical Chamber for the drastically inadequate stock of vital remedies, branding them "rather indifferent, sometimes hostile in supplying medications so needed in the ghetto."[153]

The entrepreneurs Moryc Kohn and Zelig Helle, who operated the Society for Omnibus Transport, were also granted by the Germans a

---

147 L. Grynberg-Donat, "Apteki w getcie warszawskim," Jewish Historical Institute Archives, ref. 333–575 (bequest of Bernard Mark), 1.
148 Ibid.
149 Leociak, "Służba zdrowia," 241.
150 *Gazeta Żydowska* 40 (1941): 2; 110 (1941): 2.
151 Leociak, "Służba zdrowia," 241–242.
152 *Gazeta Żydowska* 46 (1942): 2.
153 L. Grynberg-Donat, "Apteki w getcie warszawskim," Jewish Historical Institute Archives, ref. 333–575 (bequest of Bernard Mark), 2.

concession to sell medicines in the ghetto. It is possible some orders for medication were forwarded to the Transfer Office on Królewska Street, which was tasked with regulating economic activity in the ghetto by controlling imports from the Aryan side and exports from the ghetto to the outside world. The Transfer Office also supervised activities of industrial and artisanal manufacturers. Medical supplies were delivered to a railroad ramp on the *Umschlagplatz*.

The Germans handicapped the functioning of the ghetto in ways large and small. Because they considered the ghetto an "exterritorial customs zone," a fifteen-percent tariff was imposed on all pharmaceuticals.[154] Because the *Judenrat* Self-Help did not receive permission to purchase medicines from wholesalers, it was forced to rely on gifts from abroad.[155] *Judenrat* officials were the only ones exempt from paying the forty percent tax the Department of Pharmacies imposed on the sale of medicines.

The continuous shortage of bandages and medicines led to the creation of a black market, with products smuggled into the ghetto by Heniek Grynberg, who travelled to Lviv on false documents, bringing back supplies ordered by well-off Jews.[156] In July 1941, the price of an ampule of anti-typhoid vaccine was several hundred zlotys.[157] Henryk Fuks, the owner of Pharmaceutical Wholesalers, also smuggled unobtainable goods and medicines into the ghetto.[158]

In addition, small quantities of medical supplies trickled in with new arrivals from abroad. Prof. Hirszfeld tried to meet the highest ethical standards, even in desperate circumstances. He wrote that "the only capital German Jews possessed was their stock of medicines. The German

---

154  Ringelblum, *Kronika getta warszawskiego*, 261.
155  Memoir of Michał Weichert, Jewish Historical Institute Archives ref. 302/25.
156  M. Berg, *Dziennik z getta warszawskiego* (Warsaw: Czytelnik, 1983), 91–92. Mary Berg, neé Miriam Wattenberg (October 10, 1924–April 2013) was a survivor of the Warsaw Ghetto and author of a Holocaust journal, which contains her personal entries written between October 10, 1939, and March 5, 1944, during the occupation of Poland in the Second World War, see "Mary Berg," Wikipedia, https://en.wikipedia.org/wiki/Mary_Berg.
157  Berg, *Dziennik z getta warszawskiego*, 91–92. Hirszfeld gives an amount of 1,000 zlotys, while Ringelblum mentions 400–500 zlotys for two people. Considering that a vaccination cycle consisted of three injections, one ampule probably cost 500 zlotys.
158  W. Gran (Grynberg), *Sztafeta oszczerców. Autobiografia śpiewaczki* (Paris: Wiera Gran, 1980), 26, http://warszawa.getto.pl, accessed October 17, 2017.

authorities tried to convince us to requisition it for the hospitals. But we didn't want to rob paupers, even for the public good."[159]

Many of the medical supplies reached the ghetto from those beyond its walls. Mojsze Moritz Aisen recalled that his Aryan wife, who carried an official ghetto pass, brought in medicines purchased from the German pharmacy in Warsaw.[160] Jerzy Śliwczyński, an attendant at the City Tribunal, had a permanent pass and smuggled in medicines for Dr. Langleben, a dentist, for the community clinic on Krochmalna Street, and for Dr. Józef Makowski.[161] Orphanages and resettlement stations struggled to obtain the necessary medications and their situations were particularly dire.

### The Chemical and Bacteriological Institute

In June 1941, the Chemical and Bacteriological Institute was created as part of the Health Department at the initiative of Dr. Sara Syrkin-Binsztejn. At the helm of the Institute, in addition to its directors and branch managers, was a board composed of representatives from departments within the *Judenrat*: health, supplies, commerce and industry. Prof. Mieczysław Centnerszwer was the director, Dr. Eugeniusz Ritt managed the chemical branch, and Dr. Bronisława Fejgin was the bacteriologist.[162]

---

159  Hirszfeld, *Historia jednego życia*, 255.
160  An account by Mojsze Moritz Aisen, Jewish Historical Institute Archives, ref. 301/5538.
161  An account by Jerzy Śliwczyński, Ella Perkiel and Frank Perkiel, Jewish Historical Institute Archives ref. 301/6236.
162  Mieczysław Centnerszwer (1874–1944) was born in Warsaw and educated in St. Petersburg and Leipzig. From 1919, he was professor of physical and inorganic chemistry at Latvia University. In 1928, he became head of the Department of Physical Chemistry at the Faculty of Mathematics and Natural Sciences. His wife, who was German, obtained a divorce in 1940, and left behind her husband and daughter. In the ghetto, Centnerszwer presented lectures to artisan-dyers and paramedics. In his free time, he wrote a chemistry textbook. On March 27, 1944, he moved into his former wife's apartment in Saska Kępa on the Aryan side. H. Lichocka, "Mieczysław Centnerszwer (1874–1944)," in *Portrety uczonych. Profesorowie Uniwersytetu Warszawskiego 1915–1945 (A–Ł)*, ed. P. Salwa, A. K. Wróblewski (Warsaw: Wydawnictwa Uniwersytetu Warszawskiego, 2016), 163–170.

To identify possible threats to the inhabitants' health, the Institute analyzed the food available in the ghetto.[163] Between July 7 and December 31, 1941, Prof. Centnerszwer noted eighty-six analyses of bread had been done and forty-six of flour, of which forty-seven bread and seventeen flour analyses were problematic. The catastrophic quality of the bread was due to additives, such as talc powder, chalk, and magnesium. The bread contained too much water and was contaminated with larvae, husks, and other impurities. Other products were subjected to scrutiny as well: sugar, vanilla sugar, artificial honey, marmalade, sweets, meat and meat products, oils and fat, and sparkling water. Bodily fluids from the Czyste Jewish Hospital were also tested, to check for formaldehyde and formic acid when poisoning with methylated spirits or a denaturant was suspected.

The Institute's charter was formally adopted in February 1942.[164] Supplies, commerce and industry departments of the *Judenrat* contributed to the creation of the Institute, which was housed in a three-room apartment on Pańska Street. The director of a nursing school in the same building donated much-needed laboratory equipment. In February 1942, Czerniaków, through the *Judenrat*, contributed 5,000 zlotys for additional equipment, and instructed money be collected to purchase chemistry books.[165]

The bacteriological laboratory tested for typhus infections and typhoid fever. Individual tests included analyses of feces, urine, pus and suctioned fluids, cerebrospinal fluid, sputum, and nasal and aural exudates, while more than 1,021 analyses involved typhus vaccines. The bacteriological branch also conducted tests on food samples.

The Institute continued its work despite irregular supplies of gas and electricity, round ups, murders, and deportations. Investigations were commissioned by the *Judenrat* Health Department (the hospital and the six health centers), the supplies, commerce, and industry departments, and private individuals. Tests commissioned by the *Judenrat* were done

---

163  "Sprawozdanie z działalności Instytutu Chemiczno-Bakteriologicznego przy Wydziale Zdrowia Rady Żydowskiej za okres od dnia 7 lipca do dnia 31 grudnia 1941 r." (fragment), Jewish Historical Institute Archives, Ringelblum archives, Ring. I/191, Mf. ŻIH-779.

164  *Gazeta Żydowska* 21 (1942): 2.

165  Czerniaków, *Adama Czerniakowa dziennik*, 251.

at a discounted rate, while private individuals and other institutions paid according to tariffs determined by the board of the Institute.

## Medical Care for the Jewish Police

In the fall of 1940, several doctors served in the Jewish Police under German command. They were subordinate to three different institutions: the president of the *Judenrat*, the commander of the Polish Police in Warsaw and the German commissioner of the Jewish Residential District.[166] In December 1940, Colonel Józef Szeryński was appointed superintendent-commander with Jakub Lejkin, a lawyer, as his deputy.[167] The Jewish Police maintained order, regulated street traffic, and prevented misdemeanors and felonies. A special unit of thirty to forty officers, the so-called "Hospital Guard Squad," was tasked with guarding prisoners being transported to hospitals for treatment.[168]

Zygmunt Fajncyn was the principal doctor in the Jewish Police force. Colonel Szeryński's personal doctor, designated by the Jewish Police, was Dr. Henryk Makower; Dr. Ignacy Rejder was assigned to Lejkin. The ten Jewish Police doctors had the same identity cards, caps and armbands as other policemen, but instead of a star, their armbands bore the caption *Arzt* ("doctor"), and instead of stars, their caps bore the Staff of Aesculapius, the symbol of the medical profession. Their identity cards were not numbered, but bore letters, and their surnames and addresses appeared on bulletin boards in regional offices enabling police officers to call them at will. The doctors were also issued special permits.

Apart from these ten, several dozen other doctors treated policemen in their private offices or at the association's polyclinics. The right to be consulted was implied by the issuing of so-called consultation cards, handed to the sick by their unit directors and passed on to the doctor. The doctor then submitted the card to the Association's Department of Social Care and received fifty groszes for the consultation. The families

---

166 B. Engelking, "*Żydowska Służba Porządkowa*," in B. Engelking and J. Leociak, *Getto warszawskie*, 203.

167 Józef Andrzej Szeryński (Szenkman or Szynkman) was under-inspector in the State Police, and from December 1940—senior inspector (nadkomisarz) in the Jewish Police in the Warsaw Ghetto. Engelking, "*Żydowska Służba Porządkowa*," 216.

168 Diary of an unknown author, Jewish Historical Institute Archives, ref. 302/129.

of police officers were not entitled to the same medical care provided by the Jewish Police doctors.[169]

One of the police doctors, Julian Lewinson, a radiologist, was Janina Bauman's uncle. She wrote of him with mixed emotions: on the one hand, her widowed mother, Alina Fryszman, was indignant about Lewinson joining the police—apart from wearing a blue cap, he also carried a nightstick. On the other hand, she was thankful he spared no effort to save her. As Janina Bauman wrote:

> We didn't like this very much. Mother, Jadwiga, and especially Stefan, condemned those who agreed to serve in the Jewish Police. At the very beginning, soon after the ghetto was created, Stefan was offered the chance to become a policeman, but he categorically refused. Instead, he volunteered to work in a hospital as an unqualified sanitary assistant, where he did the dirtiest of jobs because he wished to be useful. He considered the Jewish Police to be collaborators and German lackeys. It must be said that, for many men, the police service was the only way to keep themselves and their families alive. But Julian was a doctor and could manage in other ways. In the end, he served in the police as a doctor.[170]

Stefan Fryszman believed that during the war, and in the ghetto especially, everyone was exposed to evil and was therefore susceptible to becoming "infected" by it. That is why he maintained extraordinary vigilance to prevent himself from descending into a morally ambiguous situation, or to prevent that from happening for as long as possible.

Dr. Makower noted that those who worked for the Germans were provided with food and received the largest rations from the Germans during the *Grossaktion*. Despite not being considered "full-fledged" police officers, the doctors in their ranks received half a kilogram of bread daily and a plate of nutritious soup.[171] Police functionaries ate at special canteens and had access to all aspects of medical care. Their

---

169  "Wspomnienia anonimowego policjanta z warszawskiego getta," Jewish Historical Institute Archives, ref. 302/129.

170  Bauman, *Zima o poranku*, 74–75.

171  Makower, *Pamiętnik z getta warszawskiego*, 58.

service in the ghetto enabled them to earn a supplementary income mostly derived from smuggling food and people.

## The Prisons

As a result of the growing terror, the prisons in Pawiak at Daniłowiczowska and Mokotowska Streets were overflowing with Jews rounded up on the Aryan side. By order of the German police, in the summer of 1941, a central detention facility was created for the ghetto. It was called "Gęsiówka," because it was situated between Zamenhofa and Gęsia Streets.[172] Dr. Johan Frendler, a prison doctor there, was assisted by the hygienist Dr. Jeszaja Bejles, who had been caught on the Aryan side.[173]

Bejles told Prof. Hirszfeld that every day several people in the prison died from hypoxia. The detention facility held three times as many people as the place could accommodate. Cells reserved for the educated had bars in the windows, while those for the working classes had tiny windows just below the ceiling. Prisoners were forced to stand, because there were too many of them in a cell.[174] Hunger and filth added to their suffering. Many of the incarcerated soon developed typhus, dysentery or tuberculosis. A Jewish welfare organization (*Żydowski Patronat nad Więźniami*), managed by Felicja Czerniaków and Councilor Bernard Zundelewicz, was able to provide some provisions and medications to the prison hospital.

## Christian Convert Doctors

In his memoirs, Hirszfeld, a Catholic convert, wrote that Czerniaków offered him the position of chairman of the Health Council, following requests by several delegations. Hirszfeld's resentment towards Orthodox Jews was obvious, and for their part, they did not accept his conversion. As Adina Blady-Szwajger wrote:

---

172 In the Ghetto there was a prison hospital, created by transforming the St. Zofia Maternity Hospital on Żelazna Street.

173 Michał Grynberg, ed., *Pamiętniki z getta warszawskiego. Fragmenty i regesty* (Warsaw: PWN, 1993), 67.

174 Hirszfeld, *Historia jednego życia*, 259.

Professor Hirszfeld and his wife were not popular in the ghetto because of their manifest relationship with the Catholic parish. Despite there being undeniable respect for their scholarly achievements, between us and them there was a kind of gulf. It was obvious that they felt duped, because they had been knocked off the pedestal that had led them to believe they belonged to a *better part of society.*[175]

At the beginning, Hirszfeld could not find his feet in the ghetto because, as he put it, he did not know the Jews or the way to their hearts.[176] He believed people's reluctance to accept him stemmed mainly from the fact he was a Christian. But people in the ghetto remembered Hirszfeld had once removed almost all the Jews from the Hygiene Institute and had applied an antisemitic policy there before finding himself in the ghetto.[177]

People knew he came from a very wealthy family, which had owned many Warsaw restaurants. They believed that his conversion was a career move because he wanted to become the director of the Hygiene Institute.[178] It was easier for the Jews to accept converts who, long before the war, had changed their faith based on a deep conviction. Dr. Adina Blady-Szwajger demonstrated this in her writings about Dr. Zofia Rosenblum-Szymańska:

> Before the war she worked in *Kasa Chorych*. One of her patients was a herring vendor, Mrs. Chana Ogórek, a mother of six. Those days, house calls were expensive. One day, Dr. Rozenblum came to the office and learned that Mrs. Ogórek bought house-call cards for her six children, who had all taken ill on Friday. The doctor, worried that it could be diphtheria, went there immediately. She entered the room to find a white tablecloth and challah on the table, Mrs. Ogórek in a festive wig and dress. "Mrs. Ogórek, what happened?"
>
> "Doctor, if I asked you to come to a poor Jewish woman for a fish [meal], would you? No! But I bought six visitation cards,

---

175  Blady-Szwajger, *I więcej nic nie pamiętam*, 69.
176  Ibid., 214.
177  Ringelblum, *Kronika getta warszawskiego*, 225.
178  A. Grupińska, *Ciągle po kole*, 175.

for half an hour each, so you have three hours for us. You will sit down and eat our Friday supper with us."

Then Dr. Szymańska explained, "You see, I tried various philosophical systems, but when all of this happened, to carry on living I had to believe that my sister, my family, Mrs. Ogórek with her six children, were somewhere, living somewhere, and that I might meet them again. And this I found in Christianity."[179]

As was the case with other assimilated Jews in the ghetto, Hirszfeld was met with biting comments and references for accepting prominent positions offered by "proselytes." As noted in the Ringelblum archives:

> Many talented people in the world of medicine occupied managerial positions in Polish society but now aspire to manage Jewish lives. The sentimental Dr. M., a *meches*, told me that it is because of an inferiority complex towards Christians and megalomania towards Jews. We can give them bread, and share the last [bite], but they will not rule the lives of the Jewish people.[180]

The statement was apparently wrong considering the number of converts in the Health Department—Christians held key positions: Ludwik Hirszfeld, Józef Stein, Aleksander Wertheim, Mieczysław Kon, and Tadeusz Ganc. Czerniaków believed that the good of the whole was more important than antagonism toward the converts. "The ghetto is not a Jewish state, but terrain occupied by converted Jews as well, and for this reason they must be treated equally."[181] The converts' case was not helped by the unfortunate memo they wrote while the ghetto was being organized, asking for a separate ghetto to be created for them with the help of the Central Welfare Council and Count Adam Roniker. Ringelblum noted: "Several days ago (February 23–27), a welcoming ceremony was held for over twenty convert families on Roniker's list. Among them were

---

179 Ibid., 177–178.
180 Ringelblum, *Kronika getta warszawskiego*, 214–215. *Meches* is a term used to designate Jewish converts to Christianity. Here the reference is probably to Dr. Izrael Milejkowski.
181 Ibid., 260.

Benedykt Hertz, Prof. Hirszfeld, Dr. Wertheim, and others. Armbands were made for them at the Jewish Association."[182]

In a way, Hirszfeld was his own worst enemy. His pronouncements betrayed the fact he had an inflated opinion of himself and his work, while he belittled efforts of others and responded to his critics derisively. He dismissed all attacks directed at him as the work of Jewish nationalists.[183] His wife, Dr. Hanna Hirszfeld, tried to dissuade him from accepting the chairmanship in the Ghetto Health Council, arguing he would be ruined, his hands sullied with allegations of corruption, that "Jewish nationalists would think he was positioning himself to join them."[184]

What made him accept the position? Was it the expertise he knew he had, even if it was undervalued in the ghetto? Or was it his compassion for the needy masses? During a conversation with Czerniaków, Hirszfeld apparently asked about the Health Council's powers, and said he had no time to give advice no one would follow.[185] Czerniaków answered that the council would have as much power as he was prepared to accept. Hirszfeld demanded that all decisions the Health Council made—and the chairman approved—be adhered to by the *Judenrat* departments.

## Mental Health in the Ghetto

In documents in the Jewish Historical Institute Archives, suicide is listed as a cause of death from the very outbreak of the war. In 1939 there were four such cases, seven were noted in 1941, but an investigation of the circumstances surrounding other deaths is likely to reveal several dozen more.[186] Dr. Chain recalled that despite "certain cases of

---

182 Ibid., 236. Among the well-known Christian doctors who came to the ghetto were Józef Stein, Aleksander Wertheim, Mieczysław Kon, Tadeusz Ganc and Wilhelm Szenwic.

183 J. Szapiro, "Tajne studia medycyny w getcie. Szczypta narracji, garść refleksji," http://www.tlw.waw.pl/index.php?id, accessed: May 5, 2017.

184 Hirszfeld, *Historia jednego życia*, 238.

185 Ibid.

186 M. Janczewska, "Dokumenty urzędowo-medyczne jako *źródło do badania* losu warszawskich *Żydów 1939–1941*," *Zagłada Żydów. Studia i Materiały* 9 (2013): 282. The author rightly notes that drawing conclusions about the number of suicide

post-traumatic nervous breakdown" because of their horrific ghetto experiences, he could not recall ever needing to send a patient to a lunatic asylum.[187] Dr. Ebin believed that more and more people with mental disorders could be found on the ghetto streets as the months passed. He reported people were laughing nonstop on street corners or talking or crying uncontrollably. An attractive woman stood in the front of a court building on Leszno Street cradling an infant and singing sentimental songs in a rather good, strong voice. After two weeks her voice became croaky, while she became swollen from malnutrition; two weeks later she disappeared.[188]

Acute psychosis was also noted among those hiding on the Aryan side, undoubtedly from lingering stress and the fear of being denounced, tortured and killed. Dr. Wertheim, who left the ghetto before the major *aktion* and settled on the Aryan side with the help of his daughters-in-law, began to show symptoms of pathological fear. In Dr. Waller's opinion it might have heralded the onset of schizophrenia.[189] When the Gestapo knocked on his door, he opened immediately and straight away admitted he was a Jew and revealed where his sons were hiding. They were all arrested and executed.

Apathy and resignation—which Dr. Noemi Makower refers to as "the poison of hopelessness" in her memoir—also affected doctors, despite being relatively well-to-do. "Resignation consumed the hungry and the sated, young and old, the once audacious and the weaklings. At the time, I considered resignation to be a contagious mental illness. Its pathogens floated in the poisonous air of the ghetto. Resignation was much more than just pessimism."[190] A similar tone permeates Helena Szerszewska's writing about "the strange weakness pervading one's soul when the danger of losing one's life was close. Only in some people, did the sense of self-preservation become sharper. The majority experienced only resignation."[191]

---

victims on the basis of death certificates is difficult, because in a medical sense, suicide is not a cause of death.

187  An account by Icchok Chain, YVA O.3/2358.
188  An account by Leopold Elbin, YVA O.3/440.
189  An account by Stanisław (Shmul) Waller (Walewski), YVA O.3/2358.
190  Makower, *Miłość w cieniu śmierci*, 68.
191  Szereszewska, *Krzyż i mezuza*, 207.

Suicide was often the result of depression and despair, though there was another reason in the ghettos, camps and concentration camps: the decision by an inmate to control their own fate and take their lives into their own hands instead of giving the enemy satisfaction. Symptoms of deepening depression led to an increase in suicidal tendencies and attempted suicide. Some were saved in time, in other cases cyanide, which had expired, failed to act. Dr. Polisiuk recalled hospital wards housed many attempted suicide cases, among them doctors Teichner and Lewin, who were resuscitated.[192] Dr. Adina Blady-Szwajger described her own suicide attempt: she took ten Luminal tablets and washed them down with alcohol. Luckily, she was found by Dr. Helena Keilson. Dr. Makower described how, one day, he saw the mutilated face of a man admitted to hospital, wheezing and howling with pain. "It was Landsberger, a well-known insurance company doctor, whose wife was a famous dentist. . . He left the hospital and soon afterwards took his own life."[193]

## The Threat of Labor Camps

Dr. Makower, who worked at the Commission, described how, in the fall, the Germans revoked all previous declarations and ordered the Labor Department to organize repeat examinations with doctors being paid only three zlotys for an hour's work.[194] Examinations that were ordered to select people for labor camps took place at the School of the Chamber of Commerce. The exams were obligatory, but even under these circumstances, exam takers had to pay a registration fee. Every individual was examined by two doctors to prevent bribery, and not without reason, because officials frequently accused doctors of corruption. In turn, the doctors accused the officials of being responsible for numerous irregularities. Eventually five doctors were dismissed, which was disagreeable to everyone, but "even more disagreeable was the very work of the Commission itself."

---

192 An account by Adolf Polisiuk, "Pamiętnik w kolekcji Abrahama Adolfa Bermana" (section "Ostatnia blokada"), Ghetto Fighters' House Museum, ref. 3182.

193 Makower, *Pamiętnik z getta warszawskiego*, 68.

194 Ibid., 52.

The sick, who turned up in huge numbers, were subjected to remarkably quick examinations, amid the noise and bustle of the hall—none of which was conducive to forming an objective assessment of someone's health. Conditions in the labor camps were horrendous, and people returning from work to the ghetto complained of being beaten by the guards, of starvation, and of doing inhuman labor. "In their eyes was fear and suffering, they looked like overworked, hunted animals."[195]

---

195  Ibid., 55.

Chapter 7

# The Great Deportation (*Grossaktion*)

## Events leading to the Great Deportation

Spring 1942 saw significant increases in looting and murders. Marek Edelman, the Bersohn and Bauman Children's Hospital runner, wrote that the turning point in the life of the ghetto was April 18, 1942, a few days after the Jewish holiday of Passover, when there was a wave of mass executions by the SS.[1]

> Until that day, no matter how difficult life had been, the ghetto inhabitants felt that their everyday life, the very foundations of their existence, were based on something stabilized and durable. . . On April 18 the very basis of ghetto life started to move from under people's feet. . . By now everybody understood that the ghetto was to be liquidated, but nobody yet realized that its entire population was destined to die.[2]

By Friday afternoon, residents became aware that the Germans were planning something. It happened after a meeting with Karl Brandt, head of the SS and the Jewish Police. The Jewish policemen were screened for their ability to speak German and those that were chosen had to report to

---

1   A. Kilian, "Bloody Friday," April 17/18, 1942, http://1943.pl/en/bloody-friday-17-18-april-1942/.
2   Ibid.

Pawiak Prison. Czerniaków's diary on April 17 reported: "There is panic in the district. The shops are being closed. The population is gathering in the street in front of the houses. I went out onto the street and walked through several streets to calm the people down."[3]

Cars filled with German "hunters" drove through the streets of the ghetto with a Jewish chauffeur and a Jewish Police officer. Using prepared lists, they politely picked up unsuspecting victims and asked them to take along documents, a toothbrush and a towel, and drove them away. The person they sought was not found, they would take whoever was available. When the Germans had driven them a few blocks from their apartments, they would order the passengers—often husbands and wives together—out of the vehicle, line them up against a wall or in a stairwell and shoot them dead—through the eye, the heart, or in the back. The Jewish Police were ordered to get rid of the bodies.[4]

Many of those murdered that night were people involved in the resistance. When it was finally over on the following morning, fifty-two people were dead. They were buried in the Jewish cemetery. The German authorities ordered Czerniaków to announce, "The action of the night of April 17 to 18, 1942, was sporadic in its nature in order to punish those who do not mind their own business. It is recommended to the population to calmly deal with their normal affairs and then such action will not happen again."[5]

The Jewish Police who helped the Germans on that bloody Friday night had to die as well. They were considered collaborators from Group 13, also called the "Jewish Gestapo" from 13 Leszno Street. Only VIPs had their death sentences deferred until after July 23, 1942, when the *Grossaktion*, the Great Deportation, was launched. Those same police were among those who charged huge sums of money to free those headed for Treblinka at the *Umschlagplatz*.[6] On the other hand, doctors who were working in the hospital adjacent to the *Umschlagplatz*, did whatever they could to help people escape, trying, from their first days in the ghetto, to do the best they could to save lives.

---

3    Ibid.
4    Ibid.
5    Ibid.
6    Ibid.

The Gestapo invaded ghetto apartments, leading residents outside one by one (or even in groups, on occasion), to kill them in the streets.[7] At other times during the day, Jews captured on the streets were taken to Pawiak Prison.[8] Abraham Lewin described these events in his diary:

> Recently, there have been more cases of Jews being rounded up on the streets and taken to Pawiak, where they are subjected to unheard-of terrors. . . Two Jews were dragged to Pawiak, one of them was handed a plank and forced to hit the other. After torturing them for a long time, one was released at around nine in the evening and still made it home in time. The other was released at 11 at night [after curfew], only for the poor wretch to be shot dead by a German patrol.[9]

During the night of May 29–30, the Nazis shot eighteen people—they were becoming more brutal than they were during the *aktion* on the night of April 17–18.[10] Soon the Germans went from apartment to apartment, beating and killing people and ordering the janitors to dispose of their bodies. Among those killed were three employees of the JES (Red Services). In June 1942, almost seventy people were led out of their apartments and shot dead in the street. In his chronicle, Emanuel Ringelblum noted that the night of June 10–11 would forever be written in bloody letters in the annals of the ghetto. That night, the Germans resolved to deal with smugglers. The carnage at the ghetto walls continued into the next day. One of the German gendarmes, SS-Rottenführer Josef Blösche, also known as Frankenstein, dressed as a Jew, discharged an automatic rifle hidden on his person. Such incidents took place on Krochmalna

---

7   "Pamiętnik Sabiny Gurfinkiel-Glocer. Szpital Żydowski w Warszawie (na Czystem) w czasie okupacji (1939–1943)," Jewish Historical Institute Archives, ref. 302/160.

8   During the Nazi occupation (1939–1945), the prison on 24 Dzielna Street was commonly known as the Pawiak (from neighboring Pawia Street). It was subordinated to Hitler's Security Police (*Sicherheitspolizei—SIPO*, part of which was the Secret State Police, *Geheime Staatspolizei—Gestapo*) took particular care of the prison, whose official name was "Gefängnis der Sicherheitspolizei, 24 Dzielna Strasse."

9   A. Lewin, "Dziennik z getta warszawskiego," trans. A. Rutkowski, *Biuletyn Żydowskiego Instytutu Historycznego* 3–4, nos. 19–20 (1956): 173. One may add that this incident demonstrates the perfidy of the Nazis who condemned the man to death by the very act of releasing him after the curfew.

10  Ringelblum, *Kronika getta warszawskiego*, 385.

and Ciepła Streets.[11] By Noemi Makower's account, smugglers, children, politicians and doctors were among those killed.[12]

## The Murder of Dr. Franciszek Raszeja

On the night of July 21–22, yet another murder took place in the Warsaw Ghetto, that of Dr. Franciszek Raszeja, a famous Polish orthopedic surgeon from Poznań. His death was a prelude to the events of the next day.[13]

Professor Raszeja was highly regarded in the Jewish community for firmly opposing the "bench ghetto" before the war. He practiced in Poznań, where he lived with his family until the war started. In August 1939, he was drafted as commander of the Łódź Military Hospital in Kowle, a small town in Wolyn province in Eastern Poland and was assigned to build a local school.[14] In November, his landlord warned him the Russians were planning to liquidate the hospital and deport its employees to the depths of the Soviet Union. Raszeja packed his possessions without delay, loaded his family and one suitcase into a horse-drawn wagon and headed to the banks of the Bug River, crossing to the Polish side by boat. His daughter, Prof. Raszeja-Wanic, remembers they hired a wagon to take them to Warsaw.[15] On December 5, 1939, Raszeja went to the Ujazdowski Hospital and reported to its commander, a colonel and professor of medicine, Dr. Teofil Kucharski. He was assigned to the Surgical Department of the Polish Red Cross Hospital at 6 Smolna

---

11  Ibid., 393.

12  Makower, *Miłość w cieniu śmierci*, 74.

13  Many people have given accounts of what happened on July 21, 1942, but no one witnessed it personally. Conflicting opinions were advanced as to why Raszeja came to the ghetto, with whom he consulted, what transpired and how many were killed. Also, the address where the murder took place changes from one account to the next. It probably happened in a tenement building on 26 Chłodna Street, but numbers 6 or 20 are given with equal frequency, and sometimes even number 18. One thing is certain: Raszeja was murdered with two shots to the head. Also killed were Dr. Kazimierz Pollak (1903–1942), his assistant in the Polish Red Cross and (when the ghetto was established) a surgeon at the Czyste Jewish Hospital.

14  Letter from Prof. Bożena Raszeja-Wanic (Raszeja's daughter) to the author, dated December 18, 2016.

15  Ibidem.

Street. With his wife, Stanisława, and their two daughters, Bożena and Ewa, they found a place to live on Rozbrat Street.[16]

As a head of a department in the Polish Red Cross Hospital, Raszeja later created a surgical sub-department with classes for students enrolled in the Underground University of the Western Lands and the Warsaw Underground. In 1941, cooperating with the secret Consensus Committee of Democratic and Socialist Doctors, he established and led the Bone and JDC Tuberculosis Clinic at 2 Karowa Street.

A patient remembered Raszeja:

> He was at the clinic every day, from the very start getting involved in more complex cases. I remember this tall, strong, and manly figure. His expression was always serious, you never saw him smiling, but you could see he was elated at seeing his patients improving. He had black eyes, dark hair, and large, strong hands. He was universally respected—by the hospital personnel, doctors, nurses and patients. I owe my life to his care, my hands, and the fact that I am not an invalid.[17]

In the ghetto he organized a clandestine blood donation center for Jews, entrusting it to Prof. Hirszfeld. In 1941, the Consensus Committee granted him permission to maintain contact with Jewish authorities and organizations inside the ghetto, which also allowed him to consult Jewish patients behind the ghetto walls.

In 1942, the ghetto was divided into two parts, which differed in location and the material welfare of the residents. In the southern part, a so-called "small ghetto" was created, home to the more prosperous inhabitants. *Judenrat* President Czerniaków lived in 29 Chłodna Street with other influential and affluent residents of the ghetto. The area was joined to the large ghetto by a wooden gangway built between two

---

16  Prof. Franciszek Raszeja's personal file in the Warsaw-Białystok Medical Chamber archives (Special Collection, Akta Izby Lekarskiej, ref. 4007) indicates he registered with the chamber on December 13 and gave his address as 11 Śniadeckich Street. The file also contains Raszeja's petition to not confiscate his private practice at 3 Rozbrat Street (document dated October 14, 1940).

17  W. Lisowski, "Franciszek Raszeja (1896–1942)—wybitny chirurg ortopeda," *Skalpel* 4 (2016): 26–29.

tenement buildings. The "small ghetto" was incorporated into the larger one in December 1941, after the boundaries were redrawn.

Before noon on July 21, 1942, Raszeja went to this section of the ghetto with permission from the Germans and bearing a valid pass. In the opinion of Tadeusz Bór-Komorowski, Raszeja was apprehensive about the visit. "He questioned whether he would be able to accede to this request because to enter the ghetto one needed a special pass. But his sense of duty as a doctor did not abandon him, so he called the Gestapo and was surprised to hear that there would be no obstacle to his entering or exiting the ghetto."[18]

A doctor from the Polish Red Cross Hospital, Zbigniew Lewicki, warned Raszeja not to expose himself to danger. Some say a Jewish policeman guarding the gate that day also warned him but Raszeja believed the Germans would keep their word and he would be safe.[19] During Raszeja's consult, the Gestapo burst into the room.[20] As Estera Rozin recounted, when asked whether he knew he was operating on a Jew, Raszeja responded that the religion of his patient was of no consequence to him.[21]

Some people think that Raszeja came to the ghetto to operate on Abe Gutnajer, an antiques dealer who lived on Chłodna Street and still had some valuables in his apartment. It is supposed his wife contacted the noted orthopedist through Dr. Kazimierz Pollak, who worked in the ghetto. But Maria Zalejska-Komar testified that the reason for the visit was to examine Albert Szulberg, also a well-known antiques dealer.[22]

In her view, Raszeja obtained a pass to enter the ghetto "through various means available to the wife of former minister Leśniewski, an Aryan, and the owner of an antiques shop on Mazowiecka Street."[23] Estera Rozin

18  T. Bór-Komorowski, *Armia podziemna* (Warsaw: Bellona, 2009), 117. General Tadeusz Bór-Komorowski was a Polish military leader, appointed commander-in-chief a day before the capitulation of the Warsaw Uprising.

19  S. Dembowska, *Na każde wezwanie* (Warsaw: PAX, 1982), 127–128.

20  Polish Blue Police guarding the ghetto walls were replaced with Ukrainians, Lithuanians, and Latvians from the auxiliary squads. It is possible that some of them were present during the murder of Prof. Raszeja.

21  An account by Estera Rozin, Jewish Historical Institute Archives, ref. 301/4511.

22  Statement by Maria Zalejska-Komar, Jewish Historical Institute Archives, ref. 349/24/2432.

23  Ibidem.

confirmed this, as she identified 18 or 20 Chłodna Street as the site of the murder.[24] A Madame Leśniewska also maintained the patient was Albert Szulberg. Yet by all accounts, Abe Gutnajer could also have been the patient, because he, too, had an antiques shop on Chłodna Street.[25]

The Gestapo executed everyone in the apartment, including Gutnajer's family—his wife Regina, his daughter Stefania, her husband and daughter, and several others, including Dr. Pollak and his surgical assistant. Raszeja was shot twice in the head at point blank range.

Was the doctor in the ghetto to consult or operate? Was it possible to operate on a patient at home? Of course, it was, since Dr. Kazimierz Pollak, a surgeon from the Czyste Hospital and a nurse were present. Reports by Dr. Zbigniew Lewicki use the term *konsylium* (consultation) time and again—but he also wrote Raszeja had X-rays in his pocket, as a possible reference for a surgical procedure.[26] Why were all those present in the apartment killed, including a doctor who was there legally? The possible motive for murder might have been looting valuables from an antique dealer's apartment. After all, no witnesses lived to tell the tale.

A similar scenario had unfolded on July 4, 1941, during the slaughter of academic staff at Lviv University. They were executed by the special unit of the Third Reich's Security Police and in this case, too, all eyewitnesses were "taken care of." It is difficult to estimate how much was stolen that day, but plunder can be confirmed as a motive, since the portrait, "A Young Man Reading or Singing" by Dutch artist Pieter Fransz de Grebber, went missing and was featured in 2006, in a Christie's catalogue, fifty-five years later. It was put up for sale by an anonymous Latvian owner.[27]

As Dr. Jan Przedborski noted in his memoirs:

To more efficiently execute their orders, the "resettlement" command, consisting of no more than 15–25 people from the

---

24  An account by Estera Rozin, Jewish Historical Institute Archives, ref. 301/4511.

25  N. Cieślińska-Lobkowicz, "*Śmierć* antykwariusza na Chłodnej,"*Zagłada Żydów. Studia i Materiały* 5 (2016): 262–278.

26  S. Wesołowski, *Od kabaretu do skalpela i lazaretu* (Warsaw: Awes, 2006), 190.

27  W. Kalicki, "Świadek tylko czyta," ("Duży Format"), *Gazeta Wyborcza*, April 22, 2008, http://wyborcza.pl/duzyformat/1,127290,5134852.html, accessed: November 22, 2016. On the intervention by The Lost Register of Art company, which searches for stolen and looted artefacts, the painting was withdrawn from the auction and the Ministry of Foreign Affairs became involved in negotiations with its current (anonymous) owner.

Lublin Gestapo, ordered one of the most modern buildings in the ghetto, at the panhandle of Żelazna Street, to be emptied of its residents only. Let's be clear: the interiors had to remain intact. In addition, to complete the decor in the building and make the rooms "livable and cozy," the instruction was given to select the most beautiful furniture, carpets, lamps, crockery, porcelain, and glass from upmarket apartments on other streets.[28]

On the night of the murders, Dr. Ludwik Hirszfeld called Dr. Sabina Dembowska and asked her to inform Raszeja's wife of his death as soon as possible, so she could petition the authorities to have the body removed from the ghetto. Hirszfeld feared it might be buried in a mass grave at the RKS "Skra" Stadium, adjacent to the ghetto. As Dembowska recalled: I called the hospital. Dr. Lewicki was on duty and he knew Hagen's temporary replacement, Health Commissioner *Reichsdeutsche* Dr. Krakowski.[29] He promised to instigate immediate efforts to retrieve the bodies from the ghetto. "But who will inform his wife?" Lewicki asked. I told him I would do it. I would tell her that her husband had been severely injured and that she had to take care of everything personally. She was an intelligent woman, a Poznań University professor and, as I had been told by her husband, a strong and courageous person.

> . . . In the morning, I went to see her. She was composed and calm. Having deduced the true state of affairs, she asked what to do. "I will take you to the Health Department," I said, "Dr. Lewicki and Dr. Krakowski will meet you there. You will talk and decide what needs to be done." I had to repeat everything Prof. Hirszfeld told me. After that, Prof. Raszeja's brother took care of his sister-in-law and two nieces: one was ten, the other sixteen at the time, and today a great doctor herself.[30]

---

28  Memoir of Jan Przedborski, Jewish Historical Institute Archives, ref. 302/172.

29  The term *Reichsdeutsche*, in contemporary usage, refers to German citizens, the word signifying people from the German *Reich*, that is, the Imperial Germany or *Deutsches Reich*.

30  Dembowska, *Na każde wezwanie*, 128. Dr. Dembowska recalled going to Raszeja's apartment the next morning, whereas his daughter recalled it as the evening of the same day. An account by Bożena Raszeja-Wanic, Jewish Historical Institute Archives,

Dr. Zbigniew Lewicki's testimony written soon after the war corroborates this. He said Raszeja received an official pass to enter the ghetto from the German authorities. When he did not return on time, Lewicki became worried and called the Jewish Police station. A policeman on duty was not specific but mentioned that it would be dangerous to look for the professor during the night curfew and warned that he might not come back. The next day Lewicki managed to obtain a ghetto pass. At the office on Nalewki Street where passes were checked, he was given the address where Raszeja had gone the day before. S. Wesołowski retold Lewicki's account:

> I went to the address on Chłodna Street, near Karol Boromeusz church. The building was completely empty; I only found the janitor, a woman who showed me to the second floor and to the apartment where Raszeja and Dr. Kazimierz Pollak were killed, after having been called for a consultation. From what she said, it transpired that all those present had been shot dead, including the patient. That heralded the first day of the mass killing of the ghetto Jews.
>
> To look for the bodies, I went to the Jewish cemetery. There, a watchman showed me a pit where several people who had been shot dead had been brought the day before. All the bodies were covered with lime, but after a brief search we found the professor's remains. He was clothed but wore no shoes and had no documents on him; in his pocket we found several reduced X-ray negatives, possibly showing the bones he was to operate on. Clearly, his death could be attributed to two gunshot wounds: one in the center of his forehead, the other above the right eye socket. The professor, a tall man, had apparently been shot while seated. I could not see any exit wounds. Removing the bodies was no easy feat—a task made possible only with the help of workers from the City Waste Management Services who had the right to enter the ghetto.
>
> I called their office and they sent a "garbage truck" we used to transport the remains to the Polish Red Cross Hospital on

---

ref. 349/24/2432. Raszeja had only one surviving brother, Aleksy; his other brothers, Leon and Maksymilian, were killed in 1939.

3/5 Red Cross Street. At the entrance to the hospital there was a small chapel, where we laid Prof. Raszeja's body. Before going to the cemetery, I called the hospital to notify staff of our arrival. All the personnel gathered at the chapel at around 5 p.m. Also present was Surgeon Bolesław Hryniewiecki.

. . . In conclusion, I must mention that I undertook the expedition alone, against the advice and warnings of everyone, including my medical colleagues and a German clerk who, upon issuing my pass, warned me of the danger of entering the ghetto, especially on the day the mass murders started.[31]

Prof. Bożena Raszeja-Wanic described the circumstances of her father's funeral:

On the morning of July 22, 1942, my mother and a doctor from the Polish Red Cross Hospital went to the ghetto to collect father's remains. She never wanted to tell us where and in what state they found him. The funeral was at Powązki Cemetery in Warsaw. Residents and representatives from the underground combat organizations turned up en masse. The day after the funeral, the Germans ordered us to immediately vacate the apartment on 9 Rozbrat Street, where they planned to establish a German residential district. My sister and I moved, with our mother, to her parents' apartment at 11 Śniadeckich Street, where we stayed until the Warsaw Uprising.[32]

## Hostage Taking

Dr. Icchok Chain of TOZ said that in July 1942, the Jewish Police barged into a meeting of the Tuberculosis Prevention League and took three doctors as hostages. Two volunteered—Chain and Schwalbe. The policemen

31 Wesołowski, *Od kabaretu do skalpela i lazaretu*, 190–191.
32 An account by Bożena Raszeja-Wanic, Jewish Historical Institute Archives, ref. 349/24/2432. Prof. Franciszek Raszeja is buried in Powązki Cemetery, section 108, row 6, grave 6. He was awarded the Gold Merit Cross twice (in 1937 and 1938) and the Commander's Cross of the Order of Rebirth of Poland posthumously (1957). In 2000, the Yad Vashem Institute awarded him the title of Righteous among the Nations.

took them to the station where they detained them for two days. When the mass deportations started, the policemen guarding the prisoners ran away in fear. Using the opportunity presented by the momentary chaos, both doctors escaped. It was pointless because once the officers' initial panic passed, the doctors were rearrested and incarcerated again. They were released only following the *Judenrat*'s intervention.

Helena Szereszewska believes that those arrested in July 1942 were the so-called Ghetto VIPs. They were taken directly from *Judenrat* premises, while others, like Dr. Jerzy Gladsztern, were arrested in the street.[33] Usually, those who were better dressed were targeted.[34]

Noemi Makower and Marek Edelman believed the Germans' intention was to terrorize the community on the eve of a deportation and to urge them not to resist the planned action.[35] It is possible that *Judenrat* officials were arrested to force them to sign documents sanctioning the mass deportations. On July 21, 1942, Czerniaków noted in his diary: "Before noon, Jewish policemen were ordered to detain all councilors present in the building. They also requested a list of all other councilors. Soon all of them were arrested in my office."[36]

On that day, sixty people were held hostage, mostly from the *Judenrat* and the Jewish intelligentsia. Nobody knew what the arrests meant, including those under arrest. Among the arrested was a Czyste Hospital gynecologist, Dr. Adolf Polisiuk.[37] A day before the Great Deportation/ *Grossaktion* started, he was at a meeting to designate two doctors to work in the Bobrujsk labor camp. The proceedings were interrupted when they heard that key *Judenrat* people were arrested. All the doctors left for home, while vehicles laden with SS cruised the streets. Polisiuk lived on Chłodna Street where arrests were common. On his way home he

---

33 An account by Jerzy Gladsztern-Gwiazdowski, Jewish Historical Institute Archives, ref. 301/2098.

34 Szereszewska, *Krzyż i mezuza*, 131.

35 Makower, *Miłość w cieniu śmierci*, 74–75. M. Edelman, *I była miłość w getcie* (Warsaw: Czarne, 2009), 91–92.

36 Czerniaków, *Adama Czerniakowa dziennik*, 304. Czerniaków committed suicide on July 23, 1942, by swallowing a cyanide pill, a day after the commencement of the mass murder of Jews known as the *Grossaktion* Warsaw. He is buried in the Warsaw Jewish Cemetery.

37 An account by Adolf Polisiuk, "Pamiętnik w kolekcji Abrahama Adolfa Bermana" (section "Pawiak"), Ghetto Fighters' House Museum, ref. 3182.

saw one such car pass him by several times. When the SS-men entered his building, he sat out their "visit" by hiding in a store. Unfortunately, they arrested his wife. When he realized what happened, he surrendered to the Germans and begged them to release his spouse, but it was too late. He was arrested and ordered to reveal the addresses of other affluent residents living on his street, including that of Docent Brokman. Polisiuk tried to avoid naming his well-off colleagues feigning ignorance by claiming he was not originally from Warsaw. It did not help, and along with the well-known Warsaw architect and engineer Wolman, and Dr. Borensztajn's wife, he was taken to Pawiak. That was when he noticed the SS had a list of names they used to conduct their arrests.

On arriving in Pawiak, prisoners were registered. As one of the last in the queue at the prison office, Polisiuk appealed to the German officer to release his wife. The man listened, instructed that her name be crossed off the list of arrested people, and without further comment personally called her to the adjacent room and said: "You are free (to go)." Polisiuk parted with his wife in the officer's presence but was permitted to hand her his gold watch. Encouraged by the German's goodwill, other detainees began to ask for their wives to be released, but the officer refused, saying that this man willingly surrendered himself so that his wife could go free, that he took a risk.

It later was made clear that officer was SS-Untersturmführer Karl Brandt. Dr. Polisiuk commented: "It was difficult for me to understand the motives influencing his attitude towards me. He might have acted on a whim."[38] Some prisoners were released after a month, others only in September.[39] On July 22, Czerniaków wrote: "I asked for the release of Gepner, Rozen, Sztolcman, Drybiński, Winter, and Kobryner, which was agreed to. By 3:45 p.m. they were all back in the ghetto, except for Rozen."[40] The next day, Czerniaków committed suicide.

---

38 In addition to Polisiuk's wife, other persons released the next day were President Abraham Gepner, engineer Sztolcman, Councilor Kobryner, Director Drybiński (from the Provisions Department) and Winter. After eight days, Councilor Jaszuński and Director Marynower were released. An account by Adolf Polisiuk, "Pamiętnik w kolekcji Abrahama Adolfa Bermana" (see "Pawiak"), Ghetto Fighters' House Museum, ref. 3182.

39 B. Engelking, "Przebieg wielkiej akcji wysiedleńczej dzień po dniu," in B. Engelking and J. Leociak, *Getto Warszawskie*, 666.

40 Czerniaków, *Adama Czerniakowa dziennik*, 304.

Once registration was completed, the prisoners were taken to a common hall where, according to Polisiuk, there were fifty men and seven women. Among the detainees were councilors from the *Judenrat*, lawyers, engineers, rabbis, and eighteen doctors. Karl Brandt encouraged them to reveal the names of other prominent Jews in exchange for their own release. The prisoners knew that they were being held hostage and, aware of their predecessors' fate, expected to be shot at any moment. They were taken to another room in groups of five where, upon surrendering their documents, money and valuables, they were issued receipts, then taken back to their cell.

The Ukrainian guards behaved relatively well until the moment they brought the prisoners to the basement of Ward Eight, a holding area solely for Jews. Once the gates were shut behind them, the detainees were lined up with their hands raised, facing the corridor wall, then called individually for a body search and forced to strip. The prisoners were beaten with whips and fists, kicked to force them to strip faster and to dress just as quickly. After being searched and having their heads shaved, the prisoners were taken to a cell the size of an average room, to be "quarantined." By then their appearance had changed so much—with their hair shorn and their faces bruised from the beatings—they did not recognize each other. They spent the night in the cell, lying crammed in on the stone floor. After bathing and having their belongings disinfected, they were taken to cell number 260 (meant to accommodate forty-two inmates) or a smaller one (for eight). Polisiuk was placed in cell 260, in Ward Eight, which at the time housed approximately 120 men.

In addition to the hostages from the ghetto, there were those arrested for living on the Aryan side, for smuggling, crossing the *Generalgouvernement's* borders illegally or for other crimes. Colonel Szeryński, for instance, was arrested for hiding his fur coat on the Aryan side. Some "foreigners" and ghetto residents with foreign passports were also detained as was the case with Dr. Jakub Szejnberg, his wife, and son—who on the first night at Pawiak Prison were taken away and probably executed.[41]

---

41 An account by Adolf Polisiuk, "Pamiętnik w kolekcji Abrahama Adolfa Bermana" (section "Pawiak"), Ghetto Fighters' House Museum, ref. 3182.

The Germans selected three persons from the cohort of hostages to act as orderlies for various "corridor duties." Their role was to maintain order in the cells, take prisoners to a washroom at designated times, serve meals, and clean the Ukrainian guards' shoes. They were not beaten or forced to work, but had to assist in the beatings, or administer the beatings themselves. With a separate cell and larger food rations, they were permitted to move along the corridors and smoke. In many instances they tried to help their fellow prisoners, but at a cost: money was transferred to their accounts, or they appropriated food packages. Many prisoners' secret messages were passed to their families via these corridor orderlies. One orderly was Colonel Szeryński. Liaising between the prisoners and orderlies were cell representatives who spoke German and were nominated by the inmates.

The prisoners' day started with bells ringing at 5:30 a.m. Everyone had to be dressed within thirty minutes with the cell ready for assembly and inspection. An SS officer, accompanied by Ukrainian guards, would enter the cell and the cell representative would announce: "Attention! Cell 260 reporting, all forty-two Jewish prisoners are present." Everyone would stand at attention. The smallest lapses—not lining up perfectly, not facing the front, or some oversight—was severely punished by lashing the "offender" (or often the entire group) with a whip. Whippings (twenty-five or thirty lashes) involved, the inmates' bare buttocks being thrashed during assembly.

Afterwards, the inmates were led to a washroom and given only ten minutes to use the toilet and clean themselves up. For this, they had to take along a bucket of contaminated water. The second time they were allowed use of a toilet was in the evening. Cell 260 was just under a hundred feet in length, furnished with two benches, a shelf for storing utensils, and fourteen pallets, which were spread on the floor at night. Each pallet had to accommodate three sleepers. The cell was equipped with tin plates, wooden spoons, washbasins, two water buckets, and a larger bucket for waste. The prisoners' daily diet consisted of a single plate of watery soup and a small quantity of bread. Evening assembly, which was held at 6 p.m., signaled the end of the prisoners' day.

At every opportunity, the Ukrainian guards and SS alike tormented the prisoners, summoning them to labor, beating and kicking them. Prisoners were forced to offload coal from cargo trains, organize warehouses by lifting 200-pound sacks, and clean makeshift morgues. They returned to their cells beaten, bruised, and bleeding. Those who lost consciousness from exhaustion were doused with buckets of cold water. Usually, to spare their older and ailing fellow prisoners, the younger ones offered to work in their place. Sometimes the guards would round up everyone, in other instances they would pick on those they wished to torment.

Rabbis were punished for wearing *yarmulkes* with public floggings. The entire prison staff witnessed an incident when guards dragged a rabbi into the prison yard and took photographs as he was forced to cross himself in front of a goat and then kiss it under its tail. A similar incident was repeated with five Jewish prisoners, but involved a cow instead of a goat. Sometimes prisoners were forced to participate in punitive exercises: they were lined up in two rows, where they had to run over burning coals for thirty minutes. Sometimes dogs, biting and tearing at prisoners' clothing, were let loose inside a cell. The inmates were also subjected to other acts of humiliation, such as forcing the cell representative to read the most virulent anti-Jewish articles from *Der Stürmer* out loud.[42]

In his memoir, Dr. Polisiuk wrote the hostages received little information about developments outside the prison, thus their fear for their families grew with each passing day. On August 24, all hostages were lined up in the prison yard. Accompanied by several SS-men, Brandt read out a list of Jewish hostages, ridiculing their surnames as being difficult to pronounce. At one point he unholstered his revolver and fired a shot into the air, then called over a Ukrainian guard and ordered him to clean the revolver. Once this was done, he put the weapon back in the holster and said: "Now you are all free to leave." Initially, the hostages did not believe him, thinking it was another ruse, another cruel means of harassing them, and they fully expected to be taken to the *Umschlagplatz*.[43] But their possessions, which had been confiscated upon registration, were

---

42 A German political weekly connected to the NDSAP. Published from 1923 to 1945 as a Nazi propaganda tool.

43 When the ghetto was established, the Warsaw *Umschlagplatz* was a point for transferring goods between the ghetto and the Aryan side. In July 1942, it became a place where ghetto residents were loaded onto boxcars regardless of age or gender and sent to Treblinka. During the Great Deportation/*Grossaktion*, part of a building adjacent to it was emptied and designated as a waiting room for those to be gassed (*poczekalnia do gazu*), that is, people who could not be accommodated on the trains.

returned to them, and after completing all the requisite formalities, they were released through the gate to Dzielna Street, while guards lashed them with whips.

During the two months of the prisoners' incarceration, the ghetto had changed in both appearance and size: streets were no longer over-crowded. Several newly released prisoners did not know what to do, where to go, or where their families might be. The physical appearance of some had changed so much their relatives did not recognize them.[44] Helena Szereszewska noted that Councilor Eckerman returned from Pawiak with no beard or teeth.[45] Physically and mentally exhausted, the doctors were welcomed back to the hospital again located on Stawki Street. Nurse Sabina Gurfinkiel-Glocer recalled what a joy it was to see Dr. Dawid Amsterdamski in those tragic days of gloom when so many were being transported from the ghettos to the death camps.[46]

## The Great Deportation

Things in the ghetto were terrible but stable until July 19, 1942, when SS Chief Heinrich Himmler ordered Friedrich-Wilhelm Krüger, the SS com-mander in charge of the *Generalgouvernement*, to carry out the deporta-tions and destruction of all the Jews in the *Generalgouvernement* by New Year's Eve.[47] And so began the *Grossaktion*, the Great Deportation.

On July 22, Sturmbannführer Hermann Höfle called a meeting of the *Judenrat* and told Czerniaków about the deportations. Czerniaków com-mitted suicide the next day and was replaced by Marc Lichtenbaum.[48] None of the ghetto residents, including the doctors, knew what was going on. Only later that year did it become clear to them that the Jewish Police, collaborating with the Germans, were not taking them to resettle in the East, but were herding them to their deaths.[49]

---

44  An account by Adolf Polisiuk, "Pamiętnik w kolekcji Abrahama Adolfa Bermana" (section "Pawiak"), Ghetto Fighters' House Museum, ref. 3182.

45  Szereszewska, *Krzyż i mezuza*, 132.

46  Gurfinkiel-Glocer, "Szpital Żydowski w Warszawie," 104.

47  Peter Longerich, *Heinrich Himmler: A Life* (New York: Oxford University Press, 2011), 573.

48  Israel Gutman, *Resistance: The Warsaw Ghetto Uprising* (Boston, MA: Houghton Mifflin, 1994), 20.

49  Edelman, "The Ghetto Fights," 17–39.

On July 23, 1942, Tisha B'Av—the ninth day of Av, a Jewish day commemorating the destruction of the Jewish Holy Temple in Jerusalem 2,000 years earlier—*Grossaktion Warschau* began. It was the code name for the deportation of all the Jews in the ghetto, which continued until September 21, 1942, Yom Kippur/the Day of Atonement, the holiest day on the Jewish calendar. This was a form of torture, especially for the observant Jews in the ghetto.[50] There were daily roundups and people were shot in the streets even as they were marched to the *Umschlagplatz*. The Germans told them it was a "resettlement to the East." Bribed with promises of work and better food rations, the Jews of the ghetto were docile as they marched to the train platform where they were shoved into crowded cattle cars and hauled off to Treblinka, the death camp about fifty miles from the city. The *Grossaktion* was directed by SS-und-Polizeiführer Ferdinand von Sammern-Frankenegg, commander of the Warsaw area since 1941.[51]

When the *Grossaktion* began, the Warsaw Ghetto was the largest in German-occupied Europe. More than 400,000 Jewish were jammed into about 1.3 square miles and were living seven to nine people to a room. Beginning on July 23, almost 7,000 Jews a day, among them hospital patients, sick children, orphans and doctors, were packed like cattle into the trains bound for Treblinka. Approximately 300,000 residents of the ghetto were murdered in the eight weeks between Tisha B'Av 1942 and Yom Kippur 1942.[52] Dr. Janusz Korczak, an outstanding educator and pioneer in early childhood development ran a famous orphanage in Warsaw. He chose to accompany his beloved charges when they were taken to Treblinka in August 1942. He was offered a chance to stay behind but chose to comfort the children as they faced death.[53]

---

50  ". . . the so-called *Grossaktion* of July to September 1942 . . . 300,000 Jews murdered by bullet or gas." Robert Moses Shapiro, *Holocaust Chronicles* (Hoboken, NJ: KTAV Publishing Inc., 1999), 35. For more information see "Grossaktion Warsaw," Wikipedia, https://en.wikipedia.org/wiki/Grossaktion_Warsaw.

51  The Nizkor Project, Statement by Stroop to CMP investigators about his actions in the Warsaw Ghetto, February 24, 1946, Wiesbaden, Germany.

52  "Treblinka," Yad Vashem, https://www.yadvashem.org/odot_pdf/Microsoft%20Word%20-%205886.pdf.

53  Betty Jean Lifton, *The King of Children* and *"The Janusz Korczak Living Heritage Association,"* fcit.coedu.usf.edu.

## The Czyste Jewish Hospital

In July 1942, Commissioner Kublinski, the Administrator of the Czyste Jewish Hospital, informed staff that the Germans believed many of the personnel were redundant and would be retrenched. They ordered a list to be compiled of those who would stay. Hospital management faced the horrific dilemma of deciding who was needed and who was not. The list was drawn up by Dr. Stein, with the assistance of Doctors Borkowski, Szenicer, a few others and representatives of the administrative staff. The list of nurses was entrusted to Head Nurse Fryd.[54] The problem was tackled in both cases despite the glaring injustices and with the same tragic consequences. Once they worked through the list, the Germans immediately ordered it to be reduced by half.[55] The final list of approved names was placed on a bulletin board in the hall. These cutbacks saw the employment of all voluntary staff and some nurses terminated. Volunteers left to work in German workshops in the ghetto, hoping to avoid deportation, but the nurses had nowhere to go. Those who were "surplus to requirement" had to leave the hospital premises. Entrances to the wards were guarded by brutal doormen who acted in the misguided belief they were protecting the lives of those who weren't dismissed. "Surplus staff" had to assemble, with their wives and children, in the hospital backyard and were taken to Pawia Street and from there to the *Umschlagplatz*.[56]

On July 22 and 23, 1942, the staff of the Czyste Jewish Hospital was ordered to vacate the premises on Stawki Street and move into a building that was once a branch of the Bersohn and Bauman Children's Hospital—88 Żelazna Street—while procedure rooms were relocated to 1 Leszno Street. Stawki Street became an assembly point for Jews waiting to be deported. Polisiuk noted that the hospital on 1 Street Leszno looked like a large campsite: it could hold, at most, 400 patients, now it accommodated over 1,000.[57]

The hospital, which had mainly specialized in different procedures thanks to three surgical departments (gynecology

---

54 An account by Stanisław (Shmul) Waller (Walewski), YVA O.3/2358.
55 Gurfinkiel-Glocer, "Szpital Żydowski w Warszawie," 104.
56 An account by Stanisław (Shmul) Waller (Walewski), YVA O.3/2358.
57 Account by Adolf Polisiuk, "Pamiętnik w kolekcji Abrahama Adolfa Bermana" (section "Czworobok"), Ghetto Fighters' House Museum, ref. 3182.

and obstetrics, ophthalmology, and laryngology) before the *aktion*, suddenly became a general hospital.... Patients with contagious diseases now lay next to surgical patients or patients from internal diseases, even from gynecology and obstetrics. All passages, every free corner was taken up by beds.... Beds were arranged alongside other beds, making it difficult for us to reach the sick. Apart from the patients, most personnel, including their closest family (400–500 people) spent the night in the hospital, wherever they could find space—in doctors' rooms, laboratories, or offices, in spaces designated for surgery, in the backyard or in any other open space on the floor.[58]

The branch on Żelazna Street, where only children had been treated, now had several wards for adult patients.[59] As the forced hospital relocation began, panic erupted, prompting parents to take home even seriously ill children. The majority of patients came from shelters and refugee centers and had nowhere else to go.[60]

Staff and patients were not threatened with deportation until mid-August.[61] Through the upper floor windows of the hospital on Żelazna Street, personnel occasionally glimpsed people being herded like cattle towards the *Umschlagplatz*, among them (not infrequently) their family or friends. Dr. Makower recalled: "I looked through a window at this incredible procession. In the full sun it made for a horrifying spectacle, with doctors dragging their feet and sending despairing looks our way."[62] Through the window, he saw Administrator Kroszczorsaw, in a crowd of deportees, Dr. Etel Kleniec, the manager of the Mother and Child Center, with her daughter Mirka, as well as medical students and surgical assistants from the hospital on Śliska Street.[63]

Initially the hospital staff were spared further deportations, but eventually they, too, received an order to reduce patient numbers. Dr. Marek Balin recalled how the hospital management at 1 Leszno Street had to whittle down the number of patients to 150. The remainder were to be

---

58 Ibid.
59 An account by Judyta Braude, YVA O.3/2360.
60 Makower, *Pamiętnik z getta warszawskiego*, 64.
61 An account by Judyta Braude, YVA O.3/2360.
62 Makower, *Pamiętnik z getta warszawskiego*, 71.
63 Kroszczor, "Szpital dla Dzieci," 40.

sent "for labor" in the East. As the deportations were in full swing, the doctors were faced with choiceless choices that challenged their notion of medical ethics—above all, to do no harm—and human ethics. Could the doctors voluntarily condemn their patients to certain death? How could they conduct such a selection, knowing full well what awaited them? And what criteria did they apply?

> The hospital was drowning in despair. Everyone understood the tragedy of this situation; Jews were being forced to send their brothers to their deaths! To give up on invalids or the infirm, for whom the slightest movement was anguish! Not only Jews, but also doctors, their charges, and their patients whose lives they had tried to prolong, whose pain they had tried to lessen, whose limbs they had tried to save, and whom they had tried to offer peace of mind. The sick, on whom they had spent nights operating in the dim light of carbide lamps, performing difficult, life-saving procedures. . . A final verdict was to be taken on the evening of this fateful day, condemning most patients to death, the verdict being pronounced by doctors themselves.
>
> Usually, in the evenings, the doctor on duty plus a few volunteers did ward rounds. This time, the heads of departments undertook that task: Doctors Rothaub, Borkowski, and Szenicer from our department—for Amsterdamski was absent, having been taken hostage by the Germans. These distinguished doctors had to decide; they carried a list of names. Next to a name, a plus sign meant deportation, a minus sign meant the patient could remain in hospital.
>
> The doctors spent a long time at each bed. They spoke quietly, in almost inhuman, hoarse voices. They discussed each case in Latin, so the patient would not suspect the perilous significance of this consultation. The director entered an orthopedic ward, where emaciated bodies with stiff limbs hung from pulleys and rails. Dr. Szenicer used his handkerchief with increased frequency. . . Ashamed, he avoided the eyes of the sick and his colleagues. He walked through the wards with his head down, hiding his face in his handkerchief. . . Other doctors, too, began to use their handkerchiefs more often. Suddenly, our

departmental chief left the ward. I never saw him again. The commission did not complete its work. The Germans completed the selection themselves the next day, filling five trucks with patients and driving them away.[64]

From the very beginning of the mass deportations, the *Judenrat* tried to do whatever it could to save its officials—as Makower put it, "valuable" community representatives—from the *Umschlagplatz*. Particular care was taken with medical personnel, left in the hands of doctors Milejkowski, Ganc, and Makower. At first it was not too difficult, with individual doctors being led away.

Courage took many forms in the ghetto, the most famous instance of that was the decision of Dr. Janusz Korczak, who was offered asylum on the Aryan side, and rejected it in order to accompany his orphan charges to Treblinka. The doctor was "an idealist, who devoted his entire life to care for abandoned children, who slept with them, ate with them from the same pot" had an opportunity to save himself, but "in this tragic hour [he] refused to relinquish this care."[65] The day after Korczak's orphans were deported, another boarding house was taken.

Makower, who was present on the *Umschlagplatz*, saw the commander of the Jewish Police, Józef Szeryński (who was responsible for organizing deportations) perfunctorily observing events on the square from his rickshaw. At one point, a young nurse standing with several children approached him to ask whether personnel had to accompany the children. "His answer was decisive and unemotional: 'Korczak showed you the way.' She blushed and joined the other nurses and children on the road to the unknown."[66]

When doctors began to appear in numbers on the *Umschlagplatz*, it was no longer possible to lead them all to safety. Every inch of free space on the walled square was filled with people waiting for deportation. At night they were let into the three adjacent buildings which had housed the Czyste Jewish Hospital and no longer resembled a place of healing. The flooded floors were dirty, sticky and muddy, the taps had no water,

---

64  M. Balin, *Selekcja w szpitalu*, manuscript from the family archives of Balin's sister, Halina Birenbaum.
65  Makower, *Pamiętnik z getta warszawskiego*, 78.
66  Ibid.

and the toilets were blocked. The pervasive stench of sweat, urine and feces was oppressive. As Makower wrote:

> When I came to *Umschlag*, before the hospital was relocated, I was told that on the fourth floor, in a separate room, there were a few doctors. I ran there and saw some of my acquaintances, I remember only Fitsztain. . . The small room is filled to capacity, all standing. They jump at me and speak all at the same time. I assured them that I will do everything I can (there really was little I could) that I will communicate with Dr. Milejkowski and Dr. Ganc whether it would be possible to free them. . . They all were deported and probably railed at me because I did not keep my word.[67]

Despite the *Grossaktion*, the nurses and doctors used everything at their disposal to rescue people from the *Umschlagplatz*. They smuggled in uniforms, used ambulances, handcarts, stretchers and did whatever they could to smuggle people through the building and away from the *Umschlagplatz*.

At first, the nurses were able to bring water to those waiting for the death trains. Hidden under their uniforms, they carried doctors' uniforms and armbands, and with their use, were able to rescue several doctors and ordinary citizens. As time went by, a small first-aid station was established in a wooden cabin on the *Umschlagplatz* itself. Nurses and doctors who worked there were relieved when shifts changed in the morning and evening. They, too, smuggled out people dressed as medical staff. In the same cabin where patients were treated, several elderly people "with connections" had their limbs broken without anesthetics, before being transported to the ghetto hospital as unfit for work.[68]

The Germans allowed them to return to the ghetto to give credence to their propaganda that people were only being deported to labor camps in the East. However, most patients treated at the clinic were infants, abandoned in the square by their parents, who hoped they might

---

67  Ibid., 69–70. It might have been Dr. Mieczysław Ganc, because Dr. Tadeusz Ganc survived the war.

68  M. Edelman, "Getto walczy (Udział Bundu w obronie getta warszawskiego)," in W. Bartoszewski and M. Edelman, *Żydzi Warszawy 1939-1943* (Lublin: Towarzystwo Naukowe Katolickiego Uniwersytetu Lubelskiego, 1993), 139–142.

miraculously survive. When the trains departed, the nurses collected the stranded children and gave them water—there was nothing else at their disposal. Babies tended to be quiet and calm, probably utterly exhausted, and up to twenty or even thirty of them could be accommodated in the cabin at a time, under the care of Nurse Fryd and Dr. Halina Szenicer-Rotstein. But every time a transport left, those babies had to be given away. Sometimes the nurses managed to smuggle several of the children left behind out of the *Umschlagplatz* by pretending they were their own children.[69]

Dr. Makower recalled that when he needed help during the September roundups, Dr. Bieleński, as head of the Internal Diseases Department at the Czyste Hospital volunteered. As Makower noted:

> In the morning, I went to the community office and met Doctors Braude-Heller, Bieleński and Fajncyn. My director [Braude-Heller] could not tell me much. Dr. Bieleński took my situation to heart and said it would be an unheard of evil if Szeryński left me out in the cold. Of his own volition, he wrote a letter to him, which he tried to send to Ogrodowa Street. I don't know whether he succeeded. In any event, he was the only person who tried to help me.[70]

Even though his wife and daughter lived on the Aryan side, Dr. Bieleński had opted not to settle there.[71]

## The General Hospital on Stawki Street[72]

In the first half of August 1942, after the "small ghetto" was liquidated, patients and personnel were ordered to vacate the premises of the Bersohn and Bauman Children's Hospital on Śliska Street. Some children were sent home to their parents, the rest were transported to the branch on Żelazna and Leszno Streets. Administration Manager Henryk Kroszczor ran through the streets, looking for wagons to take them there. Only the

---

69  Sabina Gurfinkiel-Glocer, "Szpital na Czystem i ja," YVA 0.3/396.
70  Makower, *Pamiętnik z getta warszawskiego*, 122.
71  Dr. Bieleński's daughter was a student at Luba Blum-Bielicka's nursing school in the ghetto.
72  Name used by Henryk Kroszczor. See Kroszczor, "Szpital dla Dzieci," 42.

most indispensable items and linens could be taken. The most valuable apparatus from radiology and the analytical laboratory were left behind, along with the books in the library.[73] Moving the Children's Hospital to the large ghetto took two days, from August 10–12. The next day, the Germans gave the doctors twenty-four hours to move all patients from Żelazna to Stawki, to buildings which, before the *aktion*, housed Czyste's departments for infectious and internal diseases.[74]

Fortunately, the wagons were still available, but there were not enough people to help. The move was difficult, exhausting and enervating, because nobody knew what fate would befall the hospital.[75] They suspected this was another devilish idea from the SS, and everyone—staff and patients alike—would be loaded into boxcars at the *Umschlagplatz*. To convince the patients they were safe, most personnel remained in the hospital for the night.[76]

The premises on 6 Stawki Street were in catastrophic conditions. There were no adequate lavatory facilities for the large numbers of people waiting for deportation. The floors were coated in a sticky substance, the windows were broken, and there was no equipment whatsoever. Nurses and managers of the hospital kitchen on Śliska, Rosa Gilerowicz-Odesa and her staff, tried to clean the wards, and thanks to their superhuman efforts, the buildings were made ready to welcome patients. Dr. Stein became the director of this hospital, created by merging Czyste and the Children's Hospital. Dr. Braude-Heller served as his deputy. The personnel, who lived at 22 Pawia Street, had to walk to the hospital.[77] This daily trip gave the staff a chance to spirit people away from the *Umschlagplatz* by leading them into the hospital through a door on the side of the square. Lilienstein, the regular guard at the door, allowed people in white

---

73 Ibid.
74 Makower, *Pamiętnik z getta warszawskiego*, 73.
75 Ibid., 74.
76 Ibid., 73–74.
77 An account by Judyta Braude, YVA O.3/2360. Similar information given by Sabina Gurfinkiel-Glocer. Izrael Rotbalsam mentions two adjacent buildings, 20 and 22 Pawia Street. Stanisław Waller mentions 18–22 Pawia Street. Mordechai Lensky reported that 250 doctors were employed in public healthcare (buildings 2–22), with doctors housed in numbers 18–22. M. Lensky, *A Physician Inside the Warsaw Ghetto* (Jerusalem: Holocaust Survivors' Memoirs Project, Yad Vashem, 2009), 125.

uniforms to enter. Those smuggled out of the square could go back to the ghetto once personnel returned home after their shift.

The *Umschlagplatz* was guarded by Germans, aided by Ukrainian and Latvian auxiliary units, and by the Jewish Police. The commander of the guards was a Jewish policeman, Mieczysław Szmerling, notorious for his brutality and diligence in carrying out the Germans' orders. He personally collected enormous bribes for releasing people from the *Umschlagplatz*, but any other policeman who allowed someone to escape was summarily dismissed. From time to time, the Germans checked personnel cards, meaning that those making a bid to escape had to wait in the building until the next shift change.

"Sometimes the groups being led out of the hospital were not checked at all, especially in the morning when Szmerling's temporary workers were in control. No one knows why, but the most important documents were the green personnel cards bearing a little bird without an identifying photograph—the so-called Kubliński cards (they bore the signature of the then Czyste Hospital commissioner, Dr. Kubliński). Thanks to these cards, it was relatively easy to smuggle "living goods.""[78]

Another chance of leaving the *Umschlagplatz* was via an ambulance traveling between the surgeries of the remaining hospitals on Stawki and Leszno Streets. Dr. Rotbalsam said the Germans respected ambulances and allowed them to pass through even the tightest cordons. But before a transport left, a gang of Latvians or Ukrainians would invade the hospital to search for those in hiding.[79] An officer in the Jewish Police, Stanisław Gombiński, remembered:

All sorts of people came: Jewish Police officials came to the *Umschlag* "on official business"; officials from the Health Department showed up because their people, the "column inspectors," were on duty checking the levels of cleanliness, delivering water and bread, carrying out the bodies of the dead; officials from provisioning came to inquire about food supplies; officials from the Hospitalization Department also visited the hospital. An ambulance came, the white coats of doctors and nurses mingling with people in the crowd. . . There was one

78 Makower, *Pamiętnik z getta warszawskiego*, 75.
79 An account by Izrael Rotbalsam, YVA O.3/2357.

purpose to this commotion: to pull out yet another person from behind the wires, to free them, to smuggle him or her back to the ghetto. The methods and the means varied; sometimes money changed hands, sometimes it was done without the need to pay.[80]

It was obvious the hospital had become an asylum for many doctors, nurses and auxiliary personnel, pharmacists, dentists and their kin. At intervals, huge numbers of people hid there. This troubled management: on the one hand there was the desire to save as many people as possible, on the other these acts exposed the hospital to danger. Szmerling, who was aware of this practice, tried to prevent "free riders" from escaping. Word circulated that he was colluding with a well-known nurse from the Czyste Jewish Hospital, and that together they "made a killing." This, however, was the exception—mostly, hospital staff acted selflessly.

The final act in Warsaw's *Grossaktion* took place between September 6 and 11, on Miła Street. On September 5, an announcement ordered all ghetto residents to gather in the vicinity of Smocza, Gęsia, Zamenhofa, and Szczęśliwa Streets and Parysowski Square before 10 a.m. the next morning, where the final selection would take place. Of the 100,000 who assembled in the designated area, 30,000 were permitted to remain— people who worked for the Germans and had certificates of employment. The rest were to be deported.

This time, the hospital was not spared. On September 6, 1942, the surgery departments in the hospital were closed. The order for personnel to evacuate immediately came from the *Judenrat* at 4 a.m. Dr. Stein was ordered to have all the hospital personnel—under threat of death— report for duty before noon at 19 Zamenhofa Street for final selection. Everyone knew it was a death sentence. People began to weigh their options. Nobody knew what to do, most were at a loss. Jewish Police led personnel from the Leszno Street hospital's surgery departments to Zamenhofa Street in groups of four. Dr. Polisiuk recalled "taking only our rucksacks. We stood in a line, and under the Red Cross banner, we moved along Leszno, then Karmelicka Street in the direction of Zamenhofa Street. Almost all of us went, with our director in the lead, as

---

80  Memoirs of Stanisław Gombiński (Jan Mawult), YVA O.33/2010.

the final group left the hospital."[81] In his rucksack, Dr. Stanisław Waller carried his one-year-old son.

After arriving at their destination, they were told to wait in the building at 21 Zamenhofa Street, but several people squatted outside on the street. Everybody was resigned yet agitated. In the afternoon, news came that a general selection would be performed by officials of the *Judenrat*, while in the workshops, the Germans handled the selection.

On the instruction of the head of the Hospitalization Department, Dr. Milejkowski, the group consisting of the management of all the hospitals gathered. In a secret meeting, they compiled lists with the names of those who would remain in the ghetto. This group, consisting of five individuals, had to decide the fate of 800 people. Those selected had to be viable for the possible future hospital, they were to receive temporary right to live in form of "tickets," the rest were to be deported to Treblinka.[82]

Dr. Polisiuk also recalls that the commission consisted of Doctors Stein and Braude-Heller, engineers Tempelhof and I. Sztabholc, and a Mr. K. With the exception of Mr. K., they all died or were killed. The commission favored bachelors and the childless, although Makower, who was subjected to the selection on Wołyńska Street as a Jewish Police doctor, remembered it differently. He wrote the commission made the 500 "life tickets" available to adults only, whereas the hospital also issued them to children.[83] A similar scenario unfolded in Dr. Waller's account:

> When Dr. Stein appeared in the backyard, he was immediately surrounded by hundreds of people. He was one of those compiling the list of those eligible for "tickets to live." I caught up with Dr. Stein in the crowd and asked him whether I could count on such vouchers for myself and my family (wife and son). He told me I would not receive any. In despair, I caught him by his jacket lapels with such force that I tore them and began to emphasize my value to the hospital. Thereafter, he promised I would receive the tickets. Others had no such luck.

---

81 An account by Adolf Polisiuk, "Pamiętnik w kolekcji Abrahama Adolfa Bermana" (section "Czworobok"), Ghetto Fighters' House Museum, ref. 3182.

82 Ibid.

83 Makower, *Pamiętnik z getta warszawskiego*, 125.

In the yard of the building on Dzika Street, I met the shattered Doctors Markusfeld and Rotstadt, who had no chance of receiving vouchers because of their advanced age. They told me that, being young, I was more deserving, while they, being old, had no chance, since Dr. Stein believed old people had nothing to look forward to if they carried on living.[84]

Dr. Waller also emphasized other criteria: "Those who were converts, high up in the hospital hierarchy, Secretary Tempelhof, Second Secretary Wajnbaum, Third Secretary Poznański, Provisioning Director I. Sztabholc and Director Mrs. Szejnman, heads of departments and friends of Director Stein, could all count on "tickets to live.""[85] Dr. Adina Blady-Szwajger, in turn, emphasized that Dr. Braude-Heller wanted no part in deciding who was deserving of "tickets to live," but was convinced only after Blady-Szwajger warned her that Stein would allocate all the vouchers if she refused to participate. "It was ignoble of me," Dr. Blady-Szwajger wrote, "because none of us wanted to decide who deserved to live and who did not, but we demanded this of her."[86] Dr. Waller, who talked to Dr. Braude-Heller about this several weeks later, wrote that when the "tickets to live" were assigned, she admitted to being prejudiced towards technical staff, and that in assigning the tickets she was concerned more with doctors and their wives than with nursing and auxiliary staff.[87]

In the hospital building at 6 Stawki Street, a handful of people remained behind to care for patients, trying to find space to accommodate those who were brought in on flatbed trucks from the surgeries on Leszno Street. Due to a shortage of beds, the sick were carried into the building and laid on the floor. After ferrying patients all night, nurses Sabina Gurfinkiel-Glocer and Franka Isserelis and paramedic Rubinstein created a makeshift surgery and wound-dressing station. Among the new patients were some who required immediate operations, and others whose injuries were treated and dressed (amputations and abdominal

---

84  An account by Stanisław (Shmul) Waller (Walewski), YVA O.3/2358.

85  Ibid.

86  Blady-Szwajger, *I więcej nic nie pamiętam*, 98.

87  An account by Stanisław (Shmul) Waller (Walewski), YVA O.3/2358.

gunshot wounds).[88] The two female doctors in charge of these procedures—Drs. Halina Szenicer-Rotstein and Danuta Strasman-Frejman—were assisted by a number of nurses.[89] Dr. Szenicer-Rotstein also took charge of securing meals for patients. She placed a woman on guard to prevent food from being pilfered from one of the storerooms. Each patient's daily rations consisted of soup and two slices of bread.

At 5 a.m. on September 7, people were rounded up and a list of names was read out.[90] For the 500 employees, there were 200 "life tickets." Because nobody in management wanted to read out the list, Dr. Stein ordered Dr. Adolf Polisiuk to do it. The list contained the names of twenty-five or thirty doctors, ten clerks, a dozen or so nurses, and several laborers. The remainder were children and wives who later would replace auxiliary personnel. It was, as Dr. Polisiuk wrote, the most tragic moment of his life, because while reading the list he was, in a way, pronouncing death sentences on innocent people, close friends, colleagues, coworkers, and even his own boss. He read the list several times, because people could not believe that they had been excluded. Some imagined they had not heard correctly, that their names had been omitted by mistake. In the afternoon, people whose names were on the list were issued with orange "tickets to live."[91]

According to the accounts of several survivors, the tickets were handed out in the yard of a former prison on Zamenhofa Street. Dr. Adina Blady-Szwajger, however, remembered receiving her "ticket" at the hospital.[92] The "tickets" had to be pinned to the bearer's clothing in a conspicuous place, before they were made to stand in four lines, according to their departments.

88 Gurfinkiel-Glocer, "Szpital Żydowski w Warszawie," 104.
89 Sabina Gurfinkiel-Glocer also mentions Dr. Najburzanka, an assistant in the Surgical Department on Leszno Street. Unfortunately, her personal file could not be found. Sabina Gurfinkiel-Glocer, "Szpital na Czystem i ja," YVA O.3/396.
90 An account by Judyta Braude, YVA O.3/2360 and an account by Stanisław (Shmul) Waller (Walewski), YVA O.3/2358. In Henry Fenigstein's recollection, the "tickets to live" were distributed a day earlier, on September 6, while personnel left "the infamous 'kettle,'" that is, the roundup, the next day, waiting for an end to the Germans' action on Pawia Street. Fenigstein, "The History of 'Czyste,'" xxviii–xxx.
91 An account by Judyta Braude, YVA O.3/2360.
92 A. Grupińska, *Ciągle po kole*, 198.

This happened amidst Dantean scenes. Everyone wanted to be one of the "lucky" ones who managed to secure a ticket. But it happened differently from what they had imagined. K[arl Georg] Brandt did not check whether someone had a ticket: he just mechanically counted several hundreds of people, the number which he designated and reserved for the hospital, the rest were left in the yard. This way, many people who had earlier procured a voucher by any means possible were left out.

One of the more devilish hoaxes came to light during these roundups: to create chaos and dissent in the Jewish community. Although a list was compiled by hospital representatives and the *Judenrat*, it was ignored, and it was back to business as usual. Those "tickets to live" which had been fought over so ardently during the selection carried out by Brandt, proved to be nothing but miserable pieces of paper with no significance whatsoever.[93]

Dr. Stanisław Waller did not receive the "tickets to live" for his wife and son, which Dr. Stein had promised him. He decided to inject his son with a large dose of pantopon[94] and carry him, sleeping, in his backpack. Unfortunately, it had unexpected results. After the injection, the child began screaming, drawing unwanted attention. Mother and baby were saved by the ambulance driver, who drove them to the hospital on Stawki Street, where they were later joined by Waller who had gotten a ticket.[95]

The day after the selection, nurse Luba Aronson-Tenenbaum committed suicide. She chose to give her card to her daughter, thus gifting her a few months to live. Twenty-two-year-old Deda Tenenbaum died several months later, during the last blockade of the ghetto hospital on Gęsia Street.[96] Dr. Blady-Szwajger wrote that a few days after the selection, some staff sent their "tickets" back to the hospital, to save several more people.

---

93 An account by Izrael Rotbalsam, YVA O.3/2357.
94 Pantopon is a potent opiate (see B. Koskowski, *Nauka o przyrządzaniu leków i ich postaciach* [Warsaw: F. Herod, 1927], 205).
95 The ambulance could only accommodate one child at a time. Since Dr. Askanas's son also needed help, the fathers decided to draw lots. Dr. Waller won, but, fortunately, Aleksander Askanas was also saved. An account by Stanisław (Shmul) Waller (Walewski), YVA O.3/2358.
96 An account by Judyta Braude, YVA O.3/2360.

Early in the morning of September 10, Doctors Jan Goldstein and Stanisław Waller and student Marek Balin arrived at the hospital on Stawki Street with the news that Karl Brandt, the senior officer of deportations, had ordered several hospital personnel to be moved to German workshops. Those taken were to receive special cards authorizing them to stay in the ghetto.[97] Among them were Doctors Owsiej Bieleński, Zdzisław Seidenbeutel, and Józef Teszner.

On September 12, all patients and remaining hospital personnel boarded the boxcars. Even those who had "tickets" and stayed in the hospital on Stawki Street to tend to their patients to the very end were also deported. Among them was Dr. Halina Szenicer-Rotstein who, despite being permitted to leave the *Umschlagplatz*, chose to accompany her patients.[98] Dr. Adolf Polisiuk remembered that "she went to a wagon voluntarily, to be with those needing her help; this is how she understood her duty. To many such a gesture seemed abnormal, for the will to survive was so strong. Her behavior was very poignant in its heroism."[99]

To the very end, Dr. Makower tried to save the doctors working in the Stawki Street hospital. He took those he convinced to leave the *Umschlagplatz* to the front of the building and arranged them in a column but was unable to convince Szmerling to let them walk out of the square. When he returned at around 3 p.m., the hospital was being "evacuated," using wagons. It was too late.[100] According to Dr. Henry Fenigstein, 900 patients and fifty staff members were deported to Treblinka that day.[101]

Many children walked on their own, but some were carried. Sick adults were transported on stretchers. "It was horrendous, incomparably more terrifying than the procession of healthy people led away for

---

97  Gurfinkiel-Glocer, "Szpital Żydowski w Warszawie," 104.
98  An account by Adolf Polisiuk, "Pamiętnik w kolekcji Abrahama Adolfa Bermana" (section "Czworobok"), Ghetto Fighters' House Museum, ref. 3182, 25–26. Dr. Halina Franciszka Szenicer-Rotstein (born Kon, 1907–1942) graduated from the Medical Faculty of Warsaw University in 1930. She had four children: Robert, who was seven, twins Helena (Wanda) and Jan, six, and two-year-old Staś. The children were hidden on the Aryan side and, as Judyta Braude stated, they all survived the war.
99  Ibid.
100 According to the account by an anonymous Jewish Police officer, on that day, Szmerling led several doctors and nurses out of the *Umschlag*. Jewish Historical Institute Archives, ref. 302/129.
101 Fenigstein, "The History of 'Czyste,'" xxx.

execution."[102] Doctors Anna Margolis and Adina Blady-Szwajger went to the children's ward to inject their young patients with morphine before the *Szaulis* (Lithuanian police) and Germans came to shoot those who were too ill to be transported.[103]

> And, as I had done during the two years I worked in the hospital, I again leaned over the cots in the same way, pouring the last dose of medicine into those tiny mouths. Only Dr. Margolis was with me. Screams reached us from below, where the *Szaulis* and Germans were taking patients to the wagons. Next, we went to the older children, and I told them I would give them medicine to relieve the pain. They believed me and drank it, as much as necessary. Later, I told them to undress and lie down. After several minutes (I do not remember how many), when I entered the ward again, they were asleep.[104]

Her worst fear was that some of them would wake up before the killers entered the ward.

Dr. Adina Blady-Szwajger referred to the drama ghetto doctors faced in making certain choices "superhuman medicine"[105]—superhuman, because it meant facing challenges which went above and beyond human capabilities, including euthanizing children and the elderly.

## Doctors during the Great Deportation

After getting permission to practice in the ghetto, many doctors continued to treat patients to the bitter end. Dr. Alina Brewda, a gynecologist, and her dentist mother, Zofia Wysok-Brewda, saw patients in one of two rented rooms on 32 Elektoralna Street. After her mother's death in the spring of 1942, Dr. Brewda moved to 2 Chłodna Street, where her pre-war employer, Dr. Zygmunt Endelman, rented her a spot in his kitchen, where she slept and saw patients. While Brewda attended to her patients, Dr. Endelman's wife would cook dinner.

---

102  Makower, *Pamiętnik z getta warszawskiego*, 133–134.
103  Blady-Szwajger, *I więcej nic nie pamiętam*, 100–101.
104  Ibid.
105  Ibid., 31.

In August 1942, while performing a gynecological procedure on a woman who was anesthetized, the Germans and the Jewish Police surrounded the building and its residents were ordered to leave. On her way to the *Umschlagplatz*, the train platform where the cattle cars were loaded and took the Jews to Treblinka, Dr. Brewda expressed concern about her unconscious patient. She managed to escape from the *Umschlagplatz*, thanks to the doctors working there, but was unable to return to her patient on Chłodna Street, because the building had been completely evacuated.[106]

Janina Bauman recalled that while waiting for her mother to return home on Nowolipki Street, a stranger rushed in with a sack on his back. He asked whether the Rejders had returned, and learning they had not, carefully placed the sack on the floor and demanded it be opened immediately. Inside was the Rejders' two-year-old daughter in a drug-induced sleep. Dr. Rejder and his wife returned from a roundup that evening and found their daughter in one piece.[107]

Helena Szereszewska recalled an incident involving a relative, Dr. Lichtenbaum, a sector doctor, who could easily have been spared deportation, but knowing full well what he was doing, voluntarily boarded the train at the last moment, waving his wife farewell.[108] Dr. Jadwiga Baumberg-Benkl committed suicide during the *Grossaktion*.[109] Her brother, Ignacy Baumberg, could have saved himself, but did not want to leave his wife and accompanied her to the railway wagon.[110] Dr. Benkl had a chance to leave the ghetto, but took cyanide instead: Dr. Zofia Szymańska wrote that she could not shake off the horror of Dr. Benkl's death and simply could not believe that her vivacious colleague had committed suicide.[111]

September 1942 witnessed a veritable suicide "epidemic." In a report detailing the work of the *Judenrat* in Warsaw during that time, sixty-nine instances of death by suicide were recorded.[112] Clearly, those

---

106  Minney, *I Shall Fear No Evil*, 52.
107  Ibid., 105.
108  Szereszewska, *Krzyż i mezuza*, 95.
109  An account by Judyta Braude, YVA O.3/2360.
110  Szereszewska, *Krzyż i mezuza*, 100.
111  Szymańska, *Byłam tylko lekarzem*, 169.
112  *Tak było*, 101.

were connected to the tragic events of the September round up on Miła Street, during which many people survived the *Grossaktion*, but had not received tickets to live," and so chose to commit suicide rather than die in the gas chambers of Treblinka.

When he learned his name was not on the list, the head of the Department of Dermatology and Venereal Diseases, Dr. Stanisław Markusfeld, committed suicide with his wife by jumping from a fourth-floor window.[113] Dr. Anna Meroz noted that at the time, "Doctors from the emergency services would typically note that the deaths were by suicide."[114]

## Emergency Services during the Great Deportation

During the *Grossaktion*, between July and September 1942, if they could not assist them on the spot, Self-Help's Doctors' Emergency Service (DES) collected the wounded and brought them to a hospital. Many people required prompt assistance having been beaten or shot. When the deportations ended in September, the DES staff was deployed to the Többens textile manufacturing facilities under German control,[115] where they were forced to work as factory personnel.

## Pharmacists during the Great Deportation

Initially, the pharmacy staff felt safe during the deportation. With the passing of time, however, pharmacy staffers were dragged outside during street roundups, and well-stocked facilities faced the threat of being requisitioned by the Germans.[116] Helena Szereszewska recalled:

> At the corner of Lubecki and Gęsia Streets, the Union of Pharmacies opened their own drugstore. One of its employees was Seret,[117] who previously managed the pharmacy in the

---

113   An account by Adolf Polisiuk, "Pamiętnik w kolekcji Abrahama Adolfa Bermana" (section "Czworobok") Ghetto Fighters' House Museum, ref. 3182.

114   Meroz, *W murach i poza murami getta*, 25.

115   *Szopas* (*shopn* in Fenigstein) were production workshops in the ghetto that worked for the benefit of the Germans and were under their supervision.

116   Bryskier, *Żydzi pod swastyką*, 140.

117   Probably Izaak Izydor Sereth, born 1896, holder of an MSc in Pharmacology (1925), a Warsaw resident who lived at 11 Mazowiecka Street. *Urzędowy spis lekarzy*, part 4:

"small ghetto" at the corner of Prosta and Twarda Streets. One day, his wife and ten-year-old son were taken. When he learned about this, he ran to the *Umschlagplatz* and did not return.[118]

The pharmacies at 20 Zamenhofa and 28 Nalewki Streets were the first to be closed. Along with other ghetto residents, their employees were taken to the *Umschlagplatz*. The pharmacies were boarded up and posted with signs reading "SECURED." As the residents in other areas of the ghetto were evicted, the ownership of pharmacies fell under the management of the workshops run by the Germans.

Towards the end of the *Grossaktion*, during the round-up on Miła Street, a small number of "life tickets" were distributed to pharmacy staff by Henryk Gliksberg.

## Doctors in the Jewish Police during the Deportation

The *Grossaktion* allowed the Jewish Police to unleash villainy and tyranny on the population. Under Szeryński's orders, the Jewish Police made sure that children and the sick were first to be deported as they were the weakest. Although Szeryński was caught smuggling furs over the wall and temporarily relieved of his duties during the Great Deportation, Lejkin, his deputy who took over from Szeryński, was considered incapable of handling the job and Szeryński was subsequently put back in charge of deportations by the Germans. Szeryński was considered a Nazi collaborator and traitor by the Jewish resistance fighters in the Warsaw Ghetto, who tried to assassinate him but failed. He stayed with the Jewish Police until the *Grossaktion* was over, and then committed suicide right after the deportations in January 1943.[119]

Anyone resisting arrest was beaten with a nightstick. Beatings were followed by the looting of deserted lodgings, with the excuse that nothing was to be left for the Germans. Many "respectable" Jewish Police

---

*Felczerzy*, 74.

118 Szereszewska, *Krzyż i mezuza*, 117. "Small ghetto" (*małe getto* in Polish) was the southern part of the Jewish District, remaining after the 1942 *aktion*.

119 "Józef Andrzej Szynkman-Szeryński," Warsaw Ghetto database, archival records, bibliography, and citations, Centrum Badań nad Zagładą Żydów (Centre for Jewish Holocaust Studies). Czerniaków, *Adama Czerniakowa dziennik*; also see Stanisław Gombiński, "Moje wspomnienia."

officials secured considerable assets for themselves through nefarious means. Such behavior occurred on a massive scale, and even decent people bragged that they "became rich thanks to this *aktion*" or lamented that they had not seized the moment by failing to accumulate riches in this way.[120]

In a matter of days it became clear that the deportations could not be carried out by the police alone, despite the force being several hundred strong. Therefore, Brandt demanded the *Judenrat* provide supplementary services. The next day, civilian units led by the Jewish Police and wearing white armbands marked "Resettlement Action" went out to do their dirty work.[121] Doctors were among the civilians. As someone on the hospital staff recalled:

> Once, the Germans used their rifles to motion to us—the hospital doctors—to catch the Jews. Each of us had to deliver five of them to the *Umschlag*. We had to do it, there was no way out. Several days later, one of my colleagues, who had been absent from the hospital that day, made scathing comments. However, had he been in our position, he would have done the same. Did he have the right to portray himself as a hero, and a nobler person than us? Many people believe they are better only because they were not there, they were not faced with making that choice.[122]

Dr. Makower encountered one of his colleagues, a doctor working for the Jewish Police, who was forced to participate in the *aktion*, noting that (to his knowledge) it was the only time a doctor was forced to participate in "such abominable work." After everything he went through, his colleague was exhausted and suffered a complete breakdown.[123] Street roundups using civilians as police ended once Szeryński resumed his position as head of the Jewish Police. He knew only too well the crackdowns on

---

120  Makower, *Pamiętnik z getta warszawskiego*,62.
121  Ringelblum, *Kronika getta warszawskiego*, 405. *Umsiedlungaktion* (Germ.)— resettlement action.
122  B. Engelking, *Zagłada i pamięć. Doświadczenie Holocaustu i jego konsekwencje opisane na podstawie relacji autobiograficznych* (Warsaw: IFiS PAN, 2001), 181.
123  Makower, *Pamiętnik z getta warszawskiego*, 146–147.

*Judenrat* officials would soon begin which meant it was not the right time to be using the same officials for such a task.[124]

Halina Birenbaum, a Warsaw Ghetto survivor, commented extensively on Jews serving in the Jewish Police. A direct witness and sister of Marek Balin, a medical student working at Czyste, she could speak with authority. Her uncompromising attitude toward Jewish collaborators is why, for many years, her work was not published in Israel. At the end of the 1960s, in the pages of *Daily Courier*, she wrote:

> "I parted with my father on the *Umschlagplatz*, never to see him again, when surrounded by Jewish policemen and suffering blows inflicted with their nightsticks, he was dragged to a train to be murdered in Treblinka. I also remember that he had a large sum of money with him and other valuables, and he could have escaped their hands, returned to the ghetto, and hidden in a cellar or an attic. Not for long, of course, because the German capturers and their helpers found almost everyone in the end. This, however, does not justify their diligence in following orders (sometimes more assiduously than their Hitlerite masters demanded), as was evident during various stages in the ghetto and death camps.[125]

On the morning of July 22, Julian Lewinson, the radiologist who worked in the Jewish Police came to Alina Fryszman's apartment to warn his sister-in-law that their street was to be "liquidated." He took her and her daughter to his place and, using the influence of highly placed officials (as well as paying a considerable bribe), he had Alina's name included on the list as his wife. He did it because the wives of police employees in the JES received worker registration cards permitting them to stay in the ghetto. Dr. Makower noted that Lewinson had received a "life stamp" (also called a "ticket to life" or a "life number") from one of his friends, Izrael First, a German collaborator and employee in the *Judenrat*'s Department of Economics.

---

124  Ibid., 62.
125  A fragment from personal correspondence with Halina Birenbaum, who recalled that the original appeared in the Polish-language paper, *Nowiny Kurier*, published in Tel Aviv. No further details are available.

Unfortunately, Lewinson did not manage to secure such stamps for his two nieces, Janina and her sister Zofia. At the last moment, he managed to transfer his own mother to the Aryan side. He survived the *aktion* by driving an ambulance between the *Umschlagplatz* and the hospital. Odds are he smuggled out people who wished to return to the ghetto from the *Umschlagplatz*; Janina Bauman recalled seeing him and his fellow police officers counting money in the casualty section's duty office adjacent to the hospital building.[126] She wanted to believe that, despite the money being collected from *Umschlagplatz* escapees, it was destined for acquiring arms intended for upcoming active resistance action planned by the Jewish Combat Organization (ŻOB).

In September 1942, not all Jewish Police employees had received work passes, also known as "life tickets," despite receiving assurances from their German supervisor, Brandt. Dr. Zdzisław Seidenbeutel saved himself only because he was assigned to a team of streetcar engineers. Jewish Police also did not receive "life tickets" for their children, because it was believed that parents would manage to smuggle them out.[127] Dr. Ignacy Rejder, for instance, concealed his little daughter in the trunk of a car as it was leaving the selection point. The SS officer in charge saw the child but pretended not to.[128]

According to Henryk Makower, during one of the *Grossaktion* roundups on Miła Street in September 1942, personnel of the so-called "Red Service" heard a "short and sweet" announcement informing them their numbers would be reduced by half, and the remainder, with all their wives and children, would be deported. As policemen escorted the protesting assembly to Stawki Street, some addressed their escorts, saying: "Today us, tomorrow—you." Nevertheless, the people walked on stoically as the policemen carried out their despicable task.[129]

---

126  Makower, *Pamiętnik z getta warszawskiego*, 124–125.

127  Ibid., 125. *Numerki życia*, here translated as "tickets to live," were small cards with a stamp declaring that the bearer was entitled to live. The Germans issued 40,000 such tickets when the mass deportations from the ghetto began.

128  Bauman, *Zima o poranku*, 104–105.

129  Makower, *Pamiętnik z getta warszawskiego*, 195.

# Chapter 8

# Healthcare after the Great Deportation

## The Hospital on 6–8 Gęsia Street

After the September selection, life in the ghetto meant the "constant threat of deportation to the afterlife devoid of any trust in humanity and goodness."[1] Doctors and nurses were directed to the building on 10 Pawia Street, where an infirmary was set up in a three-room apartment on the first floor, in a backyard away from the main entrance. Nurses Fryd, Gurfinkiel-Glocer, Isserlis, Mebel, Prużańska and Ickowicz immediately started to care for the ailing who worked in the German-owned production facilities.

The twelve-bed infirmary was too small to accommodate all comers, so Doctors Milejkowski and Stein obtained permission to move the patient overflow to premises on 6 Gęsia Street. The two tenement buildings which had been allocated to the hospital before the war housed a warehouse and offices, while the outbuildings consisted of private apartments. The hospital personnel made the move on September 21. Working in primitive conditions, during the first two weeks they established small departments with operating theaters. All personnel helped to clean the premises: windows, doors and floors were thoroughly washed, as were the lavatories. Useless furniture was thrown out of the windows, wooden

---

1   An account by Adolf Polisiuk, "Pamiętnik w kolekcji Abrahama Adolfa Bermana" (section "Ostatnia blokada"), Ghetto Fighters' House Museum, ref. 3182.

remnants were chopped up for firewood to be used in the kitchen and for heating wards. There were no complaints as everybody wanted to create some semblance of a hospital. There were no cleaners or other helpers; during the selection, doctors' wives had remained behind in their stead. Sabina Gurfinkiel-Glocer remembered how exhausting the work was for women who had never done manual labor.[2]

Professionals on staff repaired the water and sanitation system and furnished spaces designated as procedure rooms. Some equipment was brought from Leszno and Stawki Streets. Stein remained the director and Braude-Heller his deputy, while the hospital administration was in the hands of Ignacy Sztabholc and Henryk Kroszczor. Personnel were accommodated in the left wing and outbuildings. One apartment on the third floor housed eleven people including Dr. Anna Margolis and her daughter, Dr. Helena Keilson and her parents, Dr. Adina Blady-Szwajger and Marek Edelman (hospital messenger). The doctors initially hoped their professions and the fact that they were useful would give them a chance to survive. Alina Margolis-Edelman, Dr. A. Margolis's daughter and a nursing student of the ghetto nursing school, noted: "Hospital personnel were placed in one outbuilding, the second one was opposite the infirmary. . . All the doors bore name plaques: Dr. Wohl, Dr. Penson, doctor, doctor, doctor. . . But that title protected no one from anything."[3]

Departments were established to accommodate 400 beds:[4] internal medicine, infectious diseases, two surgery departments, and (the smallest) one for pediatrics, located in three rooms on one of the floors.[5] Children were not needed in the ghetto, because it officially became a labor camp[6] and only toddlers aged three to four years were treated.[7]

---

2  An account by Sabina Gurfinkiel-Glocer, "Szpital na Czystem i ja," YVA O.3/396.
3  A. Margolis-Edelman, *Ala z "Elementarza"* (Warsaw: FZL, 2011), 45.
4  Kroszczor, "Szpital dla Dzieci," 44.
5  An account by Izrael Rotbalsam, YVA O.3/2357.
6  The so-called "residual ghetto" (*getto szczątkowe*), created after the September *aktion*, was de facto a huge labor camp. From the 34,000 registered inhabitants, over ninety percent were in a productive age group. In the ghetto territory there were also people (*dzicy*—the "wild ones" as Fenigstein calls them, see Fenigstein, "The History of 'Czyste,'" xxx) who did not receive "tickets to live" but managed to survive the *aktion* in hiding. It is estimated that there were some 65,000 Jews in the "residual ghetto": "Getto szczątkowe," Delet, http://www.jhi.pl/psj/getto_szczatkowe, accessed March 19, 2017.
7  An account by Izrael Rotbalsam, YVA O.3/2357.

Dr. Rotbalsam believed that, in addition to various diseases decimating the youngest ghetto residents, the total absence of babies in the ghetto was the saddest thing pediatricians faced. Women were not becoming pregnant because they refused to bring children into a nightmarish existence and their bodies reacted to physical and psychological suffering. During the final days of the hospital's existence, the neonatal department shut down almost completely.

Dr. Wilk had a small surgery where frostbitten feet became his "daily bread." Toes, blackened by gangrene, were often amputated directly in the patient's bed, without surgical gloves—the mere washing of hands had to suffice.[8] At the time, the hospital received food allocations from provisions, which resumed operations. The rations were barely sufficient for the patients' needs but Dr. Blady-Szwajger noted hunger edema was no longer an issue.

Sick people arrived at the hospital every day, even from outside the ghetto. These were people who, for some reason, were *sent* to the ghetto barracks.[9] The great majority of cases were directed to surgical departments where major operations were carried out from time to time, usually in emergencies (mainly gunshot wounds).[10] Many cases of typhus were reported, with an upswing in the winter of 1942/43. One of the patients in the infectious diseases department was Natan Żelechower, a dental technician working in a broom-making workshop, who noted in his memoir:

> The next day, loaded onto a hand-drawn cart, I bid a heartfelt and teary goodbye to friends, without any hope of seeing them again, and left the workshop grounds. My means of transport was exceedingly uncomfortable, but fortunately my destination was not very far. . . I was placed in a ward with eight other people. The first impression fully corroborated the rumors circulating in the ghetto about the state of the hospital. Broken windows provided ventilation in the room where I lay, but this was not

---

8   Blady-Szwajger, *I więcej nic nie pamiętam*, 111.
9   For people who could not be admitted on Gęsia, especially the "wild ones," an outpatient clinic was opened at 24 Franciszkańska Street. Fenigstein, "The History of 'Czyste,'" xxxi.
10  An account by Stanisław (Shmul) Waller (Walewski), YVA O.3/2358.

enough to drive out the choking stench emanating from the sick. The hospital had no water. Unwashed for weeks, patients lay between dirty linens, soiling them mercilessly.

. . . There were mainly cases of typhus, typhoid fever and scabies, and patients looked like lepers with their bodies covered in pustules. Scabies plagued everybody, with the problem spreading as it moved from one person to the next. . . The hospital had no light, I lay in darkness, listening to moans and complaints, to fervent prayers for help, to the throat-clearing and spitting of those who were choking, to the wheezing of the dying. Late at night the voices subsided, the narcosis of heavy air, saturated with a foul stench, put everyone to sleep.

In the grey morning light, those who were awake looked for signs of life in the faces of those who were still asleep. The dead, their mouths half-open, baring yellowed teeth, were carried out to the vestibule. Not quite cold yet, without their bedding being changed after their removal, their places were taken by the latest arrivals.

. . . I was the only one who started fighting for everything: for a sheet, for a pillow, which was brought for me from an apartment that had been emptied, for warm water for washing, better food, disinfectants, and slowly I succeeded in getting everything I needed to prevent myself from dying immediately, but the rest—the scarcity of medicines—I left for my body to deal with. . . I managed to establish contact with a nurse who lived on the premises. In exchange for some jewelry which I still had, she procured all I needed, cooked special dinners for me, and tried to make my life easier in every way possible in this shabby hospital. . . All nine weeks were equally hopelessly long and sad, filled with news about ghetto workshops closing down. I was filled with fear that every patient would die once the hospital was shut down.[11]

---

11  "Pamiętnik Natana Żelechowera (Jana Kurczaba)," Jewish Historical Institute Archives, ref. 302/139.

During its final days of operation, students and graduates of the nursing school were also employed at the hospital.[12]

## Doctors after the Great Deportation

A number of doctors left the ghetto to hide on the Aryan side but not everyone found the promised help on the other side. Those who decided to remain in the ghetto began preparing bunkers and hideouts. The gynecologist, Dr. Adolf Polisiuk, hid in a shelter under the hospital building, and also hid a supply of medicine in the bunker.[13]

When the fate of ghetto doctors was decided in September 1942, hospital director, Dr. Bieleńki received a "ticket to live" and moved to Muranowska Street, where he worked as a doctor in the dispensary at the Többens and Schultz workshop in the Nowolipie district.[14]

After the September *aktion*, Feliks Majnamer-Mrozowski, a ghetto emergency services doctor, was forced to do physical labor. Together with his doctor wife, he worked in Wiktor Nuss' workshop. Nuss "wore jackboots; his bloated and red and ruddy face, fat neck and self-satisfied expression were proof he feasted on so-called German butter. The ubiquitous whip in his hand was in constant motion, threatening laborers."[15] Work in "his" workshops involved cleaning apartments and collecting all the abandoned possessions of those who were murdered, sorting through their things and depositing them in German-designated storehouses, which sent the sorted items to Berlin. Dr. Makower's wife, Noemi, also collected and sorted the property of the dead.[16] Every couple of days, she

---

12 Blady-Szwajger, *I więcej nic nie pamiętam*, 112. The Nursing School in the Jewish Orthodox Hospital was opened on July 8, 1923.
13 An account of Adolf Polisiuk (Ghetto Fighters' House Museum, ref. 3182), Jewish Historical Institute Archives, ref. 301/5061.
14 Többens und Schultz & Co. was a Nazi German textile manufacturing conglomerate making German uniforms, socks, and garments in the Warsaw Ghetto and elsewhere during the occupation of Poland in the Second World War. It was owned and operated by two major war profiteers: Fritz Emil Schultz from Danzig, and a convicted war criminal, Walter Caspar Többens, from Hamburg. See "Többens and Schultz," Wikipedia, https://en.wikipedia.org/wiki/Többens_and_Schultz.
15 Meroz, *W murach i poza murami getta*, 63.
16 *Werterfassung* (acquisition/procurement) was a branch subordinated to the SS and, apart from the *Szopas*, it was the most dynamic ghetto institution, commanded by Obersturmführer Franz Konrad.

would walk the empty street of the ghetto to enter yet another designated building in the so-called "neutral belt" dividing different workshops. This is how Dr. Noemi Makower recalled those days:

> Pavements clanked softly under our feet, no trace of life anywhere, only houses, one after another, empty, dead. . . The façade of an average, large apartment looked like this: door smashed, human feces on the floor, linens ripped, lots of down and feathers everywhere. A few pieces of furniture . . . in the drawers—papers, photographs, some scattered on the floor . . . piles of books. It was obvious that before we *cleaned*, the apartment had already been *cleaned* by those looking for some kind of treasure. . . In every fourth or fifth apartment on Chłodna Street, I found a doctor's armband amidst heaps of odds and ends.[17]

Dr. Henryk Makower, who collected medical books from the deserted apartments, once came to the apartment of a former colleague from Łódź. The door bore the name Dr. Zausmer. The apartment was in disarray and empty, its owner, his wife and their sick daughter had been deported to Treblinka. As Makower put it: "These two dirty, messy rooms made a greater impression on me than the entire rest of this huge building. The rest was impersonal; I didn't know anything about those other people."[18]

After the Great Deportation, the plundering and beatings followed by killings continued. From the window of the Linas Hacedek Hospital on 20 Nowolipki Street, Dr. Feliks Majnamer-Mrozowski saw two Gestapo officers order Dr. Zygmunt Sztajnkalk, a pediatrician, to walk in front of them, in November 1942, and even though he obeyed, they shot him.[19] The event was also witnessed by Dr. Zofia Rozenblum. In her words:

> The old and distinguished pediatrician, Dr. Steinkalk [sic], had been walking peacefully to visit a patient. Something about his figure was not to the liking of the two Gestapo officers. One shot him in the head, and he crashed down onto the pavement. Nobody looked back, nor did anyone rush to help him. I

17  Makower, *Miłość w cieniu śmierci*, 94–95.
18  Makower, *Pamiętnik z getta warszawskiego*, 188.
19  Meroz, *W murach i poza murami getta*, 62.

informed his wife and two daughters. When night fell, they removed the body. With utter indifference, adults and children alike passed by corpses covered with newspapers as if they were mere things lying in the street.[20]

Between January 18 and 21, 1943, on Heinrich Himmler's orders, another *aktion* was initiated in the ghetto. For the first time, an *aktion* met with armed resistance organized by the Jewish Combat Organization (*ZOB*). A group of fighters commanded by Mordechai Anielewicz joined forces with a column of Jews and headed for the *Umschlagplatz*, where they attacked German escorts on the corner of Zamenhofa and Niska Streets. Most of the Jewish fighters were killed, but several dozen managed to escape. The deportation was largely discontinued after this act of active resistance, and "only" 5,000 people were transported to Treblinka, among them patients from the hospital on Gęsia Street.

During this January 1943 *aktion*, Dr. Julian Fliederbaum killed himself after pushing his little son and wife from a fourth-floor window.[21]

After the first physical resistance against the Germans in January 1943, which temporarily stopped a deportation, ZOB, the Jewish Fighters' Group, merged with Betar, the Revisionist Zionist fighting group, and they had approximately 750 members between them. Earlier, in October 1942, ZOB had convinced the Home Army to get them some weapons— some pistols, rifles, and a few automatic weapons. They encouraged people to build bunkers and shelters because they knew there was going to be another deportation.[22]

## Nurses after the Great Deportation

Initially, the nursing students were overlooked, but once deportations started, they were randomly sent to the *Umschlagplatz*. Thus, the numbers of the nursing students were considerably reduced after the September

---

20  Quoted in Szymańska, *Byłam tylko lekarzem*, 139. (Reference to Dr. Zelman Zygmunt Sztajnkalk.)
21  Hirszfeld, *Historia jednego życia*, 325.
22  "Warsaw Ghetto Uprising," USHMM Holocaust Encyclopedia, https://encyclopedia. ushmm.org/content/en/article/warsaw-ghetto-uprising, accessed March 30, 2020.

*aktion*.[23] Some left to live with their parents; others were employed in the German ghetto workshops as paramedics or laborers.[24] Those who stayed in the hospital worked the day or night shift, where their main duty was to care for gravely ill patients.[25]

## Pharmacists after the Great Deportation

Towards the end of the *Grossaktion* in 1942, during the round up on Miła Street, a small number of "life tickets" were distributed to pharmacy staff by Henryk Gliksberg. When the *aktion* ended, what was left of the Department of Pharmacies occupied the corner of Gęsia and Lubecki Streets.[26] As early as the fall of 1942, fighters of the Jewish Combat Organization, the Jewish resistance group in Warsaw, began to appear, requiring bandages, disinfectants and medication. When the *Grossaktion* ended in September 1942, according to a report on the work of the *Judenrat*, only three pharmacies remained and two had to evacuate and relocate (see appendix 6).[27] The chairman's report of the *Judenrat*'s activities in January 1943, after that month's deportations, referred to another pharmacy on 30 Zamenhofa Street.

Some pharmacists and staff left the ghetto to seek help on the Aryan side. In 1941, Jerzy Śliwczyński, among others, helped Dr. Makowski and Jakub Kleniec (MSc Pharmacology) leave the ghetto with their families.[28]

## Emergency Services after the Deportation

Henryk Bryskier said that during a January 1943 *aktion*, emergency service staff who remained in the ghetto were without their wives and

---

23 Luba Blum-Bielicka states that in September there were nineteen students ("Szkoła Pielęgniarstwa przy Szpitalu Starozakonnych w Warszawie (1923–1943)," *Biuletyn Żydowskiego Instytutu Historycznego* 4, no. 40 [1961]: 75). Blum-Bielicka maintains that "only six or seven remained" after the roundup on Miła Street. The school received twenty "tickets to live."
24 Szereszewska, *Krzyż i mezuza*, 131.
25 Blum-Bielicka, "Szkoła Pielęgniarstwa," 74.
26 Ibid., 143.
27 *Tak było*, 101.
28 An account by Jerzy Śliwczyński, Ella Perkiel and Frank Perkiel, Jewish Historical Institute Archives, ref. 301/6236.

children.[29] Juliusz Sirota probably died in a fire with his family in a bunker on Wołyńska Street during the uprising and Dr. Mejłachowicz was deported to Bergen-Belsen, and later to Auschwitz, where he was murdered.

## The Fate of the Gęsia Street Hospital

The first rumors of planned deportations reached the hospital at midnight on January 17-18, 1943. A policeman, Bronisław Girszlak, warned personnel that selections would be conducted at the hospital:

> He came to the surgical department and motioned to nurse Gurfinkiel-Glocer to join him outside. He did not want to speak in front of my patients. The news was bad. There was a plan to liquidate the rest of the ghetto. The policeman advised me to inform people, so they would hide wherever they could. Dr. Amsterdamski, administration directors Kroszczor and Sztabholc, nurse Gurfinkiel-Glocer, and a few other officials all gathered in the office, while runner Gurwicz, on his bike, went to check the veracity of the information with the gendarmes at the gate.[30]

The nurses decided patients who could walk would be informed, so they could hide. The rest had no chance of being saved. At 4 a.m., the nurses handed out thermometers to the patients, to distract them.[31] Sleeping personnel were woken up. At approximately 6 a.m., Luba Blum-Bielicka came to the hospital to relieve head nurse Fryd. At 7 a.m. the trucks arrived and parked in front of the hospital. Two Germans, Obersturmführer von Bloescher and a German army doctor, entered the building, shouting "Deportation!" and ordered patients to be loaded onto the trucks.[32]

---

29 Bryskier, *Żydzi pod swastyką*, 233.
30 An account by Sabina Gurfinkiel-Glocer, "Szpital na Czystem i ja," YVA O.3/396. According to Tadeusz Stabholz, at that time, his uncle had pneumonia and remained bedridden in his room. Stabholz, *Siedem piekieł*, 89.
31 An account by Sabina Gurfinkiel-Glocer, "Szpital na Czystem i ja," YVA O.3/396.
32 Szereszewska, *Krzyż i mezuza*, 214.

Dr. Stein was on the other side of the wall, visiting his seven-year-old daughter, Ludwika, who was hiding on the Aryan side.[33] Instead, Tadeusz Stabholz, the medical student, met the Germans. The German doctor asked how many patients there were and when he received no answer, he slapped Stabholz across the face several times. The confrontation ended when the driver of one of the trucks reported that 320 people had already been loaded. The German shouted: "My God, surely I can't drink that much alcohol!" Apparently he had been promised one liter of alcohol for each patient he killed.[34]

Amidst great chaos in the wards, Dr. Braude-Heller dressed the children who were being deported. Other personnel carried seriously ill patients on stretchers and loaded them onto the trucks.[35] The majority of the staff hid. Several people jumped out of windows, and those who were not yet dead were shot by the Germans. Some patients refused to leave, saying: "They must shoot me here, in my bed." Von Bloescher and the German army doctor did exactly that.[36] The same fate befell infants not taken to hideouts.

Not trusting the nursing staff, the Germans ran around the hospital, searching and asking where the rest of the personnel were. Engineer Sztabholc explained that when their shifts ended, the staff had all gone home, and were probably already taken. From time to time, he surreptitiously raised a panel leading to a hideout to tell those behind it what was happening and to console them. But there were not enough hands to do the work, so he went to the cellar where some were hiding, including several men, and asked them to help carry the sick. Initially nobody wanted to leave, but he personally requested male nurse Rubinstein to lend a hand along with a colleague. The men's wives cried, trying to restrain them, but they finally let them go.[37]

Dr. Stanisław Waller, his wife, and their one-year-old child hid in the cellar of a nearby shop with Luba Blum-Bielicka, several children and nurses Gurfinkiel-Glocer and Isserlis.[38] There were a number of small

33  Stabholz, *Siedem piekieł*, 89.
34  Blum-Bielicka, "Szkoła Pielęgniarstwa," 75.
35  Makower, *Miłość w cieniu śmierci*, 104.
36  Szereszewska, *Krzyż i mezuza*, 215.
37  An account by Stanisław (Shmul) Waller (Walewski), YVA O.3/2358.
38  Ibid.

children in three rooms filled to capacity. It was feared the children might betray the location of the bolt-hole by talking or crying. Some doctors suggested injecting them with small doses of morphine so they would sleep. These "injections of silence" saved them all because in one instance the Germans stood above a trapdoor and asked what was below. Masking his anxiety, Sztabholc said he had just admitted typhus patients, and the nearby containers were bedpans used by infected patients. Hearing that, the Germans left in a rush. The hospital personnel spent three full days in the cellar, from Monday morning to Thursday afternoon (January 18–21, 1943).[39]

The second group of personnel, including director Kroszczor and his family, spent their first day hiding in an attic. Because of the freezing weather and cramped conditions, over the next two days some moved to an enclosure obscured by a wardrobe. Even though the Germans passed the wardrobe several times, opened it and prodded the back wall with the muzzles of their rifles, they did not find the hidden door.[40] Inside there were so many people that a candle would only burn for an hour before dying due to a lack of oxygen. The distant sounds of doors being smashed, one after another, reached the group, who were engulfed in complete darkness. Dr. Blady-Szwajger wrote that, for the first time in her life, she felt real fear when she heard the wardrobe being moved.[41]

On Thursday, Ignacy Sztabholc lifted the trapdoor and said, "You may come out, this time you were lucky."[42] The group emerged to find a deadly silence hanging over the wards, and almost all the beds empty. Some beds still held dead bodies of those shot in the head or chest. Some dead patients still had their limbs suspended on pulleys or in splints. Babies lay in pools of congealed blood unmoving in their beautiful white cots.[43]

On the first day of the deportations, the Germans rounded up the doctors and nurses occupying the apartments on Kupiecka Street,

---

39  An account by Sabina Gurfinkiel-Glocer, "Szpital na Czystem i ja," YVA O.3/396.
40  An account by Izrael Rotbalsam, YVA O.3/2357. According to Rotbalsam, there were twenty people, Adina Blady-Szwajger stated it could have been thirty, while Stanisław Waller maintains fifty people were hiding there.
41  Blady-Szwajger, *I więcej nic nie pamiętam*, 113.
42  An account by Sabina Gurfinkiel-Glocer, "Szpital na Czystem i ja," YVA O.3/396.
43  Blum-Bielicka, "Szkoła Pielęgniarstwa," 76.

including Dr. Izrael Milejkowski, the head of the *Judenrat's* Health Department and Dr. Sara Syrkin-Binsztejn.[44]

Stripped of their clothing, the hospital's patients were taken to the *Umschlagplatz* and detained there. Despite being a sunny day, it was extremely cold. Helena Szereszewska saw people dressed only in their hospital nightshirts, wrapped in blankets. Among them were those infected with typhus—their eyes were dull, their faces purple with fever.[45] Dr. Syrkin-Binsztejn and Dr. Milejkowski were there. Milejkowski, in a soft voice, shared the latest news from the front with the others. The crowd just stood there, absorbing his words.[46] Apparently on the way to Treblinka, Dr. Sara Syrkin-Binsztejn injected some people with deadly doses of morphine.[47] Other doctors did the same.

When the hospital had been emptied of all its patients, most of the nurses and paramedics were taken away, as were Doctors Glauternik and Gelbfisz. Dr. Stein, his wife, engineer Sztabholc, Doctors Braude-Heller and Wortman, Mrs. Rochman, and nurses Irena Szereszewska and Sabina Zenderman were spared deportation.[48] During the last night of the deportations, Dr. Amsterdamski, the head of surgery at Czyste, died unexpectedly.[49]

---

44  Kroszczor, "Szpital dla Dzieci," 45.
45  Szereszewska, *Krzyż i mezuza*, 210.
46  Ibid., 211.
47  Ibid., 325.
48  Blum-Bielicka, "Szkoła Pielęgniarstwa," 75.
49  Kroszczor, "Szpital dla Dzieci," 45. According to Stanisław Waller, Dr. Amsterdamski died in an attic hideout (YVA O.3/2358).

# Chapter 9

# The Ghetto Uprising and Its Aftermath

The Germans had intended to start the final deportation and liquidation of the ghetto on April 19, the eve of the Jewish holiday of Passover. When they came into the ghetto, the streets were deserted. Everyone had taken shelter. Led by Mordecai Anielewicz of the ZOB, on the first day of fighting they forced the Germans to retreat to the other side of the wall. The Germans, who lost 12 men, were stunned, but within three days broke the core of the resistance, which continued, piecemeal, for the next three weeks. On May 8, they discovered the main ZOB bunker at 18 Mila Street, and destroyed it, killing Anielewicz and those who were with him.[1] After initial setbacks, the Germans returned to the ghetto in force, but instead of fighting building by building and block by block, they chose to destroy the entire ghetto by setting it aflame.

## The Last Hospital in the Ghetto

Once the January *aktion* ended, many hospital employees went to the Aryan side; others went to work in the German workshops, seeing them as a means of survival. A small group stayed in the buildings on 6–8 Gęsia Street, and for the third time set out to establish a hospital. Once again, the devastated interiors were cleaned and made habitable. The Provisioning Department supplied the hospital with food and patients

---

1   Ibid.

were admitted again. But there was nobody to do physical labor, since everyone had been deported. Some posts were filled by "illegals"—people who had no right to be in the ghetto. This way, Jacek Goldman became the hospital cook.[2] Engineer Sztabholc helped by peeling potatoes and onions. As Sabina Gurfinkiel-Glocer wrote:

> Everyone who had worked in the hospital was now staying there, it looked like we were all one family: doctors, nurses, casual staff, we were all together. Together we mourned those who had been taken from us. . . The next day, patients started arriving at our hospital: those who had jumped out of the wagons and those who had been shot by the Germans, they all begged for help. A handful of doctors and nurses returned to their posts and resumed carrying out their duties.[3]

Immediately preparations began to get hideouts and shelters ready. The "room behind the wardrobe" was deemed ideal. With this in mind, a bathtub and an additional tap and basin were placed in the corridor leading to it. Under the basin was an opening someone could crawl through to the concealed room, after which screws were bolted onto the basin. Another group built a large bunker under the pharmacy at 3 Gęsia Street. This bunker connected to another one on Nalewki Street, which was in a hospital basement. All hideouts quickly filled up during the first few days of the Ghetto Uprising that began on April 19, 1943.[4]

In April, helped by the Jewish Police, the Germans discovered the shelter after a couple of days and called for everyone to leave their shelters voluntarily, promising them safe exit to the East. In the bunker under the ruined building at 3 Gęsia Street (bombed in September 1939) there were 130 people, including Dr. Józef Stein with his wife, Doctors Anna Braude-Heller, Antoni Wortman, Jakób Munwes, Adolf Polisiuk, Tobias Gitler, Owsiej Bieleńki, Ignacy Borkowski, Maurycy Brandwajn and Henry Fenigstein, student Tadeusz Stabholz, several nursing staff,

---

2  Kroszczor, "Szpital dla Dzieci," 45.
3  Gurfinkiel-Glocer, "Szpital Żydowski w Warszawie," 107.
4  The uprising in the ghetto started on April 19, 1943, and lasted until mid-May that year.

head nurse Stanisława Rochman, stewards Ignacy Sztabholc and Ignacy Fliderbaum, and several laborers.[5]

The person in charge of this hideout was the head of the medicine dosage unit, Górwicz. On April 21, Drs. Owsiej Bieleńki, Ignacy Borkowski and Henry Fenigstein and their wives, responded to the Germans' call. They exited their hiding places, among them the completely demoralized and exhausted Dr. Bieleńki and were searched and brought to the *Umschlagplatz*.[6] Those who defied the command were immediately shot.

According to postwar accounts, Dr. Bieleńki was sent to Trawniki, where he worked as camp doctor. In his 1943 testimonial, Paweł Rajman wrote that during the fall of 1943, under the pretext of being released from the camp and going abroad, Bieleńki was transferred by car to Majdanek where he was shot, most probably during the November *Erntefest*, the "Harvest Festival," a German code name for the mass killing of Jews in Majdanek in November 1943.[7]

Fenigstein's situation was somewhat peculiar. He bribed an SS officer, offering him his collection of postage stamps and a commitment to complete it with the missing pieces, in exchange for a promise to be sent to a labor camp instead of Treblinka. And so it happened.[8]

In the morning of April 22, 1943, on the fourth day of the uprising, the hospital was set on fire. Those who opted to lock themselves in probably burned to death. A handful of hospital personnel, some fifteen people, and Dr. Rotbalsam, laboratory assistant Fajga Ferszt and Dr. Rywka

---

5 An account by Adolf Polisiuk, "Pamiętnik w kolekcji Abrahama Adolfa Bermana" (see "Ostatnia blokada"), Ghetto Fighters' House Museum, ref. 3182. Ignacy Fliderbaum was a long-time purser in the Czyste Jewish Hospital, and he was a director of the community's Hospitalization Department in the ghetto.

6 An account by Adolf Polisiuk, "Pamiętnik w kolekcji Abrahama Adolfa Bermana" (sections "Ostatnia blokada" and "Czworobok"), Ghetto Fighters' House Museum, ref. 3182.

7 An account by Paweł Rajman, YVA O.3/439.

8 Dr. Henry Fenigstein was sent to work in an aircraft workshop. In May 1944, he was transferred to SS Arbeitslager Radom (a workshop on Szkolna Street) and when it was liquidated—to Auschwitz, afterwards to Vaihingen an der Enz, Durchgangslager—Krankenlager München—Allach (a sub-camp of Dachau), Hessental and, finally, Dachau. His wife, Ala Fenigstein, was murdered during *Erntefest*, in November 1943. After the war, Fenigstein worked in the Munich UNRRA hospital, in the Gynecology Department of the University Hospital. Subsequently, he immigrated to Canada where he specialized in psychiatry. See Fenigstein, "The History of 'Czyste.'"

Elbinger, with her family, went to the shelter in the cellar. Initially they tried to cover the entrance with sand, but without success. Because one wing of the hospital was still undamaged, they decided to go there. Running through the wards, they saw patients shot dead in their beds. On the first floor they found a way out into the yard and from there searched for other bunkers. Following a hazardous route, they reached a cellar where some hospital patients found shelter, and agreed to let them in. They remained there until May 11, leaving the shelter only under cover of darkness, to get to the storage facility at 20 Gęsia Street, owned by the *Judenrat*, to gather anything that was edible (mainly beets).[9]

By mid-May, almost all the houses in the area were in ruins. Those found hiding in shelters were taken to the *Umschlagplatz*, to a prison called Gęsiówka (from the street name), and to the Jewish cemetery where many of them were executed. Those who refused to leave the shelter were either shot on the spot or suffocated when gas was pumped into the cellars. On May 11, some SS-men threw a grenade into the bunker where Dr. Rotbalsam was hiding. Luckily people backed away immediately, and only one person was injured. The bunker was shown to the Germans by a Jew who had been hiding nearby, and he was rewarded with a bowl of soup. Two days later, he, too, was brought to the *Umschlagplatz*.

When the large shelter under the pharmacy was revealed, fourteen people managed to run away and hide in the vicinity of the hospital. Among them were doctors Braude-Heller, Polisiuk and Gitler.[10] Facing the magnitude of their tragedy, they lost all hope of surviving. Expecting that their sanctuary would be revealed, they dispersed.[11] Dr. Polisiuk succeeded in reaching the Aryan side on May 27, but his friend Gitler was most probably caught by extortionists.[12]

---

9   An account by Izrael Rotbalsam, YVA O.3/2357.

10  An account by Adolf Polisiuk, Jewish Historical Institute Archives, ref. 301/5061. In archives of the Jewish Historical Institute the date of this account being written is given as 1945, while in the Ghetto Fighters' House Museum the date stated is 1943 (ref. 3182). It is known that Dr. Adolf Polisiuk moved to the Aryan side and hid for some time, writing his memoirs. The narrative stops at the time that gives credence to the date given by Ghetto Fighters' House Museum.

11  An account by Adolf Polisiuk, "Pamiętnik w kolekcji Abrahama Adolfa Bermana" (section "Ostatnia blokada"), Ghetto Fighters' House Museum, ref. 3182.

12  Ibid.

Little is known about the fate of Dr. Anna Braude-Heller. According to an account included in the memoirs of Luba Blum-Bielicka, the shelter where she was hiding burned down. Friends of Dr. Braude-Heller tried to save her, preparing fake documents and offering her a safe house, but she declined their help. Dr. Blady-Szwajger remembered that, in her final letter from the ghetto, dated March 1943, Dr. Braude-Heller wrote: "Do not worry about me. I have made plans."[13] Today it is impossible to establish under what circumstances and when she died. Her sister, Judyta Braude, wrote that she had cyanide with her, and hoped she had a chance to use it. It is possible that Dr. Braude-Heller died with her other sister, Róża Aftergut.[14]

## The Fate of Jewish doctors after the Deportation

The Jewish doctors working in Warsaw, as well as their families and patients, were savagely murdered in the gas chambers of Treblinka. To the very end, they were searched for jewelry and beaten by the Ukrainian and German guards on the *Umschlagplatz*. They were transported to their final destination in overcrowded, sealed boxcars sprinkled with lime, which made it difficult to breathe. Marek Balin was one of the few who managed to jump out of the moving train and survived. Some chose to end their lives by committing suicide or they helped others to die.[15]

In Treblinka the boxcars were emptied of all people who were lined on a station ramp. Children and women were separated from the men and sent directly to the gas chambers. In 1943, those deemed fit for work were transported to Lublin in the same trains.[16] The trip from Treblinka to Lublin usually took several days, with many dying from exhaustion or thirst. When they arrived at the transit labor camp in Lublin, the so-called *Flugplatz*, the prisoners were subjected to another selection

---

13  Blady-Szwajger, *I więcej nic nie pamiętam*, 116.
14  An account by Sabina Gurfinkiel-Glocer, "Szpital na Czystem i ja," YVA O.3/396.
15  One of the two medical students who were on the wagon injected his wife with morphine at her request. Later, the unconscious woman was carried out by Ukrainians and shot. Then, the same student injected his friend. When they arrived in Treblinka, the unconscious man was carried on a stretcher to a gas chamber. An account by Izrael Rotbalsam, YVA O.3/2357.
16  The first selection resulted in 320 men being sent to a Lublin *Dulag*; there was place in Treblinka at the end of April. The transport was sent on April 29, 1943, to Budzyń near Kraśnik and to other camps in Lublin region.

before being loaded onto trucks and transported to other camps in Lublin province. Warsaw Jews were sent to camps at Poniatowa, Trawniki, Budzyń, Dorohucza, and also Lublin (to Lipowa Street, *Flugplatz*, and Majdanek).[17] Of the fifty Jewish doctors sent from the Warsaw Ghetto to Lublin to work in the prison hospital, only a few survived.[18] The majority of Jewish doctors were killed during the November *action* known as *Erntefest*. Those who were lucky to leave alive survived after being transported to other camps, or because they had false Aryan documents.[19]

## Help for Jewish doctors and life on the Aryan side

Teresa Prekerowa, historian and author of the monograph *Underground Council Aiding Warsaw Jews Between 1942 and 1945*, writes that from the beginning of the war, there was assistance for Jewish residents in Warsaw.[20] As early as the second half of 1942, a clandestine Consensus

---

17  An account by Ilie Chryzman, Henry Fenigstein, Marek Feinstein, and Aleksander Grunberg. Information concerning the fate of Jews after April 1943 deportations. Jewish Historical Institute, ref. 301/509.

18  The figure of fifty doctors was given by Izrael Rotbalsam.

19  Dr. Henryk Halpern-Wieliczański, who lived outside the ghetto with his wife Teodozja Maria and their daughter Zosia, survived in this way. He was a principal hygienist in the Union of Polish Syndicalists (ZSP), a Polish civilian-military conspiratorial organization, active between April 1941 and mid-1945 in Nazi-occupied Poland. In the Home Army his code name was "Zygmunt." He worked in the Central Toxicological Laboratory. He was arrested on January 8, 1943, and imprisoned by the Gestapo in Pawiak Prison. On January 17 of that year he was transported to Majdanek in Lublin, where he was assigned to work in a prison hospital. There, on behalf of the Home Army, he organized a resistance movement and was the commander of Field V. He was well known among the prisoners as a Samaritan who did much more than his duties required. See Maria Ciesielska and Marta Grudzińska, "Biogramy lekarzy-więźniów pracujących w obozie koncentracyjnym na Majdanku," Lekarze w pasiakach. Służba medyczna na Majdanku, http://lekarze-w-pasiakach.majdanek.eu/pl/, accessed September 01, 2017.

20  T. Prekerowa, "Pomoc lekarska ukrywającym się *Żydom (w Warszawie 1942–1944),*" *Przegląd Lekarski—Oświęcim* 40, bk. 23, no. 1 (1983): 113. The Council to Aid Jews (Rada Pomocy Żydom, also translated as Council for Aid to Jews), known by its code-name "Żegota," became one of the most active and dedicated underground resistance organizations in occupied Poland; it started operating in September 1942, and continued until after the ghetto was liquidated. It was a Christian organization, which mainly helped Jews in hiding on the Aryan side, providing means for their upkeep and certificates of baptism along with false documents. The rescued children were usually hidden in public orphanages and convents (such as Maryans

Committee of Democratic and Socialist Doctors was established in Warsaw gathering well-known representatives of the Polish medical fraternity. They organized medical help for those who decided against moving to the ghetto and those who lived in the ghetto.

The underground periodical, *Medical ABC*, published by the committee, appealed to doctors to resist harmful anti-Jewish propaganda based on pseudoscientific premises (questions around race, typhoid fever epidemics, etc.). The activists who initiated the periodical and were members of its editorial board were Doctors Ludwik Rostkowski, Jan Rutkiewicz and Tadeusz Stępniewski. The periodical was distributed in Żurawia Street and in Andrzej Trojanowski's receiving rooms on Marszałkowska Street.[21] With the passing of time, efforts to help the Jews were considerably hampered by a lack of resources and by the growing terror and severe penalties meted out to those assisting them. One entry warning that the death penalty would befall anyone who "consciously offered shelter to Jews," appeared in Governor General Hans Frank's decree, October 15, 1941.[22]

The first large wave of refugees moving from the ghetto to the Aryan side took place in the summer of 1942 during the *Grossaktion*. While it was happening, and in the aftermath, many people who had "good Aryan features" and financial means fled beyond the walls and hid in Warsaw or on the outskirts of the city. An estimated 8,000 people left the ghetto that way. Dr. Rotbalsam wrote that many of the Jewish intelligentsia, who had difficulty coping with conditions in the ghetto, and who had friends or acquaintances on the Aryan side, moved even earlier.[23] As Vladka Meed, a courier who survived, noted:

---

or Ursulines). The Żegota division in Warsaw was managed by Irena Sendler. Żegota operated under the auspices of the Polish Government in Exile through the Government Delegation for Poland. The codename "Żegota" was conceived by Zofia Kossak-Szczucka. It comes from the name of Konrad Żegota, one of the characters in *Dziady*, part 3, by Adam Mickiewicz, who conspired to overthrow the Tsarist regime.

21 W. Bartoszewski and Z. Lewinówna, *Ten jest z ojczyzny mojej. Polacy z pomocą Żydom 1939–1945* (Kraków: Znak, 1966), 131.

22 Such harsh penalty for aiding Jews was in place not only in occupied Poland, but also in Serbia and in the province of Podole. Feliks Tych states that there were 700 (according to other sources 900) documented cases where Poles were killed by the Germans for trying to help Jews. It must be remembered that, in some cases, Poles were imprisoned by the Gestapo or were sent to death camps, where they were murdered, as was the case with Dr. Zofia Garlicka. F. Tych, *Długi cień zagłady* (Warsaw: Żydowski Instytut Historyczny, 1999), 116.

23 An account by Izrael Rotbalsam, YVA O.3/2357.

The majority of those who escaped from the ghetto worked as so-called free professionals before the war. Among them were doctors, lawyers, engineers, teachers and state administration officials. Some smuggled large amounts of money to the Aryan side, well ahead of time, hoping this would allow them to live relatively normally. Some even had plans for the future, trusting their Polish acquaintances. Unfortunately, many of those plans proved futile, while money and trust were irrevocably lost. Under the new rules, assimilated Jewish intelligentsia—once rich and influential people—became desperate and helpless paupers.[24]

Regardless of how dire the situation became, doctors working in the Czyste Jewish Hospital and the Bersohn and Bauman Children's Hospital, especially heads of departments, determinedly carried out their duties. But when the hospitals were turned into places where patients came to die, they saw no sense in continuing the struggle. Dr. Jakub Penson, the head of the internal diseases department, wrote:

> By mid-August 1942 there was no longer one ghetto, but streets and alleys, divided by fences and walls, surrounding the workshops. More or less at that time I decided to leave the ghetto and go to the so-called Aryan side. I saw it as my only one, small, chance to survive. Nothing was holding me back. My immediate family, closest colleagues and friends had all died, and the hospital as I knew it no longer existed. As long as there was work in the hospital, or even a semblance of normality, I had considered it my duty to stay. Now it was a parody of a hospital, because there were no patients as such. Only the victims of Hitler's hangmen remained, who did not have enough strength to walk to the wagons and were left dying in the hospital.[25]

Dr. Polisiuk noted that during the first days of the deportations, several department heads made it through to the other side and on September 5, Dr. Szenwic, his superior, left, and soon thereafter, so did Dr. Hanna

---

24  W. Meed, *Po obu stronach muru* (Warsaw: Jaworski, 2003), 211.
25  Małecka, *Jakub Penson*, 92.

Hirszfeld.[26] Dr. Henryk Makower remembered that she received a coded warning "from the other side" to hide immediately. The next day she and her family were gone.[27] They were helped by Stanisław and Maria Popowski.[28]

The next wave of those seeking refuge left during and after the January 1943 *aktion*. This time Dr. Waller left the ghetto with his wife and son on January 23. He wrote: "A leader of the Jews who worked outside the ghetto walls, who knew we were escaping, received a bribe of 500 zlotys per head."[29] They were helped by Dr. Dobrowolska (a dentist) and her husband, an army doctor.[30] Dr. Waller and his young family hid in Zielonka, in the house of a railway employee named Mroczkowski (a monthly stay there cost between 1,000 and 3,000 zlotys), and later they moved to the attic of a wooden house belonging to the Ławrynowicz family.[31]

Helena Szereszewska was convinced anyone who had the money could leave the ghetto.[32] That money went to pay the guards and leader of the checkpoint who smuggled small groups of people out among those working outside the ghetto walls. He needed to bribe the guards, but also worked to earn money for himself. In this way, Dr. Adina Blady-Szwajger passed through. In her book, she wrote her escape was just the beginning. Apart from the cost of living, those in hiding had to pay crooks and extortionists. Soon after leaving the ghetto Dr. Blady-Szwajger found herself at a crossroads, in a bustling crowd. Among them were tradesmen, waiting to buy items from those escaping the ghetto, and crooks searching for

---

26 An account by Adolf Polisiuk, "Pamiętnik w kolekcji Abrahama Adolfa Bermana" (section "Czworobok"), Ghetto Fighters' House Museum, ref. 3182. The author does not specify how many heads of departments left the ghetto at the time.

27 Makower, *Pamiętnik z getta warszawskiego*, 64.

28 Hirszfeld's daughter suffered from an incurable pituitary gland disease and died on the Aryan side in February 1943.

29 Sabina Gurfinkiel-Glocer gave a similar amount in payment for being led out by a guide. Dr. Polisiuk stated he paid 8,000 zlotys in May 1943. Jews employed outside the ghetto were called *placówkarze*, see Agnieszka Latała, Jakub Gutenbaum, and Wiktoria Sliwowska, eds., *The Last Eyewitnesses: Children of the Holocaust Speak*, transl. Fay Bussgang and Julian Bussgang (Evanston, IL: Northwestern University Press, 1998), https://books.google.co.za/books?isbn=0810115115.

30 Dr. Dobrowolska's name was not established.

31 Dr. Mordechai Lensky said the price for a hideout on the Aryan side was 5,000–7,000 zlotys a month for one person. Lensky, *A Physician Inside the Warsaw Ghetto*, 194.

32 Szereszewska, *Krzyż i mezuza*, 213.

potential prey and demanding a ransom.[33] "I heard them 'meowing'"—Dr. Blady-Szwajger wrote, "which is how they let their accomplices know a Jew was coming, but I immediately removed my armband and looked straight into their eyes with such confidence, nobody bothered me."[34]

The extortionists also looked for Jews already in hiding. Doctors—especially those who were popular before the war—had to be particularly vigilant. Sabina Gurfinkiel-Glocer wrote that Dr. Wertheim, though very well hidden, was recognized and blackmailed by a doorman at Omega Clinic, where Wertheim had worked for many years as co-owner.[35] A similar case was that of Dr. Chain, who was tracked down by extortionists after escaping from the ghetto and had gone into hiding with former patients. He admitted that although he had "bought himself out with a large sum of money, the place was no longer safe."[36]

Dr. Leopold Ebin could, at first, find nowhere to hide. He could not join his wife, who was in hiding almost from the beginning of the war, because she lied to her landlady and told her he was in Russia. Fortunately, an acquaintance gave him shelter on the condition that he hid under the bed during the day, until he could obtain fake documents and move. Ebin spent three weeks hidden in that way.[37] Later he found a place with a Polish family in the borough of Ursus but leaving Warsaw left him with no source of income. When he could no longer pay, the owner told him outright: "I can no longer house you, you must go to Pruszków."[38] At that time, leaving the hideout meant certain death. Left with no choice, Dr. Ebin responded firmly: "Yes, I will go, but you will have to come with me." That settled things. He was left in peace until January 1945.[39] Warsaw was freed on January 17, 1945.

---

33  *Szmalcownik* (an extortionist) was a person extorting ransom from the hiding Jews, or from the Poles who were helping them, threatening denunciation. This practice took place predominantly in larger cities, where ghettos were established and where Jews sought refuge on the Aryan side. More detail in Grabowski, *Ja tego Żyda znam*.

34  Blady-Szwajger, *I więcej nic nie pamiętam*, 133.

35  An account by Sabina Gurfinkiel-Glocer, "Szpital na Czystem i ja," YVA O.3/396.

36  An account by Icchok Chain (Józef Gołębiowski), YVA O.3/2355.

37  An account by Leopold Ebin, YVA O.3/440.

38  An account by Icchok Chain (Józef Gołębiowski), YVA O.3/2355.

39  Ibid.

Dr. Jerzy Gladsztern, a laborer in Döring's workshop, left the ghetto in May 1943 with a group of Poles setting out for work in Żoliborz. He agreed to work for the streetcar driver, Karolak (who was already sheltering seven Jews behind a double wall made of board, at a daily rate of 100 zlotys). "We stayed there until October 1944," Dr. Gwiazdowski noted. "A year and five months—actually, I paid Karolak some 7,000 zlotys, and gave him some medical instruments and furniture, protected by other people, who passed them on to Karolak at my request."[40]

Dr. Süsswein rented a room in an apartment in Żoliborz. In order not to raise his landlord's suspicions as to his real identity, Süsswein rented another room a few streets away, under the pretext of being involved in research. He spent entire days there pretending to work.[41]

But not everyone had friends, honest landlords or helpful patients. Jews on the Aryan side lived in constant fear. Even if they lived under reasonably good conditions and had false documents, many chose to commit suicide. Dr. Stanisław Szenicer, helped by Dr. Andrzej Trojanowski, a colleague from the university, was employed as a paramedic in Stoczek on the river Bug. He came to Warsaw to do reconstructive surgery, working with Trojanowski to reconstitute foreskins for Jewish men.[42] He himself underwent the procedure. Not being able to cope with the pressure, he committed suicide before the end of the war.

A couple, both doctors and both in hiding, planned to end their lives and that of their five-year-old son. They made the decision when, emotionally drained, the owners of the house in which they were hiding, fearing for their own safety, asked them to leave. As they prepared the three doses of poison, the son suddenly started to scream that he wanted to live. They abandoned their plan and began looking for an alternative solution. Help came in the form of Dr. Wacław Skonieczny, who got the father a job as a doorman at a clinic in the Jerozolimskie Avenue. The job meant the family could live in a tiny room off the entrance hall, and that is where they remained until the Warsaw Uprising in August 1944.[43]

---

40  An account by Jerzy Gladsztern-Gwiazdowski, Jewish Historical Institute Archives, ref. 301/2098.

41  Szereszewska, *Krzyż i mezuza*, 317.

42  An account by Anna Szenicer-Matusiak, August 27, 1965, Jewish Historical Institute Archives, ref. 301/6147.

43  Blady-Szwajger, *I więcej nic nie pamiętam*, 237.

A suicide, especially in the case of a person who had no Aryan documents, caused serious problems for whoever sheltered him or her. Jadwiga Hennert, a famous singer and the daughter of Prof. Maurycy Hurwicz, tried to poison herself while her landlady had visitors, but was revived. Szereszewska wrote:

> Something like this was considered bad manners. Had she not been revived, what then? Police, statements, investigation. It would have been very damaging to Ada [Szerszewska's relative], even though she had a Swedish passport. At this time, a Jew or Jewess with Aryan papers would have been advised not to expose their landlords if they wished to endanger themselves. They could rather poison themselves in a field, in a secluded path in a park, on the staircase of some random house.[44]

Putting one's landlords in a position of having to organize a burial for an undocumented person was tantamount to placing them and their family in mortal danger.

Some doctors decided to send their children to live outside the ghetto. Dr. Stein placed his seven-year-old daughter Ludwika on the Aryan side, and sometimes managed to slip out to see her.[45] He planned to join her, but by the time he decided to do so, it was too late.[46] Dr. Anna Braude-Heller found a home for her son Arie, his wife, and her little granddaughter outside the ghetto. Bubi, the son of her sister, Dr. Róża Aftergut, left the ghetto with his aunt, Judyta Braude, and Dr. Bolesław Ałapin and his wife sent their two-year-old son Piotr away rather than keeping him in the ghetto.

Dr. Stanisława Ałapin-Rubiłłowicz recalled:

> I remember how Bolek [her husband] and I looked through a window in the court building (one entrance was on the ghetto side in Leszno Street, the other on the Aryan side) as a cleaner led our little son out of the building on her way home from work, holding him by the hand as she would her own child. My heart stopped when they passed a German soldier guarding

---

44 Szereszewska, *Krzyż i mezuza*, 284.
45 Stabholz, *Siedem piekieł*, 89.
46 An account by Sabina Gurfinkiel-Glocer, "Szpital na Czystem i ja," YVA O.3/396.

the entrance to the building: would he stop them? Would he kill them? . . . Our friends placed little Piotr in Milanówek, in a monastery belonging to the Order of St. Ursula, where he survived as Piotr Pietraszkiewicz.[47]

Sabina and Władysław Glocer sent their daughter, Lilusia, to live with the Wojciechowski's family. When they escaped from the ghetto, they initially lived in Mrs. Szandrowski's guesthouse, but constant visits from Polish police and even the Gestapo, forced them to move in with the family of a railroad employee, where they remained until the Warsaw Uprising began. Financially, they received some support from Franciszek Puncuch, the Yugoslavian Consul in Warsaw.

Dr. Halina Szenicer-Rotstein placed her four children on the Aryan side. The sister of her first husband, Halina Szenicer, took seven-year-old Robert and six-year-old Jan out of the ghetto; six-year-old Wanda (Jan's twin sister) and two-year-old Staś were taken out by Dr. Janina Radlińska. All four children eventually ended up in the Anusia Home, an orphanage in Konstancin for the children of deceased Polish officers.

In the second half of January 1943, Henryk Bryskier and his wife Felicja (a dentist) sent their daughter out of the ghetto as well. Felicja was killed during the Ghetto Uprising, while her husband was deported to Majdanek, where he managed to escape. He returned to Warsaw and hid in an apartment on Chełmska Street under the false name of Władysław Jankowski. Blackmailed by extortionists, in May 1944 he joined his daughter who was hidden in the borough of Praga. Both survived the war.

Some adults were forced to return to the ghetto, while children were brought back once the money for their upkeep ran out. Dr. Rotbalsam hid on the Aryan side in January 1943, where he remained for a short while only before he was blackmailed and had to return to the ghetto.[48] Helena Szereszewska described another case:

While walking along Kurza Street, I met Dr. Ałapin, our neighbor from Walicowów Street. "My wife," he told me, "moved to the Aryan side with our son, but they came back." I was

---

47  T. Nasierowski, "Bolesław Ałapin (1913–1985)," *Postępy Psychiatrii i Neurologii* 2, no. 4 (1995): 193.

48  An account by Izrael Rotbalsam, YVA O.3/2357.

surprised. Why would she come back after leaving? "Because she had nowhere to sleep." So, it sometimes happened that there was nowhere to sleep. The ground on the other side had to be prepared very thoroughly before one went there.[49]

Usually, Jews discovered on the Aryan side were shot on the spot. Such was the fate of Dr. Natalia Zylberblast-Zand, who was arrested in her friend's apartment. The friend was Dr. Zofia Garlicka, head of the Gynecology and Obsetrics Department at the Ujazdowski Hospital.[50] Dr. Garlicka's apartment was a safe haven for couriers ("the silent and unseen") and escapees from POW camps.[51] On August 11, 1941, the Gestapo burst into a house on Topolowa Street and arrested everyone present. Dr. Zand was executed in the ghetto, while Dr. Garlicka and her daughter, Zofia Jankowska, contracted typhus and died in Auschwitz. English POWs were imprisoned in Pawiak.[52]

From fall 1942 onward, Jews captured on the Aryan side were usually shot in the ghetto around Pawiak Prison. But there were exceptions. Dr. Anna Messing and her mother were led by German gendarmes to the ghetto, locked in the prison on Gęsia Street, and then taken to the *Umschlagplatz*. Because there were no regular deportations at the time, they managed to escape and after paying a bribe, made their way back to the Aryan side.[53]

In September 1942, the Government Delegation for Poland, a branch of the Polish Government in Exile, established the Provisional Committee to Aid Jews, consisting mainly of Catholic and democratic activists. This committee that provided help to 180 persons, was led by Zofia Kossak-Szczucka and Wanda Krahelska-Filipowicz. In December

---

49  Szereszewska, *Krzyż i mezuza*,. Dr. Bolesław Ałapin left the ghetto on August 1, 1942. His wife escaped as well.

50  M. Ciesielska, "Dr. Zofia Garlicka (1874–1942)—lekarz ginekolog, przewodnicząca Zrzeszenia Lekarek Polskich, więźniarka Pawiaka i obozu koncentracyjnego Auschwitz-Birkenau," *Acta Medicorum Polonorum* 4 (2014): 79–91.

51  S. Bayer, *Służba Zdrowia Warszawy w walce z okupantem 1939-1945* (Warsaw: MON, 1985), 266. "The silent and unseen" (*cichociemni*) were the elite special-operations paratroops of the Polish Army in Exile, created in Great Britain during the Second World War to operate in occupied Poland. See "Cichociemni," Wikipedia, https://en.wikipedia.org/wiki/Cichociemni.

52  Ciesielska, "Dr. Zofia Garlicka."

53  Szereszewska, *Krzyż i mezuza*, 198.

1942 the committee was dissolved, and the Council to Aid Jews, code-named Żegota, was formed with Julian Grobelny as president.[54] Its purpose was to provide wide-ranging help to Jews hiding on the Aryan side and those in forced labor camps.

To facilitate patient care, a medical section employed trusted Poles and a number of Jewish doctors who made house calls. Żegota doctors were paid directly by the council (on average 100 zlotys per visit). In the opinion of Basia Temkin-Bermano, the medical section lasted just a few months and was not particularly popular. Organizing a visit was complicated, and the waiting time was usually a couple of days. A liaison would report the patient's address to the office, sometimes using a password, and the next day, a section employee would check to see if everything was in order. Only then would a doctor arrive. Those in hiding were reluctant to acquaint strangers with the details of their whereabouts. Most often, a visit was arranged with a doctor who came recommended for his honesty and courage. Such a doctor had to know how to behave in unusual circumstances and remain discreet.[55]

> In many cases, Jewish doctors also helped. Their work was more difficult because they could not prescribe medicines. One doctor, a young Miss Rozental . . . received a stamp from her friend with a similar surname and issued prescriptions in her name. Dr. Landsberg practiced on his colleagues. When Jarosław [Roth] called him to attend to [Stanisław] Michalski, his dear friend, and landlord with a heart problem, Landsberg pretended to be a paramedic. . . Gynecologist Polisiuk performed procedures in his home, but only accepted trustworthy persons, because his stay in the apartment was not completely legal. Most Jewish doctors did not practice, because despite their acceptable appearance (fair-skinned) they were reluctant to appear in public for fear their faces would be known to too many people.[56]

Before the war, Halina Szpilfogel married Kazimierz Cetnarowicz, a Polish colleague from her years in the Scout Movement. Because she had

54  Prekerowa, "Pomoc lekarska ukrywającym się Żydom," 113.
55  B. Temkin-Bermanowa, *Dziennik z podziemia* (Warsaw: Twój Styl, Żydowski Instytut Historyczny, 2000), 130–131.
56  Ibid., 134.

"proper Aryan papers," she did not live in the ghetto. She and her husband agreed to hide Henryk Frydman, a doctor from Zofiówka, who had false documents under the assumed name of Falęcki, an officer. By then, Frydman had moved from place to place, not sleeping in one place for longer than two nights. In the end, with the help of Cetnarowicz's cousin, he found lodging with a widow on Saska Kępa. Because of his so-called "good appearance" (light-colored hair, blue eyes) he could move around the suburb, go to the library and give private lessons.[57]

Dr. Henryk Halpern-Wieliczański, an internist specializing in lung diseases at the Jewish Hospital of the Poznański Family Foundation in Łódź, was also spared the ghetto. During the German occupation he lived in Warsaw with his Polish wife, Teodozja Maria, and their daughter, Zosia. In October 1942, the Wieliczańskis employed a nanny, Sara Celnik, under the assumed name of Stefania Pabiańska. The couple befriended her and helped her materially. After the war, she wrote that many times she witnessed the couple assisting people in need.

An important aspect of a doctor's work, when helping those in hiding, was issuing death certificates, essential for burials. They also authorized medical treatment in hospital infirmaries (for a few months, Jews could obtain documents certifying them as war invalids from the Ujazdowski Hospital—documents that allowed them to leave the ghetto) and issued certificates excusing individuals from compulsory vaccinations.[58] These exemptions were important for men who, despite having Aryan documents, were not sure they could pass on their appearance and physical attributes, especially men afraid of being unmasked during physical inspections and intensive scrutiny at a vaccination station. Avoiding vaccination without a valid certified excuse meant losing one's food stamps.[59]

Another tool in the doctors' arsenal to save lives was reconstructive surgery. Rhinoplasty was most popular, as people wanted to make their noses look "less Jewish".[60] Another popular operation was foreskin

57  Szereszewska, *Krzyż i mezuza*, 314–315.
58  M. Ciesielska, "Dr. Szczepan Wacek—lekarz, żołnierz, więzień," *Acta Medicorum Polonorum* 3 (2013): 14–28.
59  Temkin-Bermanowa, *Dziennik z podziemia*, 333.
60  Rhinoplasties were performed by doctors Edmund Mroczek, Janusz Skórski, Stanisław Michałek-Grodzki, Janina Radlińska, Andrzej Trojanowski, Józef Dryjski, Mieczysław Tylicki, Wojciech Staszewski, and Stanisław Białecki. J. Skórski,

reconstruction.[61] Even before the ghetto was sealed off, Dr. Ludwik Koenigstein asked Dr. Kanabus to "uncircumcise him," and if the procedure proved successful, to do the same for his son.[62] The first procedure was performed in Koenigstein's apartment in Warsaw's Old Town, with his son as the next patient. During the surgery, Kanabus was assisted by his wife, Dr. Irena Kanabus. Later, Dr. Jan Rutkiewiczor and Adam Gutgisser (Edward Drozdowicz) stepped in—the latter was in hiding despite carrying Aryan papers. Dr. Helena Landy-Budzilewicz, Kanabus' mother-in-law, acted as anesthetist. Together, they also performed rhinoplasties—a procedure not performed at home since it was too dangerous, and in an emergency, the patient would have to be transported through the city, revealing the identity and address of the surgeon. More complicated procedures were done in the Children's Health Clinic or the hospital infirmary on Kopernik Street.[63] Dr. Kanabus performed approximately seventy such procedures. Many such operations were also performed by Doctors Janusz Skórski and Andrzej Trojanowski, who were assisted by Stanisław Szenicer, a Jewish doctor in hiding.[64]

Many Aryan doctors tried to help their prewar colleagues and acquaintances (see appendix 7). Soon after the ghetto was established in 1940, Dr. Aleksandra Rowińska, a pediatrician at the Transfiguration of the Lord Hospital in Warsaw's Praga district, took in and cared for her university colleague, Dr. Róża Herman. When Herman's presence in

---

"*Repraeputiatio glandis.* Operacje na obrzezanych. Rys historyczny i technika," *Archiwum Historii i Filozofii Medycyny* 1, no. 64 (2001): 17–35.

61 Foreskin reconstruction was performed by doctors Feliks Kanabus, Andrzej Trojanowski, Janusz Skórski, Stanisław Michałek-Grodzki, Józef Kubiak, Józef Dryjski, Wojciech Wiechno, Stanisław Grocholski, Sergiusz Boryszewski, Stefan Wesołowski, Janina Radlińska, Leszek Aleksandrowicz, Mieczysław Tylicki, and Stanisław Białecki as well as Jewish doctors Stanisław Szenicer and Adam Gutgisser. Skórski, "*Repraeputiatio glandis,*" 17–35.

62 A. Jerzmanowska, "Lekarze czasów zagłady,"*Gazeta Wyborcza*, September 18, 2014, http://wyborcza.pl/alehistoria/1,121681,16671740,Lekarze_czasow_zaglady.html, accessed: March 29, 2017. Dr. Stanisław Grocholski also performed approximately fifteen such procedures; his patients were Adam Gutgisser and Dawid Epstein. Adam Gutgisser remembered that he assisted during his own operation, during which he had to sit, and while his operation was successful, his friend's was not.

63 Anka Grupińska and Paweł Szapiro refer to the fragments of Feliks Kanabus's oral account, which was written down by Helena Kozłowska. See footnotes in Temkin-Bermanowa, *Dziennik z podziemia*, 335.

64 Skórski, "*Repraeputiatio glandis,*" 34.

her apartment drew unwelcome attention, Rowińska moved her to a village in Lublin province, where her friend eventually survived the war. Dr. Rowińska cooperated with Żegota to help others, turning her apartment into a transit point before fugitives were relocated to monasteries or other hiding places.

Dr. Emil Paluch helped Dr. Henryk Makower when he and his wife escaped from the ghetto in January 1943, while Dr. Wacław Skonieczny, who saved Dr. Dora Keilson, Dr. Feliks Kanabus and his wife, Irena, née Budzilewicz, hid many of their Jewish colleagues.[65] Dr. Ewa Rajewska, a doctor in the outpatient clinic and in the Internal Diseases Department of St. Roch Hospital, concealed her school friend, Maria Wilk, her husband Dr. Severyn Wilk, and their seven-year-old son Aleksander in her apartment. Both Dr. Rajewska and her mother, active in the resistance, facilitated contact between Dr. Wilk and Stanisław Steczkowski, a major in the Home Army, who organized false documents in the name of Wilczyński for the entire family. He found work for Dr. Wilk by introducing him as a Polish officer in hiding. Thanks to his job, the family was allocated an apartment. Dr. Seweryn Wilk-Wilczyński was sworn into the Home Army, and when the Warsaw Uprising started, he reported for duty as a doctor to Group "Gurt," at 58 Złota Street which served as a sanitary center and later became a hospital.[66]

A month before the Ghetto Uprising began, Dr. Zdzisław Askanas and his family escaped to the Aryan side. In a letter to the author, his son, Dr. Aleksander Askanas, described those times:

> My father was a tall, blond man with blue eyes, very thin when in the ghetto (like almost everyone else). He had multiple boils on his back from malnutrition and a vitamin deficiency and became ill with typhus (a patient infected him). During the *Grossaktion*,

---

65 Dr. Feliks Kanabus and his wife, Dr. Irena Kanabus (née Budzilewicz) hid Dr. Maria Tursz in their apartment for two years, while her husband was led out of the ghetto by Dr. Kanabus himself, who found him another shelter. The Kanabus couple also hid Dr. Zdzisław Askanas, his seven-year-old son Alexander, Dr. Bronisław Wiśniewski and Jan Fuerstenberg. See J. Rytlowa, *Wywiad z Martą Jerzmanowską, córką Feliksa i Ireny Kanabusów* (Warsaw: n.p., 2010); "Rodzina Kanabusów," Polscy Sprawiedliwi, https://sprawiedliwi.org.pl/pl/historie-pomocy/historia-pomocy-rodzina-kanabusow, accessed March 27, 2017.

66 B. Szerszyński, "Dr. Seweryn Stefan Wilk-Wilczyński (June 26, 1896–October 16, 1978)," *Polski Przegląd Chirurgiczny* 51 (1971): 1246–1247.

we tried to change apartments to avoid deportation to Treblinka, but towards the end of the *Grossaktion* we were captured and taken to the *Umschlagplatz*, where we miraculously managed to escape. My father designed and built many shelters and hideouts for us and others. We escaped from the ghetto a month before the uprising, on my fifth birthday, March 19, 1943. We emerged from under a bundle of rags on a large horse-drawn delivery cart. The wife of a regimental commander from Modlin, the charming Mrs. Zając, aided the families of regimental officers. She organized our first and subsequent apartments on the Aryan side, and we remained friends with her for many years after the war. After escaping from the ghetto, my father, who had a so-called "good appearance," appeared in public just as all other Poles did. Nevertheless, a university doorman denounced him. In the Home Army my father had been known as "Lieutenant Janek," and after the Warsaw Uprising, he organized a hospital near Kampinos for the local population and the large number of Home Army forces.[67]

Thanks to the help and persuasion of Prof. Edward Loth, Dr. Ludwik Stabholz escaped from the ghetto a week before the uprising. He met up with his wife Maria (a nurse and surgical assistant) and his mother (Franciszka, née Marienstrass) in a rented apartment.

After my escape from the Warsaw Ghetto in March 1943, I remained in the city as the holder of Aryan papers. Under the assumed name of Bolesław Dziedzic, I rented an apartment on Waliców Street, where I lived with my wife and mother. . . But we did not feel safe and decided to leave Warsaw. Mrs. Halina Lewandowska, a Polish woman from Otwock, helped us. She accompanied my wife as she went to rent an apartment in Miłosna, near Warsaw. Moving to a village brought new difficulties. There, where typically people know their neighbors, I had to justify my stubborn insistence on staying indoors, or I could easily have been suspected of being a Jew. Prof. Loth,

---

67  Letter by Dr. Aleksander Askanas (son of Prof. Zdzisław Askanas) to the author, dated June 1, 2017.

whose student I had been before the war, helped me. He deserves a separate mention.

Prof. Loth had been a distinguished scholar and anatomist, well known in Poland and abroad. However, this famous scientist was also widely known as a Jew-hater (żydożerca). He had been one of those at Warsaw University who fervently propagated and supported the idea of the "bench ghetto". He also embraced *numerus clausus*. And now, this enemy of the Jews became my savior. How to explain this change, this problem with Prof. Loth? I must add that, during the occupation, he tried to help me as much as he could, even before I left for the village. He offered me money, wanted to use his influence to send me and my family abroad, together with residents of the "Polish Hotel." He even tried to find a job for me.[68] With this in mind, he gave me a letter recommending me to an acquaintance, Mrs. Korsun, asking her to "find a tutor position with a Mr. Szostek for *magister* Dziedzic" (as he called me).

When I went to Miłosna, I had to justify staying indoors. I feigned having a broken leg. Prof. Loth came to Miłosna specially to put a plaster cast on my healthy leg. The arrival of such a prominent scientist to perform the procedure in person served to allay any doubts in even the most suspicious. The question still remains, though: Why did Prof. Loth do this? What changed his attitude towards the Jews? Well, as he told me during our conversation, he considered the Germans' behavior towards the Jews to be a crime against humanity and decided to oppose that with all his might.[69]

The final symbolic act of helping the Jews took place in November of 1944. Zofia Frydman and Maria Feinmesser turned to Dr. Stanisława Śwital, who

---

68 The events associated with Hotel Polski are treated in detail in Agnieszka Haska, *Jestem Żydem, chcę wejść. Hotel Polski w Warszawie, 1943* (Warsaw: Centrum Badań nad Zagładą Żydów, 2006). Germans lured the Jews who had passports of South American countries under the pretext that they will be deported to special camps in France and Germany as part of a swap deal. Among those who came to the hotel were Doctors Jan Przedborski (murdered in Auschwitz), Aleksandra Chorążycka-Wajntal and her father, Dr. Borys Chorążycki.

69 An account by Ludwik Stabholz, YVA O.3/861.

worked at the City Council Health Center no. 3, and asked him evacuate fighters from the ŻOB from a cellar on Promyk Street. During the Warsaw Uprising, Dr. Śwital had served as an ensign (code name Wronowski) in the Home Army headquarters, in Warsaw's northern Downtown District. When the insurgents were defeated, he left Warsaw with the city's civilian population, and managed a small Red Cross hospital on the outskirts of Warsaw, in Boernerowo.[70] When the Ghetto Uprising failed, the fighters remained in hiding, under exceedingly difficult conditions, exhausted and increasingly exposed to the danger of discovery. The female fighters had managed to escape a few days earlier, and after reaching the transit camp in Pruszków, met up with Dr. Anna Margolis, who worked there as a nurse. With a letter of recommendation from Dr. Lesław Węgrzynowicz (code name Bartosz), a former Sanitary Chief in the Home Army, they turned to Dr. Śwital.[71] He immediately organized a rescue mission, in which Kazimierz Syłkiewicz (real name Józef Żyłkiewicz), his wife Maria (a medical student), Barbara Kinkiel, Zbigniew Ściwiarski, Janusz Osęka, and Ala Margolis participated.[72] Among the fighters rescued from the cellar were Doctor Teodozja Goliborska and the hospital runner, Marek Edelman.[73]

---

70  Dr. Stanisław Śwital rendered help to Jews in the ghetto. In summer 1943, for several weeks he treated the burn wounds of a three-year-old Jewish boy and found refuge for him and his mother with one of his friends. He visited them frequently, bringing them food, and when the health of the boy improved, he moved them both to Blizne, the village where the child's mother worked in horticulture. See D. Polak, "Siedmioro z ulicy Promyka," http://www.goniec.net/goniec/inne-dzialy/reportaze-gonca/siedmioro-z-ulicy-promyka.html, accessed March 27, 2017; "Pamiętnik Józefa Żyłkiewicza (Kazimierza Syłkiewicza)," Jewish Historical Institute Archives, ref. 302/199.

71  D Polak, "Siedmioro z ulicy Promyka."

72  After the war it became known that only one of them were of Jewish origin.

73  Among them also were Icchak Cukierman, Cywia Lubetkin, Tuwie Borzykowski, Julian Fiszgrund, and Zygmunt Warman.

# Chapter 10

# Resistance by the Medical Fraternity

## The Underground Medical School

With the Germans determined to dehumanize and humiliate the Jews in the ghetto, preventing intellectual, artistic and spiritual activities, anyone or any group involved in lifting people out of their misery practiced a form of resistance to the German onslaught on their souls and bodies. That included learning Torah and praying, educating children, putting together theatrical performances and night club acts, and in the case of the doctors, creating an underground medical school.

When the authorities ordered paramedic training to combat epidemics and support prevention, the course developed into a *de facto* underground medical school in the ghetto.[1] The course organizer was Docent Juliusz Zweibaum.[2] Dr. Ludwik Stabholz recalled that Dr. Edward Loth, the well-known anatomist and university professor, was the first to suggest using the Germans' plans to help combat infections to organize secret educational initiatives.[3]

---

1   R. Zabłotniak, "Wydział Lekarski w getcie warszawskim," *Biuletyn Żydowskiego Instytutu Historycznego* 2, no. 74 (1970): 82.
2   An account by Juliusz Zweibaum, "Informacje w sprawie szkolnictwa wyższego w getcie warszawskim," Jewish Historical Institute Archives, ref. 301/4108.
3   An account by Ludwik Stabholz, YVA O.3/861. Dr. Loth was known to support "bench ghettos" and *numerus clausus* before the war.

Dr. Milejkowski created a teaching council to develop a curriculum. A subcommittee was elected, including Professors M. Centnerszwer, Lachs, Hirszfeld, and associate Zweibaum.[4] The official announcement was published in the *Jewish Gazette*, May 9, 1941.

> With the permission of the German authorities, a course in paramedic training to combat epidemics will be offered under the patronage of the *Judenrat*'s Health Department. Youths of both genders will be able to acquire basic knowledge and participate actively in combating the threat of epidemics. The purpose of the course is to train sanitary instructors, disinfection officers and auxiliary personnel.[5]

Those who attended the course were excused from doing compulsory work. News that the course would be similar to a medical education was passed on by word of mouth. The official launch took place in the great hall of the *Judenrat*, most probably on May 17, 1941.[6]

The *Jewish Gazette* published the following brief commentary:

> A few days ago, the great hall of the Jewish Association witnessed the formal inauguration of sanitary courses aimed at combatting epidemics. After the welcoming address by Docent Dr. Zweibaum, the inaugural lecture was delivered by Dr. I. Milejkowski, who noted the monumental importance of the courses, while the director of the Czyste Jewish Hospital, Dr. Stein, spoke about "life and death." Lecturers for the courses, who have been recruited from highly respected scientific circles, are distinguished specialists in their respective fields of medical knowledge. The courses have been met with great interest on the part of the public and are frequented by a large number of

---

4   H. Balicka-Kozłowska, "Tajne studia medyczne w getcie warszawskim," in *Tajne nauczanie medycyny i farmacji w latach 1939–1945*, ed. Aleksander Dawidowicz (Warsaw: PZWL, 1977), 246.

5   *Gazeta Żydowska* 37 (1941): 3.

6   The account of the inauguration appeared in the *Gazeta Żydowska* 42, May 27, 1941. The first sentence read: "A few days ago, the Great Conference Hall of the *Judenrat* witnessed an inauguration ceremony for courses enabling paramedics to deal with epidemics." Of the dates found in the literature, May 17, 1941, seems the most probable.

attendees. Given their popularity, the organizers have decided to institute a parallel course with an identical program, relying on the same staff. An independent course for doctors involved in combating epidemics was also introduced on May 17.[7]

Dr. Jerzy Szapiro recalled that the first-year course was the most popular, with over 200 students. Several dozen students were admitted to the second year, students from medical faculties who passed the first-year course before the war.[8] Dr. Zweibaum saw an opportunity to give young people some purpose, some hope of a better life by helping them fill idle hours plagued by stress and fear. The students hailed from more affluent families, but they, too, were affected by food shortages, fear, disease, and the deaths of their relatives. Dr. Fenigsztein, who taught elementary anatomy to first-year students and pathological anatomy to third-year students, said teaching under those horrendous circumstances gave him tremendous pleasure.

> I enjoyed teaching people who wanted to learn then, and I enjoy teaching people who want to learn now. . . In the Warsaw Ghetto, teaching those eager young people was much like an ego trip for me: that's how much satisfaction I derived from it. . . There were no artificial barriers between teachers and students. The teachers helped as much as they could, spending as much time as possible with each individual, applying a good dose of irreverent humor. We worked hard, yet we often found time to joke, chat and laugh. It was necessary to relieve the tension.[9]

The image of youths concentrating and eager to learn resonated in Zweibaum's memories.

The so-called Collegium on Leszno Street was a venue for these courses. Although formally located outside of the ghetto walls, administratively it belonged to the ghetto. To reach the building, students passed through a gate guarded by German, Polish and Jewish Police. Eventually, an overhead walkway was built to link the lecture hall with the ghetto. Lectures were held on the fifth floor in the afternoons,

---

7   *Gazeta Żydowska* 42 (1941): 3.
8   Szapiro, "Tajne studia medycyny w getcie."
9   Fenigstein, "Holocaust and I," 129, 130–131.

between 5 and 8 p.m., so students could get home before curfew. The hall was unheated, and because there was no proper lighting, candles and carbide lamps were used. Lectures were remarkably popular, so a parallel course was organized in the polyclinic belonging to the Warsaw Emergency Services.

The fee for the course was about forty zlotys, but many people relied on discounts and stipends. Lecturers were paid, some as much as 1,000 zlotys per month. Their duties included lecturing, publishing tutorial notes, preparing tables and teaching aids. Students from the Graphic Design College on Sienna Street helped prepare the teaching aids. The *Judenrat* did not support the courses financially, but in May 1942, Czerniaków contributed 10,000 zlotys to the cause. Practical classes were conducted at Czyste and in a laboratory on Stawki Street. Microscopic specimens were supplied by Warsaw University's Institute of Histology and Embryology, and textbooks were delivered from the Aryan side, thanks to Professors Loth and Bronisława Konopacka. Substantive supervision of courses on the Aryan side was provided by Prof. Witold Orłowski.[10]

Lectures on epidemiology and infectious diseases were organized to validate the character of the course and the need for practical training. As a rule, the Germans did not intrude on the lectures or practical classes for fear of contagion. During the "semester," the Germans performed just a single inspection. To deflect suspicion about the real purpose of the courses, in case of a sudden inspection, the chalkboards in the lecture halls usually featured the names of various disinfectants.

In April 1942, the *Jewish Gazette* announced a second round of recruitments for the six-month long paramedics training course.[11] Nine basic subjects were listed, along with the names of the lecturers in charge of each (see appendix 9).

The lectures were very popular and open to all. More than forty doctors and university professors participated in the underground lectures. By 1940, several professors, docents and assistants from Warsaw University, along with many renowned doctors, were living in the ghetto. Many of them were distinguished specialists in their respective fields with considerable scholarly achievements and teaching experience.

---

10  Balicka-Kozłowska, "Tajne studia medyczne," 246.
11  *Gazeta Żydowska* 39 (1942): 3.

Dr. Zweibaum, a docent of natural sciences, became associate professor of histology and embryology, teaching in two departments, medicine and veterinary medicine. He organized the first tissue culture in Poland.[12] Prof. Hirszfeld managed the State Hygiene Institute in Warsaw, while world-renowned bacteriologist and immunologist Dr. Henryk Brokman was a senior assistant in the Pediatric Clinic. Docents such as Dr. Henryk Lewenfisz worked in the Laryngology and Otiatrics Clinic, while Władysław Sterling lectured on neurology to university students and students registered with the Free Polish University.

Those who managed to survive continued their academic careers after the war, among them, Prof. Brokman in pediatrics and Prof. Aniela Gelbard (Zofia Majewska) in neurology. Prof. Wilhelm Szenwic (Włodzimierz Sowiński) became a gynecologist. Dr. Herman Eufemiusz created a department and clinic for nervous illnesses at Łódź University, and in 1953, became director of the clinic at the Warsaw Medical Academy. Prof. Hirszfeld and his wife, Dr. Hanna Hirszfeld, continued their academic careers in the Medical Faculty at the University of Wrocław. In 1945 he became director of the Institute for Medical Microbiology at Wrocław and dean of the medical faculty. Despite her painful memories of the ghetto, Janina Bauman attended one of Prof. Hirszfeld's lectures, which she remembered as lucid and fascinating.[13] It is interesting that when students first heard that Prof. Hirszfeld was going to give a lecture, they planned to boycott because they heard rumors that he believed they were believers in racial theories, which he intended to debunk. Milejkowski persuaded them to abandon both the idea of a demonstration before the lecture and of its boycott.[14]

Prof. Hirszfeld obtained Dr. Hagen's permission to present a supplementary course in epidemiology, partially financed by the *Judenrat* for students who passed the first *rigorosum* before the war, or those who completed basic sciences at the former Lviv University (which remained open until 1941). The course was meant to cover material of the third, fourth and fifth years of medical studies. The students were not divided into groups, and no formal routine was observed. The majority worked

12  "Życiorys Juliusza Zweibauma" ("Biography of Juliusz Zweibaum"), undated typescript made available by his granddaughter, Zofia Karłowicz-Perzyńska.
13  Bauman, *Zima o poranku*, 73.
14  Szapiro, "Tajne studia medycyny w getcie."

in hospitals and attended Prof. Hirszfeld's lectures, with a few dozen of them enrolled in the so-called clinical course in mid-1941. One of them was Jerzy Szapiro, who after the war wrote:

> The news was that Zweibaum's "nursery school," as the jealous older colleagues called the first and second year of underground medicine, would soon become part of a faculty. That was because third-, fourth-, and fifth-year clinical studies were to begin, in full cooperation with, and under the auspices of, Warsaw University's Medical Faculty. . . It was a revelation. The emergence of underground studies, masquerading as courses to prepare specialists to combat epidemics (mainly typhus), was manna from heaven: several hundred young people, wasting away in mediocrity and survival mode without any prospects, were given a chance to study, to obtain a medical education, and embark on a life path that would allow them to reclaim their dignity—a form of active resistance to a life of slavery under the occupation. The news was a revelation to us older students who were doing our clinical years that we were starting off in a better position than our younger colleagues. The news was remarkable, simply exciting. An inspiring vision of the road to a diploma was fashioned for us, a road we could not even dream of before: studies under the auspices of Warsaw University meant they would count, and our exams would be accepted. . . We could be useful, and at the same time we could satisfy our hunger for knowledge, develop our practical skills and gain priceless experience. We became members of a team (or teams) whose functions and existence refused to accept a mediocre life. And this was already more than a refuge. It was an oasis. It became obvious that it mattered with whom we interacted at this oasis.[15]

The first round of final exams for the students attending Zweibaum's courses were held before a commission in the spring of 1942. Successful students received certificates generally honored after the war. This was possible because the Pedagogical Council kept credits for the courses

---

15  Ibid.

and exam results up to date, passing them on to the underground faculty board at Warsaw University.

Zweibaum, who believed the lectures would be accredited in the future, kept this in mind from the beginning. Older students were not subjected to a strict time frame—they could come to the lecturer and ask to be examined whenever they felt ready. Students received credits for specific examinations by obtaining written statements from their professors, though after the war this rather informal mode of learning presented some difficulties when it came to receiving credits for a particular year of study.

About 500 students participated in the courses, among them a few pharmaceutical students, whose courses were organized by Hirszfeld.[16] More student admissions were envisioned for the academic year of 1942/1943. It was hoped that the seminar-like nature of the work would make it possible to complete the material within three years, following Warsaw University's undergraduate medical qualifications.[17]

The graduates of 1941/1942 held a dance. Soon after that, most of the students and lecturers were deported to Treblinka. Only fifty students from the so-called underground university came to Warsaw University after the war to have their credits verified.[18]

## The Blum-Bielicka School of Nursing

Some nurses were recruited from courses organized in the ghetto under the auspices of the *Judenrat*. These were mainly classes for paramedics in the Jewish Emergency Services (managed by Dr. Leon Jabłoński), courses for paramedics in the nursing division at the Jewish Health Chamber and nursing classes managed by Ala Grynberg-Gołąb, the pioneer of social nursing services in Poland.[19]

Many nurses were trained at the Blum-Bielicka School of Nursing. At the beginning of the occupation, the school had served as an administrative building of the Old Order Jewish Czyste Hospital. Once the

16 Balicka-Kozłowska, "Tajne studia medyczne," 252.
17 Zabłotniak, "Wydział Lekarski," 83.
18 Balicka-Kozłowska, "Tajne studia medyczne," 252.
19 An account by Ada Sztrumfeld, Jewish Historical Institute Archives, ref. 301/4262; Blum-Bielicka, "Szkoła Pielęgniarstwa," 75.

ghetto was established, in November 1940, the school and its boarding house were moved to the ghetto with Blum-Bielicka as director[20] who was reputed to have "ruled [the school] with an iron fist." The *Judenrat* arranged for the school to be relocated in the Social Insurance Company building at the corner of Mariańska and Pańska Streets.

"The house on Mariańska was large, so one could forget we were in the ghetto."[21] On the ground floor, one student was always on desk duty, and a portrait of Florence Nightingale hung in the corridor. The director's office was next to the entrance. It had an extra room where she lived with her two children. There was a lecture hall and a classroom for demonstrations and hands-on practice. It had a bed for practicing how to make beds, an examination table, a medicine cabinet ,and a special doll, the size of a five-month-old baby.

The students' dormitories, on the first and second floors, contained ten to twelve beds each, arranged in rows, covered with clean white linen and blankets. The kitchen and dining room were in the basement. Every morning, two students set the table, setting out white cups and plates with the day's portions of bread. Each week those portions shrank—the girls were stealing bread for their relatives in the ghetto.[22]

Classes started on January 10, 1941, with the best hospital doctors as teachers, among them Emil Apfelbaum, Ignacy Borkowski, Eufemiusz Herman, Emma Mościsker, Jan Przedborski, Sara Syrkin-Binsztejn, Dawid Wdowiński and Maria Wilk. Alina Margolis-Edelman wrote that the students were scrupulously taught an entire range of medical issues.[23]

The students, in their characteristic pink short-sleeved dresses with starched collars, white pinafores and caps, and blue capes, looked like "pink flower petals, perhaps cyclamens and, in their brightness, cleanliness and pastel colors, created the impression of being illusory creatures, apparitions that appeared out of the blue."[24] The girls protected those capes for the long term. Dressed in their uniforms, they walked the

20 Ibid., 37; A. Grupińska, "Myśmy tam żyły jak w jakimś azylu," interview with Alina Margolis-Edelman, *Tygodnik Powszechny*, May 9, 2004, https://www.tygodnikpowszechny.pl/mysmy-tam-zyly-jak-w-jakims-azylu-125305, accessed March 22, 2017.
21 Margolis-Edelman, *Ala z "Elementarza,"* 34.
22 Ibid., 37.
23 Ibid., 35.
24 Grupińska, "Myśmy tam żyły jak w jakimś azylu."

ghetto streets to the hospitals where they gained practical experience—to the Mother and Child Center on Śliska Street and to deportation stations. Thanks to their endless sacrifice tending to the sick, their place in the tragic history of the ghetto is secure. They helped wherever it was needed—something as simple as bringing a bottle of water to a patient or offering words of consolation to those waiting for deportation on the *Umschlagplatz*.

Not all nurses served in hospitals; some were forced to work in the German-owned workshops in the ghetto, as was ultimately the case with Luba Blum-Bielicka, who worked in the Schultz workshop. A few organized first aid stations.

## Studies in Hunger Disease

Doctors at Czyste studied the effects of typhus and hunger disease on adults. The departments led by doctors Jakub Penson and Emil Apfelbaum, with the anatomopathological laboratory under Dr. Józef Stein, were at the forefront of investigating these illnesses, and on a scale never seen before. Postmortems on deceased adults were performed in a building on Stawki Street.[25]

Hunger was the ever-present companion of war. The hospital's growing inability to feed its patients began in the autumn of 1939, when the Germans ordered *Kasa Chorych* to stop payments to Jewish hospitals. Food supplies were quickly exhausted. Gradually, and as far as possible with the assistance of the JDC, conditions began to improve. In February 1940, special yellow food cards—vouchers bearing the Star of David—were introduced for Jews, but their food rations were curtailed. Patients who came to the hospital seeking medical aid had to hand over several of their vouchers to help meet the needs of all the patients.

Food, the only effective remedy for treating hunger disease, was distributed by the doctors, so as not to expose the nurses to the torment of temptation. Medical personnel were in a somewhat better position concerning the rationing of spirits. Occasionally, doctors from pediatrics met for a shared breakfast in the laboratory. These meals, which were

---

25 A much larger dissection room was in the Bersohn and Bauman's Children's Hospital, where research-based postmortems into deaths from starvation were performed by Dr. Moryc Płońskier.

their main [source of] sustenance, consisted of 190 grams of voucher bread, cut into thin slices, ten grams of sugar beet jam, or fifty grams of "monkey fat."[26] This was supplemented with one twenty-five-gram tot of undiluted spirits, which did not render the drinker intoxicated, but did ease the burden of their work.

Doctors later discovered, when there was total famine, how significant this insubstantial dose of alcohol was for their calorie intake because none of them experienced starvation edema. "With a miraculous lack of after-effects," Dr. Blady-Szwajger noted, "despite depriving us of food, the Nazis continued allocating spirits to doctors."[27] Dr. Waller also referred to the rationing of spirits, saying that "at that time, during the last weeks of the ghetto liquidation, the food portions increased. Doctors were given rations of alcohol."[28] Some personal files belonging to the Warsaw-Białystok Medical Chamber contain documents confirming that spirits, denaturants and soap vouchers were given to doctors.

Prof. Hirszfeld observed that prolonged starvation led to diseases previously not known to doctors, such as a decrease in bone density described by Dr. Jelenkiewicz.[29] German and Swiss doctors were equally interested in the progression of these diseases. Dr. Szapiro recalled an incident during a visit to the hospital in Stawki Street:

My direct superior in Dr. Penson's department was Michał Lapidus; he must have been about thirty years old, a friendly and level-headed man. However, Michał was far from cool-headed when an "excursion" of several German and two Swiss doctors arrived at Stawki and he was delegated to be their guide because he was fluent in German and highly qualified. The "excursion" was specifically interested in hunger disease, and one of the doctors, possibly a Swiss, looking at a horribly emaciated seven- or eight-year-old child, asked how long it had taken to reach such a state. Michał's face became red and he growled "Too long!" The entire "excursion" froze, and this

---

26 The author was unable to establish what the so-called "monkey fat" (*małpi smalec*) was.

27 Blady-Szwajger, *I więcej nic nie pamiętam*, 50–51.

28 An account by Stanisław Waller, YVA O.3/2358.

29 Hirszfeld, *Historia jednego życia*, 241.

probably saved him. Usually, far less belligerent statements were severely punished.[30]

In November 1941, Dr. Milejkowski and Czerniaków established the Organizational Committee, to prepare research into the effects of famine on the human body. Its members were Doctors Milejkowski, Braude-Heller, Stein, Apfelbaum, and Fliederbaum. Research began in February 1942. Apfelbaum wrote that, in addition to documenting and leaving for posterity testimony to the suffering of Jews behind the ghetto walls, it demonstrated the dignified conduct of Jewish doctors in defending human rights.[31]

The effects of starvation on adults aged twenty to forty were described by a team of doctors under the leadership of Dr. Apfelbaum, while children aged six to twelve were examined by a team led by Dr. Braude-Heller. Dr. Fliederbaum, a graduate of St. Petersburg University and an exceptional internist from Vilnius, helmed the team of scientists. As Hirszfeld described him after the war, Fliederbaum was the "embodiment of subtlety and kindness, an excellent scholar and doctor."[32]

Pediatrician Dr. Izrael Rotbalsam described the circumstances leading to research into hunger disease:

The idea of writing a study entitled "Hunger Disease" was received favorably by the directors, Doctors Milejkowski (from the *Judenrat*'s Health Department), and Guzik. The JDC subsidized the work. The idea of working with the Warsaw University Internal Diseases Clinic run by Prof. Orłowski was also received favorably. Auxiliary materials were necessary for starting and continuing the work—chemicals, apparatus, and other items—and some of these were purchased, while others were received via the *Judenrat*'s Health Department and the JDC. In the [children's] hospital, we created a specialist department to carry out research into hunger disease. Children who were being treated in this department received wholesome food. Resources were obtained from the JDC and from the community.

30  Szapiro, "Tajne studia medycyny w getcie."
31  Apfelbaum, *Choroba głodowa*, 5.
32  Hirszfeld, *Historia jednego życia*, 325.

... Alas, it was impossible to save these children, because even those who improved somewhat and felt a little better, kept returning to the ghetto and falling ill again. We had young patients who would return to hospital several times and, in the end, they would die.[33]

The progression of hunger disease always followed the same course. The first symptom was starvation diarrhea, the result of changes in the mucous membrane of the large intestine. It was accompanied by constant painful urges to defecate, followed by the passing of feces, later becoming watery and filled with mucus, blood, and pus. One third of the patients developed edema because of decreased levels of protein, vitamins, and microelements, as well as an accumulation of toxins due to intensified cellular catabolism.

Edema, which resulted from protein deficiency and heart failure, was localized in the lower legs and thighs in patients who could walk, while in the bedridden, it presented in the area of the buttocks. Skin became pasty, then rough, and began to peel. Hair became lackluster and fell out, body temperature dropped, breathing slowed down to ten breaths per minute, while low blood pressure and slower heartbeats prevailed. Movements lacked coordination, with the patient suffering repeated falls.

The collapse of the body's immune system caused frequent infections and typical internal and infectious diseases; the symptoms and progression of diseases were altered, making diagnosis of the most infectious diseases difficult, especially tuberculosis. Starving people became confused, their speech was soft and slow, their interest limited mostly to activities related to finding food and dealing with sleep-related problems. Their thought processes slowed down, comprehension and memory suffered; they collapsed into states of indifference or distress. Children stopped growing; retrogression in psychomotor development set in.

Patients were carefully selected to prevent other diseases from blurring the progression of hunger disease itself. To achieve this, Doctors Einhorn, Goldberg and Lederman worked in refugee centers and at quarantine stations, choosing so-called "clean cases of starvation" from among the inmates. They were moved to the hospital and placed in special "starvation wards," where they received additional food

33  An account by Izrael Rotbalsam, YVA O.3/2357.

(on average 800 kcal per day)[34] and were monitored. The team supervisor, Dr. Milejkowski, organized monthly academic sessions in his apartment. Reports were presented on the progress of the research, and conclusions were reached and shared, followed by lively discussions.[35] The preliminary results were presented in the presence of Czerniaków, Director of Provisioning Abraham Gepner, and representatives from the Council for Provisioning. On July 6, 1942, Czerniaków noted in his diary: "Conference at Dr. Milejkowski's after dinner. Results of research into hunger."[36]

Dr. Milejkowski first reiterated the purpose of the study and emphasized its significance. Dr. Fliederbaum revealed his team's research results, and Dr. Apfelbaum presented the results of functional research into the circulatory system. Other speakers were Doctors Braude-Heller, Stein, Goliborska and Kocen. Their discussions placed emphasis on the scientific significance of the project and its social importance.[37]

The last meeting was held in August 1942.[38] Any typescripts completed before April 1943 were stored in a building on the grounds of the Jewish cemetery and, according to Dr. Rotbalsam, later handed to Dr. Milejkowski's son-in-law, Advocate Galecki (or Galewski).[39] Dr. Goliborska assumed the typescripts were buried in the Jewish cemetery. What happened to the originals remains a mystery, but a copy was handed to Prof. Witold Orłowski. According to Leonard Tusznet, the typescript (accompanied by a letter) was collected by an unnamed woman who delivered it to Orłowski.[40] In the process of formulating its final version, he reviewed the study.[41] His son, Tadeusz, played an important role in saving the manuscript: during the German occupation of Warsaw, he attended the underground medical courses, and after the war became an eminent internist and transplant professor. According to

34  Fenigstein, "Holocaust and I," 138.
35  An account by Izrael Rotbalsam, YVA O.3/2357.
36  Czerniaków, *Adama Czerniakowa dziennik*, 296.
37  Apfelbaum, *Choroba głodowa*, 17.
38  Blady-Szwajger, *I więcej nic nie pamiętam*, 64.
39  An account by Izrael Rotbalsam, YVA O.3/2357.
40  L. Tushnet, *The Uses of Adversity: Studies of Starvation in the Warsaw Ghetto* (New York and London: Thomas Yoseloff, 1966), 49.
41  J. Weremowicz, "Działalność prof. Dr. med. W. Orłowskiego w czasie okupacji," *Polski Tygodnik Lekarski* 26 (1968): 1002–1004.

his father, Tadeusz buried the typescript on the grounds of the Infant Jesus Children's Hospital. It was not easy, but he recovered it when Dr. Apfelbaum came to collect it.[42]

Thirty doctors as well as students of the underground university and auxiliary personnel participated in examining the effects of hunger disease. Only five survived (16.5 percent). In 1946, thanks to the efforts of the JDC, the book *Hunger Disease: Clinical Investigation of Hunger Conducted in the Warsaw Ghetto in 1942* appeared—a study based on surviving notes, edited by Dr. Apfelbaum.[43] The editorial board included JDC Director Dawid Guzik, Prof. Dr. Juliusz Zweibaum, Dr. Marek Koenigstein, Editor Jonas Turkow, and Doctors Józef Chain, Józef Sack, and Leon Płockier."[44]

In the introduction, written while he was still in the ghetto, Dr. Milejkowski explains:

> This work is not complete. In July 22, 1942, it was suddenly stopped. It represented a turning point in the existence of the Warsaw Ghetto, the start of the "resettlement," that is, of mass murder. Yes! Deportation, meaning mass murder—alas, in our ghetto, at this moment, these words are synonymous. It is a deed unseen in history; its monstrosity, in all its enormity and terror, will reveal itself to the world only in the future.[45]

Information about the deaths of Doctors Kocen, Raszkes, Płońskier and Blacher, as found in the book, confirms that progress on their enquiry into hunger disease came to an abrupt halt.

## Studies in Typhus

On many occasions, doctors displayed the highest level of ethical concern and bravery. One of the way they preserved their dignity was by remaining doctors and by pursing scientific discoveries, even in the ghetto. After

---

42  S. G. Massry and M. Smogorzewski, "The Hunger Disease of the Warsaw Ghetto," *American Journal of Nephrology* 2–3 (2002): 197–201.

43  The fragment of the study compiled by doctors Mieczysław Kocen and Mieczysław Raszkes was not found.

44  Apfelbaum, *Choroba głodowa*, 2.

45  Ibid., 7.

the war, Dr. Jerzy Szapiro, a staff doctor, remembered Dr. Penson as a scientist who, despite the catastrophic conditions in the ghetto, did not stop his research, and inspired his students to also get involved:

> The boss pondered the problems of non-renal azotemia in the progression of typhus, therefore, we, the brave students being his control group, drank the urea solution voluntarily and eagerly, hoping that, perhaps thanks to some juxtaposition of our blood test results with those of the patients, some tiny (miniscule even) truth would be revealed. We were bursting with pride, simply because of the times when we participated in—well, well!—scientific studies. We were also flattered about attending hospital meetings and being invited to the considerably rarer scientific sessions. We were told that this was a departure from the prewar tradition.
>
> These sessions were also attended by doctors from outside our hospital, some of whom were distressed and, by the looks of it, not well nourished. Nevertheless, we understood that we were encountering people of distinction. If you think about it—if one of us left the room (but especially they, regardless of their age) we could be beaten up, corralled into slave labor and become victims of some "casual" round-up with a view to being deported to an unspecified destination.
>
> Yet the sessions were well attended, while the mood was normal, even exalted. Those were not insignificant moments, not just "checking off" items on a list, but another modest protest against spiritual enslavement. This was uncommonly fortifying. Thus, burdening ourselves with the urea solution, or our revered participation in the sessions, might be considered yet another element of our secret studies, given their "partisan" progress and dimensions—whose framework unfolded as daily hospital duties under the watchful eye of our teachers, our superiors and asylum seekers.[46]

From Dr. Penson's postwar publications, we learn that during the winter of 1941/1942 and the spring of 1942, the first results of nitrogen

---

46  Szapiro, "Tajne studia medycyny w getcie."

metabolization in patients with typhus were presented during clinical sessions at the Czyste Jewish Hospital. This research became the topic of Penson's postwar post-doctoral study, *Clinical Characteristics of Typhus in 1940 and 1941/42 in Warsaw: Our Research into the Metabolization of Nitrogen, with a Particular Emphasis on Kidneys. A Method of early Detection.* M. Małecka quoted a fragment from the introduction to Penson's study:

> Epidemics, as we observed, had a place in the Warsaw Ghetto. Besides our daily hospital duties, despite strict bans by the German authorities, we conducted scientific research. This was possible because we managed to save and move the chemical and anatomopathological laboratory of the Czyste Hospital to the ghetto. Of the 800 doctors in the Warsaw Ghetto, a few dozen survived. Of my department, which had twenty doctors and students, four survived: Doctors Aniela Gelbard (later Prof. Zofia Majewska), Irena Sieradzka, Jerzy Szapiro and, as mentioned earlier, J. Penson.
>
> Thanks to these people, the work was reconstructed from the surviving notes. Materials on typhus disease were carefully examined, both clinically and anatomopathologically. During the liquidation of the ghetto, the entire archives were lost; they comprised the medical history of some 25,000 cases, detailed notes from autopsies, histopathological specimens, and microphotographs. Two prominent anatomical pathologists were murdered: Doctors J. Stein and Gilde, who had done tremendous work, especially in the field of histopathological studies of the brain.[47]

---

47  Małecka, *Jakub Penson*, 107.

# Chapter 11

# Conclusion

Hunger and infectious diseases were the main causes of the deaths of almost 100,000 Warsaw Ghetto Jews, one in four, between 1940 and 1942.[1] A further 265,000 Jews were murdered during the forty-six days of the *Grossaktion* from July 23 to September 1942, almost all of them in Treblinka.[2] A few doctors managed to escape death by forging a new life on the Aryan side of the wall. By studying the registration files of Jewish committees from the years 1944–1946, researchers estimate that fifteen to twenty percent of Jews survived on the Aryan side.[3] In Gunnar S. Paulsson's somewhat higher estimation, of the 28,000 Jews hiding in Warsaw, 11,500 survived.[4]

---

1   M. Janczewska, "Liczby i słowa. O śmierci w liczbach w dokumentach Archiwum Ringelbluma," in *Listy do Oneg Szabat*, ed. A. Matysiak (Warsaw: 2017), 27. The author emphasizes the growing number of Jewish deaths, from 10–11 percent a year in 1939 to 25–45 percent in June 1941, caused by a spike in typhus infections. Nevertheless, she stressed, the main reason of death in the ghetto was hunger disease.

2   J. A. Młynarczyk, "Treblinka—obóz śmierci akcji Reinhardt," in *Akcja Reinhardt. Zagłada Żydów w Generalnym Gubernatorstwie*, ed. Dariusz Libionka (Warsaw: IPN, 2004), 217. Młynarczyk relies on German sources. Barbara Engelking states that on the eve of the *Grossaktion* in July 1942, there were some 380,000 residents, of which 300,000 were murdered in two months. See B. Engelking, "Mieszkańcy getta—dane demograficzne," in B. Engelking and J. Leociak, *Getto warszawskie*, 66-67.

3   A. Stankowski, P. Weiser, "Demograficzne skutki Holokaustu," in *Następstwa zagłady Żydów. Polska 1944-2010*, ed. F. Tych and M. Adamczyk-Garbowska (Lublin: Wydawnictwo UMCS, 2012), 27.

4   He also repeats after Barbara Bermanowa that among those in hiding, the dominating group were members of the educated as well as middle classes, where doctors and other medical professionals were only five percent. A considerably large percentage were teachers (nine percent), engineers (ten percent), merchants and artisans (15.7

According to Jan Bohdan Gliński's estimates, forty-two percent of people in medical professions whether Jewish or Catholic (doctors, dentists, pharmacists, and so forth) died or were murdered during the Second World War.[5] Such a high mortality rate among individuals from a single profession is undoubtedly emblematic of the almost complete annihilation of the Jewish medical fraternity. According to the author's estimates, of the 831 Jewish doctors registered as members of the Warsaw-Białystok Medical Chamber, 103 lived to see the end of the war—a mere 12.4 percent.[6] This survival ratio shows that doctors were among the more fortunate in the ghetto. Certainly, the professional standing of doctors and their better-than-average financial situations seemed to guarantee their survival during the initial stages of life in the ghetto. Financial means and friendships with university peers and, later, their years in medical practice (including at non-Jewish hospitals) undoubtedly secured the privileged status of many medical professionals. This is confirmed by the fact that, of the twenty-four members of the prestigious Warsaw Medical Society who worked in the ghetto as doctors, ten survived (forty-one percent), which, when compared to the overall number of survivors, is a relatively high figure. But during the war, their elevated position in the ghetto lasted only as long as they were useful in combatting epidemics.

The main objective of this study was to answer principal questions about various organizations involved in providing healthcare in the Warsaw Ghetto after the outbreak of the Second World War. Thanks to the numerous accounts of survivors, it was possible to recreate the fortunes of those medical agencies and institutions established by the *Judenrat* and similar entities. While investigating the history of hospitals and outpatient clinics, it became apparent that those institutions operated until the ghetto was destroyed. Their medical personnel mainly consisted of doctors who worked full-time. Most doctors were from

---

percent). G. S. Paulsson, *Utajone miasto. Żydzi po aryjskiej stronie Warszawy (1940–1945)* (Kraków: Znak, 2009), 322.

5 J. B. Gliński, "Straty osobowe lekarzy polskich podczas II wojny światowej," in *Zagłada chorych psychicznie. Pamięć i historia*, ed. T. Nasierowski, G. Herczyńska, D. M. Myszka (Warsaw: Eneteia, 2012), 147. According to the official registry of doctors (*Urzędowy spis lekarzy*), on January 1, 1939, 2,815 practicing doctors were registered.

6 The doctors who survived the war in death or labor camps were Alina Brewda, Józef Celmajster, Henry Fenigstein, Arno Kleszczelski, Henryk Wieliczański, Izrael Rotbalsam, Tadeusz Stabholz (a student), and Dawid Wdowiński.

"non-invasive" disciplines that is, internists, podiatrists, dermatologists, neurologists and radiologists, while only one in five doctors came from more "invasive" specializations. Most of the physicians were graduates of the Medical Faculty at Warsaw University. Studying recovered documents made it possible to estimate the number of doctors who worked in the Warsaw Ghetto between November 1940 and April 1943. There were up to 1,000 of them.[7]

Hospital departments were perpetually overcrowded, medicines were chronically in short supply, as were wound dressings and food. During the typhus epidemic, hospitals overflowed with patients suffering from infectious diseases. Doctors struggled with innumerable difficulties and threats from city officials, as well as from the Germans. Many patients who sought treatment were victims of gunshot wounds received while attempting to escape from the ghetto. Conditions in Jewish hospitals and outpatient clinics worsened on a weekly basis, as did their ability to offer effective treatment. Eventually, only basic nursing care could be provided by an ever-decreasing number of medical agencies.

The most probable location of primary medical institutions was established, as well as the dates which are so crucial for understanding the history of medical services in the ghetto. Accounts written after the war by eyewitnesses tend to be contradictory, but by referring to surviving maps and notes written soon after the Liberation, it has been possible to pinpoint almost all the addresses of the medical institutions in the ghetto, along with the names of most of the serving personnel. In this way, the first aggregated list of doctors working in the ghetto was composed, featuring 831 names and basic biographical information.

The operations of the Jewish Medical Chamber was outlined as well as the first and subsequent location of its activities. Its mention in the literature has, until now, been limited to allusions to its existence, frequently confusing it with the Health Council. Furthermore, three Jewish emergency services in the ghetto were described in as much detail as possible, highlighting their different and as-yet-unexamined functions. Attention was also paid to the hitherto disregarded quarantine hospital at 109 Leszno Street. The locations of the outpatient clinics, which were

---

7    This data comes from an analysis of information gathered during research for this study.

overseen by the *Judenrat* and TOZ, were also established. The proceedings detailing the activities of the Chemical and Bacteriological Institute, found in the Jewish Historical Institute archives, outlined the functioning of this institution and its role in combating infectious diseases. Important, and in need of elaboration, were the efforts of doctors who tried to limit the spread of infections, initially typhoid fever, and later typhus and finally tuberculosis. Surviving issues of the *Jewish Gazette* made it possible to examine vaccination campaigns in the ghetto, as well as the work of the department for combating epidemics.

An analysis of memoirs and personal accounts reveals the ethical dilemmas doctors faced as well as instances of discord within the medical fraternity. This study briefly described the particularly difficult and painful episode of doctors joining the ranks of the Jewish Police, especially during the liquidation of the ghetto. Despite their different religious orientations, within the confined space of the ghetto, doctors cooperated to improve sanitary and living conditions.

These differences in outlook, which remained evident until their final days did not undermine collaboration both in the institutions run by the *Judenrat* and in other social care agencies. Undoubtedly, all staff associated with the health services in the ghetto enjoyed certain privileges. Some doctors working in the commission or tasked with overseeing the disinfection of tenement houses, accepted considerable bribes for medical certificates, which exempted the holders from forced labor, or enabled them to conceal cases of typhus infection.[8] Nevertheless, a crucial privilege was having work and documents excusing them from forced slave labor and deportation to the labor camps.

Another privilege was the ability to admit family members to a relatively safe hospital, especially important when the Germans began to liquidate the ghetto. Hospital personnel usually had contact with German doctors, who sometimes shared information about the planned "*aktions.*" If a close relative was sent to the *Umschlagplatz*, the medical staff could assist with their escape by providing medical uniforms and leading the person through the adjacent hospital grounds or spiriting them away in an ambulance. Staff also had easy access to medicines, vaccines and poisons. The upper echelons of hospital management received "tickets to

---

8    Makower, *Pamiętnik z getta warszawskiego*, 106.

live" which, in September 1942, granted them the right to remain in the ghetto.

Manual laborers and cleaners, then nursing staff, and in the end, many doctors, too, lost these privileges. When the Germans decided to liquidate the ghetto, they drew a line through the role of medical personnel. The few doctors and nurses who remained in the ghetto helped those who still worked in the workshops, while a number of their cohort escaped to the Aryan side.

The fact that Jewish doctors organized underground medical courses, that they continued scientific research, and that lecturers at the nursing school continued teaching, deserve special mention. More so, because this happened in the face of grinding poverty and utter hopelessness. Such deeds may be understood as acts of rebellion against totalitarianism but also as a desire to make sense of one's daily existence.

Soon after the war, several researchers' medical findings were published. In 1946, the editorial committee led by doctors Juliusz Zweibaum and Emil Apfelbaum (editor-in-chief) succeeded in publishing a study entitled *Hunger Disease*. Prof. Jakub Penson also published his research. For many years these books were the only sources of knowledge about prolonged periods of starvation, in addition to offering unique testimony about historical events.

Paradoxically, in this "sea of death," there also was love in the ghetto: the fact that loving families chose to face death together on an almost daily basis, brought people to tears. When caregivers or doctors made such decisions—they sacrificed their lives to accompany the dying—were they acts of heroism or unnecessary loss of yet more lives? Some believed such conduct to be abnormal, others saw it as heroic. Perhaps the conscious decision to share in another person's death should be considered an act of love. However, heroic deeds should never be taken as the norm or as a determinant of general conduct, especially since free choice in the ghetto was an illusion.

Finally, health services in the ghetto ground to a halt because of the *Grossaktion*, which was tantamount to the ghetto being liquidated when its residents were either murdered or deported to Treblinka. Up until that point, the well-organized Health Department run by the *Judenrat* had functioned against all odds, and along with other community organizations had provided medical assistance. It finally stopped operating in September 1942. In the so-called "residual ghetto," the few remaining doctors continued taking care of the sick, creating a small hospital on Gęsia Street. The definitive end of healthcare in the ghetto coincided with the Ghetto Uprising in April 1943.

Using archival material to recreate the fate of Jewish doctors who died or were murdered during the war is virtually impossible. In the remaining personal files of doctors registered with the Warsaw-Białystok Medical Chamber there is no information about their fate. Of necessity, any outline of past events must thus rely on the memoirs and post-war accounts of survivors. These allow us to recreate the history of this professional group, and to look at it as an example of the universal fate of the Jewish people in Poland during the Second World War. Indeed, the Holocaust inflicted on Jewish doctors in Warsaw did not differ from the mass-murder of other ghetto residents.

# Appendix 1

# List of Jewish Doctors Who Were Arrested and Held Hostage in 1940 Following Andrzej Kott's Escape from the Gestapo

A group of activists from the Polish People's Action for Independence (*Polska Ludowa Akcja Niepodległościowa*, PLAN) was arrested on January 14, 1940, based on a report by the provocateur Stanisław Izdebski. Andrzej Kott, a member of PLAN, escaped from the Gestapo. Mass arrests followed, including 255 Jews. According to the Ringelblum archives, ninety were released whilst 165 were executed (most probably in Palmiry or in Saski Park).[1] Among the victims were sixteen medical staff. One of the doctors arrested was a gynecologist, Dr. Izaak Szachnerowicz, taken hostage at the Czyste Old Order Jewish Hospital. When the Gestapo came for him, he was performing a medical procedure. The Gestapo said they weren't barbarians and let him finish.[2] Szachnerowicz's wife, Anna Meroz, wrote that ten doctors were arrested at the hospital that day. Unfortunately, despite the efforts of Czerniaków, the hostages were

---

1    Rutkowski, "Sprawa Kotta," 67.
2    Meroz, *W murach i poza murami getta*, 18.

executed. Dr. Antoni Wortman, the director of the Hospitalization Department of the *Judenrat*, was the only one released.[3]

This list, which is drawn from a larger list of victims from the Ringelblum archives, features the names of sixteen doctors, two dentists, and one hospital attendant. In Adam Rutkowski's opinion, all hostages were executed.[4]

1.  Altkaufer Chaim
2.  Atlasberg Abram Izaak
3.  Berliner Jan Jonas
4.  Bernstein Henryk
5.  Birenbaum Arnold
6.  Fiszel Hersz Dawid
7.  Kohn Stanisław
8.  Majner (first name unknown)
9.  Perelman Beniamin
10. Rakower Abram
11. Rajner (Reiner) Chaim
12. Rozensztrauch Karol
13. Stückgold Józef
14. Szachnerowicz Izaak
15. Trachtenberg Moszek Marek
16. Wiener Seweryn

Twelve of the sixteen names appear in the "List of Non-Aryan Doctors" in appendix 2. The names of Henryk Bernstein, Chaim Reiner, Józef Stückgold, and Majner do not feature there. Of the four, only Reiner submitted the registration questionnaire to the Warsaw-Białystok Medical Chamber in 1938. Instead, in the Official Registry of Doctors (*Urzędowy spis lekarzy*, USL) of 1939 there is the name Henryk Bernsztejn, born 1903, which corresponds in respect of age with the records in the Ringelblum archives, and explains the incorrect orthography of his

---

3   In Ringelblum's archives there are two lists of hostages who were arrested; these were delivered to the *Judenrat* in August 1940. On the first there are 165 surnames with "deceased" noted in pencil, on the second there are ninety surnames with annotations reading: "alive."

4   Rutkowski, "Sprawa Kotta," 67

surname. Józef Stückgold does not feature in any of the registries. In the "Medical Yearbook" (*Rocznik Lekarski*) of 1938, in the "Official Registry of Doctors 1938," as well as in the documents of the Medical Chamber, the first names of three doctors appear—Abram, Chaskiel, and Władysław—with Stückgold's surname. They all submitted registration questionnaires in the fall of 1940, therefore they could not have been shot dead in January or May 1940. Most doubts surround the surname Majner. In the "Medical Yearbook" of 1938, and the "Official Registry of Doctors 1938" (1939) there is a similar-sounding name, Majnemer, but it is doubtful this is the same person, because Dr. Feliks Fiszel Majnemer survived the war.

# Appendix 2

# List of Non-Aryan Doctors in Warsaw from the Archives of the Jewish Historical Institute

A copy of this document, which is dated May 1, 1940, with the list of non-Aryan doctors is deposited in the Archives of the Jewish Historical Institute. The document has the reference number of another archive, 806/I/94. No information on where the copy came from is available. Whilst it has not been established on whose order this list was drawn up, above the title there is an annotation: Warsaw-Białystok Medical Chamber (hereinafter referred to as IL-WB), Warsaw, 37 Koszykowa Street, which suggests that the list was prepared for the needs of the Jewish Medical Council.

The list below includes only the names and surnames of the persons listed, but the original list also included addresses of the 737 doctors. There is also one mistake in the original list: Malwina Biro's name is repeated twice whilst the name of Biro Maksymilian, her husband, is missing.

The list was typed in alphabetical order, with the last eight names added at the end after the list was prepared. Among these last-minute additions are Dr. Benno Aron (he died in Kharkiv), Dr. Pejsach Berendt (he was in a POW camp until February 24, 1940), Dr. Tobias Gitler (he was in a POW camp until May 8, 1940), and Dr. Jan Przedborski (he stayed in Kamień Koszyrski until May 10, 1940).

The list contains the names of people who, at the time of its preparation, would have been unable to complete the registration questionnaires, such as the aforementioned Dr. Benno Aron and the doctors arrested in January 1940 and shot soon after: Dr. Abraham Rakower, Dr. Karol Rozensztrauch, or Dr. Izaak Szachnerowicz. Perhaps the list was made before the date of their arrest or they were placed on the list because their death was not yet known.

The names of some of the doctors known to have been working in the ghetto are missing, as are the interns (such as Dr. Adina Blady-Szwajger). With three names (Dr. Michał Eliasberg, Dr. Anna Jokisz Grynbergowa, and Dr. Albert Mazur) there is a repeated annotation: "Attention Mr. Taflowicz—as far as I know, Dr. . . . left Łódź for Warsaw with the outbreak of the war; in 1942 he was brought back to the Łódź ghetto along with forty other doctors." Please see appendix 4.

The 737 first names and surnames follow:

1   Aberdam Selligowa Gusta

2   Abramowicz Łaska Anna

3   Adam Estera

4   Adelfang Dawid

5   Adler Jakub II

6   Ajgengold Jakub

7   Alter Eliasz

8   Altfeld Mieczysław

9   Altkaufer Chaim

10   Altkaufer Henryk

11   Altkaufer Kazańska Cypora

12   Ałapin Herman

13   Ałapin Stefan

14   Amsterdamski Chaim Josel

15   Amsterdamski Dawid Salomon

16   Ancelewicz Henryk Hunon

17  Anisfeld Józef
18  Apfelbaum Emil
19  Apte Felicja
20  Arkin Wiktor
21  Aronowicz Jakub
22  Askanas Rachela
23  Askanas Zdzisław
24  Aszer Makow Maria
25  Aszowa Ida
26  Atlasberg Abram
27  Augenfisz Józef
28  Ax Anna Natalia
29  Bakman Mieczysław
30  Banasz Artur
31  Baraban Chaim
32  Baranowicz Gustaw
33  Bauer Jakub
34  Baumberg Benkielowa Jadwiga
35  Baumritter Paweł
36  Beatus Jakub
37  Beim Maria Paulina
38  Beiles Jeszaja
39  Bemski Edward
40  Ber Alter Paltyel
41  Berensztejn Henryk
42  Bergazen Stefania
43  Berger Wdowińska Antonina
44  Bergman Salomon
45  Bergson Józef
46  Berkman Grosglikowa Zofia
47  Berliner Jan Jonas
48  Berlis Paweł

49   Berłowicz Matys

50   Berman Fiszel

51   Berman Jakub

52   Berman Flaksbaumowa Elżbieta

53   Berman Goldwichtowa Rachela

54   Bernstein Aleksander

55   Bernsztejn Mojżesz

56   Bezberg Władysław

57   Bieleńki Andrzej

58   Billingowa Paulina

59   Binsztejnowa Syrkin Sara Zofia

60   Birenbaum Arnold

61   Birenbaum Michał

62   Birencwejg Julian

63   Biro Malwina

64   Biro Maksymilian Maks

65   Birzowski Efraim

66   Blacher Leon

67   Blay Jerzy

68   Blay Rabinowicz Julia

69   Boczko Hipolit

70   Boczko Leonora

71   Borkowski Izaak Ignacy

72   Bornstein Roman

73   Bornsztein Maurycy

74   Boszes Rywka

75   Brand Jakub

76   Brandwajn Maurycy

77   Bregman Eliasz

78   Bregmanowa Fejga

79   Brewda Alina

80   Brochis Estera

81  Brokman Henryk
82  Bromak Szmul Jankiel
83  Bruksztein Josif
84  Brylant Kahanowa Halina
85  Bussel Mowsza
86  Cejtlin Mieczysław
87  Celmajster Józef
88  Celmajster Majer
89  Chain Abram
90  Chanarin Józef
91  Charadramo Hufnaglowa Fejga
92  Chaskielowa Romana
93   Chazan Beatrycze
94  Chorążycki Julian
95  Cohn Jerzy Georg
96  Cukier Sajetowa Noma
97  Cunge Jakub
98  Cunge Samuel
99  Cybulska Klejmanowa Ewa
100  Cygielnik Abram
101  Cygielstreich Józef
102  Cygielstreich Maria
103  Cyprys Gecel Gustaw
104  Cytter Priwa Fajga
105  Czernikow Luba
106  Dankowicz Herman
107  Datyner Herman
108  Dobryszycki Stefan
109  Dobrzyński Marceli
110  Dołkart Pizmanter Stella
111  Donatt Juliusz
112  Drutman Adam

113 Dubrow Grodzieńska Irena
114 Dynkiewicz Gilel
115 Dziewczepolski Adolf
116 Edelsburg Folmanowa Paulina
117 Edelszein Adam
118 Edelszein Zofia
119 Edilchanow Michał
120 Efros Gurfinkiel Róża
121 Egid Leopold
122 Einhorn Artur
123 Eisenfarb Jakub
124 Ejnchorn Chaim
125 Ejzenberg Abram
126 Elbingerówa Rywka
127 Eliasberg Michał
128 Elwicz Stanisław
129 Endelman Bogumił
130 Endelman Kipman Izabela
131 Endelman Leon
132 Endelman Zygmunt
133 Engel Mozes Anna
134 Engelman Eliasz
135 Epsztein Henryk
136 Erlich Anna
137 Erlich Bernard
138 Ettinger Zofia
139 Eychner Jakub
140 Fajans Tadeusz
141 Fajgenblat Ludwik
142 Fajgenblat Maksymilian
143 Fajgenblat Szymon
144 Fajncyn Zygmunt

145   Fajnzylber Chaim Henryk
146   Falkowska Roza Rebeka
147   Falkowski Dawid
148   Federman Michał
149   Fedorowski Grzegorz
150   Fedorowski Mojżesz
151   Feilchendowa Zofia
152   Feinstein Markus
153   Feinstein Stanisław
154   Fejgin Bronisława
155   Feldhusen Maurycy
156   Felhendler Jankiel
157   Fenigsztein Bernard
158   Ferber Borys
159   Fernberg Abe
160   Ferster Mendel
161   Ferszt Lejzer
162   Festensztadt Abram
163   Finkelkraut Markus
164   Finkelsztejn Leib Leon
165   Finkiel Josif
166   Finkielsztein Abram
167   Finkielsztein Pesa
168   Fiszel Gersz
169   Fiszhaut Zeldowicz Ludmiła
170   Flancman Chaim Józef
171   Flatau Helena
172   Flaum Jadwiga
173   Floksztrumpf Sabina
174   Fogel Mojżesz Symcha
175   Forbert Chil Henryk
176   Frank Józef

| | |
|---|---|
| 177 | Franz Luxemburgowa Wanda |
| 178 | Frejmanowa Danuta |
| 179 | Frendler Anatol |
| 180 | Frendler Czesława |
| 181 | Frendler Ludwika |
| 182 | Fridman Rywka |
| 183 | Friedstein Gustaw |
| 184 | Fryde Jakub |
| 185 | Frydland Chil |
| 186 | Frydman Leon |
| 187 | Frydman Leonard |
| 188 | Fryling Ela |
| 189 | Fryszberg Bronisława |
| 190 | Fuswerk Józef |
| 191 | Fux Fred Zenon |
| 192 | Gabay Baszenszpiler Helena |
| 193 | Gabryjelew Mordka |
| 194 | Gajst Izrael |
| 195 | Galewski Alfred |
| 196 | Gantz Róża Maria |
| 197 | Garfinkiel Jakub |
| 198 | Gat Juda |
| 199 | Geisler Józef |
| 200 | Gelbard Aniela |
| 201 | Gelbart Ajzyk |
| 202 | Gelbfisz Beniamin |
| 203 | Gelbfisz Jakub |
| 204 | Gelertner Bernard |
| 205 | Gerkowicz Rafał |
| 206 | Ginzburg Abram |
| 207 | Ginzburg Bella |
| 208 | Ginzburg Szpilman Franciszka |

209   Gladsztern Szymon
210   Glajchgewicht Uszer
211   Glauternik Chaim
212   Glass Bronisław Boruch
213   Glass Mieczysław
214   Glauberman Morduch
215   Gliksman Józef
216   Glocer Lewendel Ewelina
217   Glozman Salomon
218   Gocław Zofia
219   Goldband Izrael
220   Goldberg Chaim
221   Goldberg Chana Anna
222   Goldberg Edward
223   Goldberg Henryk Dawid
224   Goldberg-Górecki Julian
225   Goldberżanka Anna
226   Goldberżanka Jadwiga
227   Goldblum Natan
228   Goldblum Mackiewicowa Zofia
229   Golde Żyżmorska Chaja Zlata
230   Goldfarb Hersz
231   Goldflam Menachem
232   Goldinberg Majer
233   Goldkorn Lajwa
234   Goldman Jadwiga
235   Goldman Mieczysław
236   Goldman Maurycy
237   Goldman Rozenbaumowa Helena
238   Goldman Wilkowa Maria
239   Goldstein Józef
240   Goldszmidt Henryk

241 Goldsztein Berek
242 Goldsztein Chil
243 Goldsztein Markus
244 Goliborską Gołąbowa Teodozja
245 Gordon Karpel
246 Gordon Salomon
247 Gotlib Aron
248 Gottfryd Fabian
249 Granatsztein Moszek
250 Grodzieński Edward
251 Grodzieński Michał
252 Grodziński Hieronim
253 Grojsblat Mojżesz
254 Groniowski Antoni
255 Grundzach Ignacy
256 Grycendler Stanisław
257 Grynberg Zygmunt
258 Grynblat Szmul
259 Gutentag Stanisław
260 Guterman Józef
261 Gutman Łaja
262 Halbersztadt Szymelowa Tila
263 Hanna Eluzor
264 Hartglas Janina
265 Hejman Włodzimierz
266 Held Józef
267 Heller Brande Chana
268 Heller Maurycy Mojżesz
269 Heller Hermelinowa Berta
270 Helman Emilia
271 Hercberg Chaim Józef
272 Herman Eufemiusz

273 Hermelin Adolf

274 Herszfinkiel Jechiel

275 Hertz Artur

276 Higier Henryk Chaim

277 Higier Stanisław

278 Hindes Salomon

279 Hirsz Maksymilian

280 Hirszbajn Salomon

281 Hirszhorn Maria

282 Hochsinger Józef

283 Holc (or Hamburger) Zygmunt

284 Holendrówa Ala

285 Hufnagel Jadwiga Jenta

286 Iberbajn Mojżesz

287 Jabłoński Józef

288 Jabłoński Leon

289 Jacobius Leonardt

290 Jakubowicz Henryk

291 Janower Moszek

292 Janowski Ilia

293 Jawic Zusman

294 Jelenkiewicz Lucjan

295 Jelin Mojżesz

296 Jochelson Gitla

297 Jokisz Grynbergowa Anna

298 Judt Regina

299 Justman Stanisław Samuel

300 Kachan Aleksander II

301 Kadysiewicz Leon

302 Kahan Aleksander

303 Kahan Izaak

304 Kahanowicz Borys

305   Kajzer Abram
306   Kajzer Naftal
307   Kakiet Kroszczorowa Rachela
308   Kaltman Rozencwajg Ewa
309   Karasz Hersz
310   Karbowska Paulina
311   Karbowski Mieczysław
312   Karsz Jefim
313   Katz (or Kac) Mendel
314   Keilson Inda
315   Kenig Józef Czesław
316   Kenigsberg Dawid
317   Kigiel Izaak
318   Kipman Jerzy
319   Kirjacefer Jerzy
320   Kirszbraun Aleksander
321   Kirszenblat Migdor
322   Kiszycer Grzegorz
323   Klaperzak Jakub
324   Kleczko Chaja
325   Kleczko Majer Nison
326   Klein Kleimanowa Fejga
327   Klein Sara
328   Klejn Chaim
329   Kleniec Eida
330   Knaster Ludwik
331   Koenigstein Ludwik
332   Koenigstein Marek
333   Koenigsteinowa Ernestyna
334   Kolin Michał
335   Koliński Józef
336   Koltun Euzebiusz

337 Komarowski Mojsze

338 Kon Daniel

339 Kon Isaj

340 Kon Jerzy

341 Kon Goldszteinowa Halina

342 Kon (or Kohn) Stanisław

343 Kon Fajgenblat Janina

344 Konstantyner Zysla

345 Kopciowski Aleksander

346 Kopersztyc Dawid

347 Korman Jakub

348 Korman Kielman

349 Korman Lejb

350 Kornberg Józef

351 Kosman Ezra

352 Krakowski Isaj

353 Krakowski Mieczysław

354 Kramsztyk Stefan

355 Kranc Perlmutter Stefania

356 Krantz Ignacy

357 Krasubka Fajga Liba

358 Krejndel Rosenbergowa Eta

359 Krenicki Izaak

360 Krenicki Józef

361 Krongold Dawid

362 Krongoldowa Łaja Ludwika

363 Krukowski Gustaw

364 Krzypow Bajnisz

365 Kurchin Spielreinowa Elżbieta

366 Kurzman Izydor

367 Kustin Noe

368 Lajchter Chil

369   Landau Abram
370   Landau Alicja
371   Landau Anastazy
372   Landau Eugenia
373   Landau Gołda
374   Landau Henryk Jakub
375   Landau Jerzy
376   Lande Adam
377   Landesman Maurycy
378   Lando Boruch
379   Landowski Julian
380   Landsberger Józef
381   Landstein Ignacy
382   Lapidus Michał
383   Lastman Hersz
384   Leber Jakub
385   Lederman Symcha
386   Lejpuner Icko
387   Leneman Bencjan
388   Leński Morduch
389   Lesiński Majloch
390   Lewi Alfred
391   Lewi Margolisowa Cerla
392   Lewicki Izydor
393   Lewin Henoch Henryk
394   Lewin Izaak
395   Lewinson Julian
396   Lichtenbaum Abram
397   Lichtenbaum Szpilfogel Natalia
398   Lichtenberg Izaak
399   Lifszyc Eliasz
400   Lilienfeld Krzewski Szymon

401 Lindenfeld Berta

402 Lipowska Krejnes Sara

403 Lipsztat Paweł

404 Lipsztat Muszkatowa Natalia

405 Lipszyc Henryk

406 Lipszyc Izaak

407 Litauer Amelia

408 Litauer Wojdysławska Elzbieta

409 Liwszyc Józef

410 Lobmanówa Halina

411 London Juda

412 Lubelczyk Eli

413 Mackiewicz Paweł

414 Majnemer Fiszel

415 Makower Herman

416 Makower Łaja

417 Makowski Józef

418 Makowski Józef (II)

419 Maliniak Izydor

420 Maliniak Karolina

421 Mamrot Artur

422 Manblit Arnold

423 Manson Naum

424 Mantin Izrael

425 Margolis Anna

426 Margulies Józef

427 Markson Jelenkiewiczowa Mira

428 Markusfeld S. Abram

429 Marmor Salomon

430 Mastbaum Stanisław

431 Maszlanka Abram

432 Matecki Władysław

433  Mauer Izrael
434  Mayzner Mojżesz
435  Mazur Albert
436  Mejłachowicz Salomon
437  Mejnster Mery
438  Melzak Naftal
439  Mendelson Nachum
440  Messing Anna
441  Mesz Jadwiga
442  Mesz Natan
443  Mesz Stefania
444  Meszowa Datner Frajda
445  Mic Jakub
446  Milejkowska Gajewska Janina
447  Milejkowski Abram
448  Milejkowski Izrael
449  Miller Mendel Mieczysław
450  Milsztejn Chaja
451  Minc Ludwik
452  Mindes Juliusz
453  Miński German
454  Mintzowa Tauba
455  Miszurski Eliasz
456  Mossenkisowa Emilia
457  Moszkowicz Benedykt
458  Moszkowska Irena
459  Mościsker Emma
460  Munwez Jakub
461  Muszkatblat Paulina
462  Muszkatblat Perec
463  Nachtman Zelman
464  Nadel Ignacy

465 Nadel Izydor

466 Naftali Stok Salomea

467 Natan Feliks

468 Nejman Jakub

469 Neuman Izydor

470 Nick Bernard

471 Nissenzon Arnold

472 Nochlin Abraham

473 Olicki Michał

474 Openheim Berek Bolesław

475 Oppenhejm Szmul Samuel

476 Orensztein Froim

477 Orliński Menasse

478 Ostrowski Mordko

479 Pakszwer Ryszard

480 Papierny Kisiel

481 Pekielis Rubin

482 Penzon Jakub

483 Perelman Beniamin

484 Perl Jerzy

485 Perlman Albert

486 Petersburg Mieczysław

487 Pianko Necha

488 Pianko Pesia

489 Pinczewska Zofia

490 Pinczewski Jakub

491 Pitzele Halina

492 Plesner Jakub

493 Płocki Juda

494 Płockier Leon

495 Płońskierowa Estera

496 Polakow Rozalia

497    Polisiuk Adolf

498    Poliszczukowa Renla

499    Pollak Kazimierz

500    Ponez Ludwik

501    Potok Abram

502    Poznański Nikodem

503    Praszkier Fiszel

504    Prawda Calel Jakub

505    Prechner Hufnagel Kazimiera

506    Proszower Władysław

507    Prussak Leon

508    Prussakowa Salomea

509    Przeworska Alicja

510    Przeworski Bernard

511    Przysuska Beiles Rachela

512    Pumpiański Rafael

513    Rabinowicz Gerkes Basza

514    Rabinowicz Henryk

515    Rabinowicz Noj Wolf

516    Raciążer Stanisław

517    Rajcher Artur

518    Rajchert Maurycy

519    Rajman Pesach

520    Rakower Abraham

521    Rakowski Gerszko

522    Rall Szapiro Fajga

523    Rapiport Zelman

524    Rappel Michał

525    Raszkes Bolesław

526    Raszkes Henryk Chaim

527    Rathaus Gustaw

528    Rajner Izydor

529 Ratner Blumenszteinowa Szejna
530 Regelman Maurycy
531 Reicher Edward
532 Rejchman Pinkus Apolinary
533 Rejder Icek
534 Reiner Chaim
535 Rewucka Łącka Anna
536 Rogoziński Piotr
537 Romanowska Tamara
538 Rosenberg Jakób
539 Rosenblum Jakób
540 Rosenblum Zofia
541 Rosenthalowa Pomper Ewelina
542 Rotbalsam Israel
543 Rotbard Daniel
544 Rothaub Zygmunt
545 Rotmil Stefan Jerzy
546 Rotsztadt Julian
547 Rozenberg Nehama
548 Rozenberg Szmul Grejzman Grzegorz
549 Rozenblat Jakób
550 Rozenblum Bolesław
551 Rozencwajg Dawid
552 Rozenfeld Jakób
553 Rozengarten Celina Cyna
554 Rozensztrauch Karol
555 Rozental Samuel
556 Rozental Zofia
557 Rozenwurcel Róża
558 Rubaszew Icchok
559 Rubinlicht Mordka
560 Rubinraut Leon

561 Rubinrot Stanisław

562 Rubinstein Izrael Michał

563 Rubinsztein Borys

564 Rundstein Leniewska Zofia

565 Rundsztajn Teodozja

566 Rundsztein Moszek

567 Rybak Szołom

568 Rywlin Jakób

569 Saidman Maurycy

570 Saks Mieczysław

571 Salman Eugenia

572 Sarna Symcha

573 Schmorak Szymon

574 Schoenman Hipolit

575 Seid Dawid

576 Seidenbeutel Zdzisław

577 Serejska Perla

578 Sieradzka Irena

579 Sieradzki Stanisław

580 Sierota Salomea

581 Simchowicz Tauba

582 Simchowicz Teofil

583 Sirota Lejwi

584 Skotnicki Arkadiusz

585 Skórnik Salomon

586 Słomnicka Kahanowa Chaja

587 Słon Flamenbaum Liza

588 Sołowiejczyk Mojżesz

589 Sołowiejczyk Orko

590 Somachowa Inhorn Ruchla

591 Spielman Karol

592 Srebrny Zygmunt

593 Srebrowicz Chaja Zlata Helena

594 Stein Józef

595 Stein Wolf Natan

596 Sterling Władysław

597 Stern Filip

598 Stiller Feliks

599 Stopnicka Wizel Marta

600 Strykowska Rojza Róża

601 Stückgold Abram Bronisław

602 Stückgold Chaskiel Hillary

603 Stückgold Władysław

604 Suchotin Borys

605 Suchowczycki Eliezer

606 Sulkes Jakub

607 Swisłocki Zusman

608 Szachnerowicz Anna

609 Szachnerowicz Izaak

610 Szarogroder Ludwik

611 Szejnfajn Irena

612 Szejnman Michał

613 Szenicer Stanisław

614 Szenicerówa Halina

615 Szenkier Nik Nusym

616 Szenwic Wilhelm

617 Szer Róża

618 Szereszewska Eugenia

619 Szerman Joel

620 Szkop Mordka

621 Szlifsztein Józef

622 Sznajderman Icek Ignacy

623 Szoor Henryk Hersz

624 Szour Michał

| | |
|---|---|
| 625 | Szpechtówa Blima |
| 626 | Szper Janina |
| 627 | Szpigielman Mieczysław |
| 628 | Szpilman Neudingowa Paulina |
| 629 | Szpinak Adolf |
| 630 | Szpinak Bernard |
| 631 | Sztajnkalk Zelman Zygmunt |
| 632 | Szteinsapir Azriel |
| 633 | Sztokman Rozenblum Abram |
| 634 | Sztycer Herman |
| 635 | Szwajcer Jakub |
| 636 | Szwalberg Izrael |
| 637 | Szwarcenberg Kazimierz |
| 638 | Szwarcman Józef |
| 639 | Szyfrys Ajzyk |
| 640 | Szyk Naum |
| 641 | Śniadower Sara |
| 642 | Taube Kotler Sara |
| 643 | Taubenfeldowa Teofila |
| 644 | Teichner Izydor |
| 645 | Temerson Herman Hersz |
| 646 | Temkin Maria |
| 647 | Thursz Dawid |
| 648 | Tiefenbrunn Benon |
| 649 | Tombak Jakób |
| 650 | Tonenberg Leon |
| 651 | Torończyk Grodzieńska Klara |
| 652 | Trachtenberg Marek |
| 653 | Trachtenherc Naftali |
| 654 | Trepman Jechiel |
| 655 | Tuchendler Antoni |
| 656 | Tuchendler Maksymilian |

657    Turkus Sterlingowa Bronisława

658    Tursz (or Thursz) Mojżesz

659    Turyn Efriam

660    Turynowa Zofia

661    Tylbor Rubin Roman

662    Typograf Józef

663    Tyras Zygfryd

664    Uryson Akiwa

665    Uzdański Salomon

666    Verständig Zygmunt

667    Wajnbaum Józef

668    Wajntraub Szloma Salomon

669    Wajnsztok Samuel Szlama

670    Wajsberg Efraim

671    Wajshoff Herszlik

672    Wajsman Lejbus Leon

673    Wajsmanówa Noemi

674    Waksman Bernard

675    Waksówna Łaja

676    Waldman Goldowa Helena

677    Walfisz Artur

678    Waller Szmul

679    Warmbrum Izaak

680    Waserman Henryk

681    Waserman Hufnagel Hanna

682    Wasserman Jakób

683    Wasserthal Jakób

684    Wdowiński Dawid

685    Weinberg Izaak

686    Weinberg Perec

687    Weisblat Julian

688    Welt Roman

689  Wengerman Mordche
690  Wertheim Jerzy Aleksander
691  Wiernikowski Wolf
692  Wiesen Władysław
693  Wilk Seweryn
694  Winawer Artur Aron
695  Winer Szyja Seweryn
696  Winer Bezbergowa Sara
697  Wittenberg Leokadia
698  Włodawer Julian
699  Wohl Ichaskil
700  Wolf Ludwik
701  Wolf (or Wolff) Moisiej Maurycy
702  Wolf Gutmanowa Maria
703  Wolfowicz Izrael
704  Wołk Paweł
705  Wortman Antoni
706  Zakin Asir
707  Zaks Łazarz
708  Zaks Marek
709  Zalcman Henryk
710  Zalcwasser Robert
711  Zamenhof Zofia
712  Zamenhofowa Frenkiel Wanda
713  Zamkowy Samuel
714  Zandowa Natalia
715  Zarchi Zarhower Maria
716  Zaurman Stanisław
717  Zimmerman Aleksander
718  Zirler Maksymilian
719  Złotowaka Stefania
720  Zuckerwar Gustaw

721   Zusman Henryk

722   Zusman Pesach Lejb

723   Zweigbaum Marek Maksymilian

724   Zylberbartowa Rozalia

725   Zylberblast Nikodem

726   Żyw Izaak

727   Żabner Józef

728   Żyłkiewicz Józef

729   Aron Benno

730   Berendt Pejsach

731   Bursztyn Jakób

732   Dawidson Aron Moszek

733   Grosglik Józef

734   Gitler Tobias

735   Srebrny Jan

736   Przedborski Jan

# Appendix 3

# List of Jewish Doctors Working and Living in Warsaw in 1940–1942

The starting point for the creation of this list was the document entitled "List of Non-Aryan Doctors" (see appendix 2). To supplement the existing list, extensive archival research was made in the collections of the Old Medical Book Department of the Central Medical Library in Warsaw, searching among the questionnaires completed in 1940–1942 for the initial registration of medical professionals (*Fragebogen zur erstmaligen Meldung der Heilberufe*) covering members of the Warsaw-Białystok Medical Chamber. Some of the photographs presented in appendix 8 originate from these questionnaires. 6,693 personal files were reviewed. Undoubtedly, these files are a valuable source of personal data and should constitute a starting point for further research. From among these several thousand documents, questionnaires marked with a seal with the word *Jude* were identified. Of individual questionnaires, the first to be registered was the document completed by Dr. Maurycy Rajchert, dated April 4, 1940. As the last one, on July 3, 1942, Dr. Jakób Frajermauer was registered. In this way, a list of 831 names was created.

On the basis of all kinds of sources (books, reports, diaries) and documents collected in the personal files of the Warsaw-Białystok Medical Chamber, people who survived the war with varying probability were identified. Their names are written in bold.

The denominations were marked with abbreviations: Jewish ("j"), Roman Catholic ("r-c"), Old Catholic ("o-c"), Evangelical-Augsburg ("e-a"), Evangelical-Reformed ("e-r"), Greek-Catholic ("g-k"), and Armenian-Gregorian ("or-gr"). Several people did not answer this question or wrote that they were nondenominational. The overwhelming majority indicated that they were of Polish nationality ("p") but there were also Germans ("g") and Soviet citizens ("u").

The correct spelling of the names was determined each time on the basis of the record made by the doctors themselves at the time of filling in the questionnaire for the first registration of a medical profession. In the case of women, the first column lists the surnames taken upon marriage, and the maiden name is added to the second column. In the case of unmarried women, the maiden name is shown next to the first name. Some doctors changed their names before, during, or after the war, which, if that happened, is noted in parentheses.

The names of cities and villages are given in modern spelling, with the indication of the country to which they now belong.

| First name and surname | Maiden name | Year of birth | Day, month of birth | Place of birth | Warsaw address (at the time of fillng the questionnaire) | Religion and nationality | | Place and year the studies were completed | | Specialization |
|---|---|---|---|---|---|---|---|---|---|---|
| Abramowicz Ludwik | | 1897 | 14.01 | Chervonohrad (now Ukraine) | 13/2 Nowolipie Street | j | p | Warsaw | 1923 | laryngologist |
| Adam Estera | Podlasiak | 1886 | 18.03 | Warsaw | 81/6 Sienna Street | j | p | Lausanne (Switzerland) | 1914 | pediatrician |
| Adelfang Dawid | | 1898 | 08.02 | Warsaw | 29/2 Nowolipki Street | j | p | Warsaw | 1926 | internist, phthisiologist |
| Adler (né Feit) Jakub Wit | | 1900 | 20.01 | Ivano-Frankivsk (now Ukraine) | 8/35 Zielna Street | J | p | Berlin | 1924 | dermatologist and venereologist |
| Ajzensztat Izaak | | 1897 | 30.04 | Warsaw | 17/16 Nowolipie Street | j | p | Warsaw | 1924 | dermatologist and venereologist |
| **Ajzner Joel Julian** | | **1883** | **14.09** | **Łódź** | **8/1 Szpitalna Street** | **j** | **p** | **Kharkiv (now Ukraine)** | **1907** | **surgeon** |
| **Alter Ignacy Edward Eliasz (Ignacy Edward Kowalewski)** | | **1905** | **12.03** | **Pławno** | **29 Ogrodowa Street** | **j** | **p** | **Liège (now Belgium)** | **1931** | **surgeon, gynecologist** |
| Altfeld Mieczysław Mozes Mowsza Zbigniew | | 1889 | 02.02 | Warsaw | 41/43 Mokotowska Street | r-c | p | Tartu (now Estonia) | 1915 | dermatologist and venereologist |
| Altkaufer Chaim | | 1884 | 20.01 | Warsaw | 30/8 Twarda Street | j | p | Halle (Germany), Odesa (now Ukraine) | | pediatrician |

| First name and surname | Maiden name | Day, month of birth | Year of birth | Place of birth | Warsaw address (at the time of fillng the questionnaire) | Religion and nationality | Place and year the studies were completed | Specialization |
|---|---|---|---|---|---|---|---|---|
| Altkaufer Cypora | Kazańska | 02.01 | 1886 | Chișinău | 30/8 Twarda Street | j / p | Bern (Switzerland) 1910 | analyst |
| Altkaufer Henryk | | 07.03 | 1878 | Warsaw | 11/8 Elektoralna Street | j / p | Warsaw 1901 | gynecologist |
| **Alapin Stanisława Joanna** | **Grynbaum** | **06.02** | **1915** | **Warsaw** | **46/5 Krochmalna Street** | **r-c / p** | **Warsaw 1939** | **no specialization** |
| **Alapin Bolesław (Kowalski, Kazimierz Kościński)** | | **16.08** | **1913** | **Warsaw** | **6/27 Waliców Street** | **j / p** | **Warsaw 1937** | **neurologist** |
| Alapin Herman | | 26.01 | 1877 | Warsaw | 27/10 Królewska Street | j / p | Tartu (now Estonia) 1904 | ophthalmologist |
| Alapin Stefan | | 22.05 | 1907 | Warsaw | 119/4 Marszałkowska Street | j / p | Warsaw 1931 | surgeon |
| Amsterdamski Chaim Josel | | 12.11 | 1890 | Mariampol | 34/8 Chmielna Street | j / p | Warsaw 1923 | dermatologist and venereologist |
| Amsterdamski Dawid Salomon Chaim | | 27.03 | 1895 | Mariampol | 7/8 Złota Street | j / p | Warsaw 1925 | surgeon |
| Ancelewicz Henryk | | 04.07 | 1897 | Warsaw | 20/15 Sienna Street | j / p | Warsaw 1922 | internist |
| Anisfeld Józef | | 24.12 | 1893 | Nowy Sącz | 23 Nalewki Street | j / p | Lviv 1925 | urologist |
| Anszer Sebastian | | 28.04 | 1876 | Suwałki | 31 Zielna Street | j / p | Warsaw 1903 | dermatologist and venereologist |

| First name and surname | Maiden name | Day, month of birth | Year of birth | Place of birth | Warsaw address (at the time of fillng the questionnaire) | Religion and nationality | Place and year the studies were completed | Specialization |
|---|---|---|---|---|---|---|---|---|
| Apel Szlama | | 05.03 | 1909 | Grodzisk Maz. | 7/12 Nowolipie Street | j p | Bologna (Italy) 1937 | surgeon |
| Apfelbaum Emil (Kowalski) | | 15.02 | 1890 | Warsaw | 22/26 Senatorska Street | j p | Warsaw 1922 | internist cardiologist |
| Apt Chana Rojza | | 18.12 | 1900 | Warsaw | 14/28 Nalewki Street | j p | Vilnius 1939 | internist |
| Apte Felicja | | 11.08 | 1887 | Warsaw | 30/52 Sienna Street | j p | Geneva (Switzerland) 1913 | internist |
| Arkin Wiktor (Zalewski) | | 08.04 | 1894 | Warsaw | 64/6 Hoźa Street | j p | Rostov (Russia) 1916 | ophthalmologist |
| Aronowicz Izarael Jakub | | 10.11 | 1896 | Radomsko | 3/1 Solna Street | j p | Vilnius 1928 | internist |
| Askanas Rachela Alicja | Cajlingold | 07.09 | 1911 | Warsaw | 38/8 Nowolipki Street | j p | Warsaw 1935 | pediatrician |
| Askanas Zdzisław | | 01.06 | 1910 | Warsaw | 38/8 Nowolipki Street | j p | Warsaw 1935 | internist cardiologist |
| Asz Ida Iza | Kryształ | 27.02 | 1900 | Łowicz | 15/1 Chłodna Street | j p | Warsaw 1932 | physical therapist |
| Aszer Maria | Makow | 15.01 | 1898 | Łódź | 6/1 Pawia Street | j p | Warsaw 1927 | Paediatrician |
| Augenfisz Józef | | 16.02 | 1898 | Warsaw | 42 Ząbkowska Street | j p | Warsaw 1925 | Gynaecologist |
| Bakman Mieczysław | | 16.03 | 1886 | Nowy Dwór | 45/6 Żelazna Street | j p | Erlangen (Germany) 1912 | Internist |
| Bałaban Aleksander Zygmunt | | 17.01 | 1915 | Vienna | 38/5 Sienna Street | j p | Warsaw 1939 | no specialization |

| First name and surname | Maiden name | Day, month of birth | Year of birth | Place of birth | Warsaw address (at the time of fillng the questionnaire) | Religion and nationality | Place and year the studies were completed | | Specialization |
|---|---|---|---|---|---|---|---|---|---|
| Baraban Chaim Lajb Henryk | | 22.04 | 1900 | Warsaw | 28/2 Ząbkowska Street | j | p | Warsaw | 1929 | Internist |
| Barow Piotr | | 07.02 | 1898 | Yevpatoriya (now Russia) | 11 Orla Street | | | Warsaw | 1926 | Internist |
| Baumritter Paweł | | 15.09 | 1894 | Warsaw | 42/4 Hoża Street | r-c | p | Warsaw | 1922 | pediatrician |
| Bądźzdrów Teofila | | 15.05 | 1915 | Sompolno | 20/11 Ogrodowa Street | j | p | Poznań | 1937 | no specialization |
| Beiles Rachela | Przysuska | 01.02 | 1904 | Warsaw | 28–30/28 Senatorska Street | j | p | Warsaw | 1928 | pediatrician |
| Beim Maria Paulina | Felsen | 23.08 | 1912 | Lviv | 82/26 Wronia Street | j | p | Poznań | 1938 | no specialization |
| Bejles Jeszaja Isaj | | 20.04 | 1901 | Warsaw | 28–30/28 Senatorska Street | j | p | Warsaw | 1927 | Internist |
| Bemski Edward | | 27.02 | 1896 | Pińczów | 64/5 Wspólna Street | e-r | p | Warsaw | 1923 | dermatologist and venereologist |
| Benkielowa (or Benklowa) Jadwiga | Baumberg | 12.03 | 1898 | Warsaw | 23/11 Żurawia Street | j | p | Warsaw | 1929 | internist, pediatrician |
| **Ber (Borowski) Alter Altyel Paftych Artur** | | **26.03** | **1908** | **Płock** | **33/21 Wronia Street** | **j** | **p** | **Warsaw** | **1937** | **gynecologist** |
| Berendt Pejsach | | 20.10 | 1902 | Słupca | 20/6 Nowolipie Street | j | p | Warsaw | 1932 | gynecologist |

| First name and surname | Maiden name | Day, month of birth | Year of birth | Place of birth | Warsaw address (at the time of fillng the questionnaire) | Religion and nationality | Place and year the studies were completed | Specialization |
|---|---|---|---|---|---|---|---|---|
| Bergazen Stefania | | 11.02 | 1888 | Warsaw | 25/33 Muranowska Street | j | p | St. Petersburg | 1915 | Internist |
| Bergman Salomon | | 20.03 | 1891 | Łódź | 25/7 Złota Street | j | p | Warsaw | 1923 | Internist |
| Bergson Józef | | 02.11 | 1903 | Warsaw | 62A/9 Grójecka Street | j | p | Warsaw | 1937 | surgeon, gynecologist |
| Berlinerbau Markus Mordechaj | | 12.06 | 1901 | Warsaw | 10/4 Ceglana Street | j | p | Warsaw | 1938 | pathologist |
| **Berlis Paweł** | | **17.03** | **1897** | **Warsaw** | **56/30 Leszno Street** | **j** | **p** | **Warsaw** | **1922** | **dermatologist and venereologist** |
| **Berłowicz Matys** | | **29.03** | **1896** | **Warsaw** | **25/3 Zamenhofa Street** | **j** | **p** | **Warsaw** | **1923** | **internist** |
| Berman Wiera Irena | Krenicka | 11.01 | 1914 | Warsaw | 20/3 Sienna Street | j | p | Warsaw | 1938 | Internist |
| Berman Fiszel | | 02.11 | 1910 | Łódź | 11/28 Dzielna Street | j | p | Prague | 1936 | Internist |
| Berman Mieczysław Samuel Szmuel | | 13.01 | 1900 | Warsaw | 20/3 Sienna Street | j | p | Warsaw | 1930 | surgeon |
| Berman Rachela Raszela | Goldwicht | 31.12 | 1886 | Białystok | 3/4 Ogrodowa Street | j | p | Kharkiv (now Ukraine) | 1915 | gynecologist, surgeon |
| Bernstein (Burzyński) Aleksander Aron | | 26.11 | 1871 | Ostrołęka | 36/8 Sentorska Street | r-c | p | Warsaw | 1898 | internist |
| Bernstein Zygmunt | | 29.04 | 1906 | Skalat (now Ukraine) | 16/6 Ogrodowa Street | j | p | Lviv | 1930 | internist |

| First name and surname | Maiden name | Day, month of birth | Year of birth | Place of birth | Warsaw address (at the time of fillng the questionnaire) | Religion and nationality | | Place and year the studies were completed | | Specialization |
|---|---|---|---|---|---|---|---|---|---|---|
| Bernsztein Mojżesz Naftali | | 25.11 | 1897 | St. Petersburg | 20/5 Chłodna Street | j | p | Warsaw | 1926 | internist |
| Bezberg Sara | Winer | 20.06 | 1900 | Warsaw | 4/26 Dzielna Street | j | p | Warsaw | 1925 | pediatrician |
| **Bezberg Władysław** | | **26.04** | **1893** | **Warsaw** | **4/26 Dzielna Street** | **j** | **p** | **Warsaw** | **1923** | **gynecologist** |
| Bieleńki Owsiej Awsiej Andrzej | | 26.04 | 1884 | Cherkasy (now Ukraine) | 5/1 Szpitalna Street | j | p | Warsaw | 1913 | internist-pulmonologist |
| Billingowa Pessa Paulina | Barakan | 10.05 | 1889 | Warsaw | 16/3 Nowolipki Street | j | p | St. Petersburg | 1915 | gynecologist |
| Binsztejn Sara Zofia | Syrkin | 15.12 | 1889 | Bielsk Podlaski | 32 Elektoralna Street | j | p | Kyiv | 1915 | hygienist |
| Birencwejg Julian Klemens | | 29.10 | 1893 | Łódź | 4 Finlandzka Street | r-c | p | Warsaw | 1923 | internist |
| Birnbaum Jonas | | 22.05 | 1906 | Oświęcim | 37/9 Leszno Street | j | p | Berlin | 1939 | internist |
| Biro Maksymilian Maks | | 25.11 | 1866 | Warsaw | 124/4 Marszałkowska Street | j | p | Warsaw | 1891 | neurologist |
| Biro-Kon (Kon) Malwina | Blum | 12.01 | 1883 | Gąbin | 124/4 Marszałkowska Street | j | p | Paris | 1914 | pediatrician |
| Birzowski Edward Efraim | | 28.06 | 1890 | Vilnius | 66/3 Wolska Street | j | p | Kharkiv (now Ukraine) | 1915 | gynecologist |

| First name and surname | Maiden name | Day, month of birth | Year of birth | Place of birth | Warsaw address (at the time of fillng the questionnaire) | Religion and nationality | | Place and year the studies were completed | | Specialization |
|---|---|---|---|---|---|---|---|---|---|---|
| Blacher Leon Lejba | | 29.08 | 1894 | Warsaw | 3/3 Flory Street | j | p | Warsaw | 1922 | internist |
| Blay Jerzy | | 26.01 | 1876 | Kalisz | 37 Kozietulskiego Street | r-c | p | Warsaw | 1904 | internist, paediatrician |
| Blay Julia | Rabinowicz | 02.02 | 1886 | Warsaw | 7/78 Miodowa Street | j | p | Zürich | 1908 | dermatologist and venereologist |
| Blumstein Szejna | Ratner | 10.09 | 1883 | Kharkov | 20/8 Nowiniarska Street | j | p | Kharkiv | 1914 | internist, bacteriologist |
| Boczko Abram | | 17.08 | 1904 | Mława | 17/34 Dworska Street | j | p | Paris | 1932 | internist |
| Boczko Hipolit | | 15.06 | 1899 | Warsaw | 17/2 Nowolipki Street | j | p | Warsaw | 1925 | internist |
| Boczko Leonora | Landsberger | 26.08 | 1989 | Łódź | 17/2 Nowolipki Street | j | p | Warsaw | 1920 | paediatrician |
| Borkowski Izaak Ignacy | | 27.09 | 1888 | Warsaw | 4/1 Pawia Street | j | p | Heidelberg (Germany) | 1918 | surgeon |
| **Bornstein (Born) Roman** | | **14.01** | **1898** | **Łódź** | **8/9 Sosnowa Street** | **j** | **p** | **Warsaw** | **1923** | **internist** |
| Bornsztajn Frymeta | | 02.08 | 1906 | Łódź | 45/36 Sienna Street | j | p | Geneva (Switzerland) | 1936 | internist |
| **Bornsztajn Maurycy** | | **11.11** | **1874** | **Warsaw** | **8/11 Czackiego Street** | **j** | **p** | **Warsaw** | **1899** | **neurologist, psychiatrist** |

| First name and surname | Maiden name | Day, month of birth | Year of birth | Place of birth | Warsaw address (at the time of fillng the questionnaire) | Religion and nationality | | Place and year the studies were completed | | Specialization |
|---|---|---|---|---|---|---|---|---|---|---|
| Brand Jakub | | 11.11 | 1907 | possibly Chełm | 27/12 Królewska Street, 13/7 Nowolipie Street | j | p | Warsaw | 1933 | radiologist |
| Brandstaetter Gizela | Ritterman | 30.12 | 1889 | Tarnów | 38/10 Muranowska Street | j | p | Vienna | 1926 | neurologist |
| Brandwajn Maurycy | | 10.06 | 1898 | Warsaw | 46/7 Długa Street | j | p | Warsaw | 1930 | surgeon |
| Bregman Fejga Franciszka Teresa | Friedman | 20.05 | 1899 | Uhelno | 44/7 Chmielna Street | r-c | p | Kraków | 1929 | internist |
| Bregman Ludwik Eliasz | | 13.12 | 1865 | Vilnius | 5 Napoleona Street | j | p | Tartu (now Estonia) | 1890 | neurologist |
| **Brewda Alina** | | **14.06** | **1905** | **Warsaw** | **11/12 Miodowa Street** | **j** | **p** | **Warsaw** | **1930** | **gynecologist** |
| Brochis Estera Edwarda | | 13.02 | 1881 | Warsaw | 10/23 Chmielna Street | j | p | Kharkiv (now Ukraine) | 1917 | dermatologist and venereologist |
| **Brokman Henryk** | | **12.08** | **1886** | **Warsaw** | **28/8 Jerozolimskie Avenue** | **r-c** | **p** | **Heidelberg (Germany)** | **1911** | **pediatrician** |
| Bromak Szmul Jankiel | | 27.03 | 1890 | Warsaw | 4/4 Ks. Skorupki Street | j | p | Warsaw | 1924 | internist |
| Bruksztein Josif | | 19.11 | 1904 | Koło | 15/5 Leszno Street | j | p | Warsaw | 1934 | internist |
| Brzoza Abram Fajwel | | 17.04 | 1913 | Łódź | 15/33 Twarda Street | j | p | Genoa (Italy) | 1938 | no specialization |

| First name and surname | Maiden name | Day, month of birth | Year of birth | Place of birth | Warsaw address (at the time of fillng the questionnaire) | Religion and nationality | | Place and year the studies were completed | | Specialization |
|---|---|---|---|---|---|---|---|---|---|---|
| Bussel Mowsza Maurycy | | 11.08 | 1894 | Skidzyel (now Belarus) | 7/18 Żabia Street | j | p | Warsaw | 1922 | pediatrician |
| Bzura Józef Szmul | | 21.03 | 1914 | Płock | 44/84 Muranowska Street | j | p | Warsaw | 1937 | no specialization |
| Causmer Naum | | 04.10 | 1897 | Łódź | 28/34 Elektoralna Street | j | p | Lviv | 1928 | pediatrician |
| Cejtlin Mieczysław | | 03.02 | 1909 | Warsaw | 28/49 Świętojerska Street | j | p | Warsaw | 1935 | internist |
| **Celmajster Józef** | | **27.12** | **1901** | **Warsaw** | **23/5 Miła Street** | **j** | **p** | **Vilnius** | **1933** | **gynecologist** |
| Celmajster Majer | | 14.09 | 1909 | Warsaw | 17/4 Chłodna Street | j | p | Milan (Italy) | 1935 | no specialization |
| Celniker Zelman Zygmunt | | 19.07 | 1898 | Warsaw | 7/9 Muranowska Street, apart. 5 | j | p | Warsaw | 1924 | internist |
| **Chain Abram Icchok (Gołębiowski Józef)** | | **23.11** | **1894** | **Mogilev (now Belarus)** | **47/2 Złota Street** | **j** | **p** | **Bratislava** | **1923** | **internist-cardiol-ogist** |
| Chanarin Józef Hirsch | | 30.10 | 1897 | Daugavpils (now Lithuania) | 38/7 Nowolipki Street | j | p | Odesa (now Ukraine) | 1922 | radiologist |
| Chaskielewicz Chaskielowa Romana | Mamelok | 17.08 | 1912 | Zawiercie | 42/4 Zielna Street | j | p | Warsaw | 1934 | gynecologist |

| First name and surname | Maiden name | Day, month of birth | Year of birth | Place of birth | Warsaw address (at the time of fillng the questionnaire) | Religion and nationality | Place and year the studies were completed | Specialization |
|---|---|---|---|---|---|---|---|---|
| Chazan Beatrysa | | 25.06 | 1902 | Moscow | 17A/5 Nowolipie Street | j / p | Zürich / 1928 | neurologist |
| Chorążycki Borys | | 28.08 | 1871 | Šiauliai (now Lithuania) | 17a/31 Górczewska Street | j / p | Tartu (now Estonia) / 1896 | laryngologist |
| Chorążycki Julian | | 19.08 | 1885 | Šiauliai (now Lithuania) | 31/18 Nowogrodzka Street | r-c / p | Kharkiv (now Ukraine) / 1921 | laryngologist |
| Chosgelert Zelik | | 03.07 | 1910 | Warsaw | 49/1 Miła Street | j / p | Brussels / 1938 | internist |
| Chudy Nechemia | | 26.11 | 1912 | Warsaw | 30/45 Pawia Street | j / p | Bologna (Italy) / 1939 | internist |
| Cukier Abraham Chaskiel | | 04.01 | 1909 | Warsaw | 6/6 Twarda Street | j / p | Montpellier (France) / 1937 | no specialization |
| Cunge Samuel | | 18.09 | 1865 | Konin | 34/4 Chłodna Street | j / p | Warsaw / 1893 | surgeon, internist |
| Cunge (or Zunge) Jakub Mieczysław | | 04.03 | 1908 | Warsaw | 34/4 Chłodna Street | j / p | Warsaw / 1947 | neurologist |
| Cygielnik Abram Nusyn | | 23.10 | 1911 | Biała Podlaska | 53/19 Nowolipie Street | j / p | Vilnius / 1936 | no specialization |
| Cygielstreich Maria | Michels | 12.05 | 1887 | Kazimierz | 95A/3 Żelazna Street | j / p | Geneva (Switzerland) / 1913 | internist |
| Cygielstrejch Józef | | 22.02 | 1889 | Warsaw | 95A/3 Żelazna Street | j / p | Geneva (Switzerland) / 1915 | internist |
| Cyprys Gecel Gustaw | | 04.07 | 1906 | Płock | 46/6 Puławska Street | j / p | Montpellier (France) / 1932 | ophthalmologist |
| Cytter Priwa Fajga | Lichtenberg | 01.04 | 1881 | Warsaw | 24/2 Nowolipki Street | j / p | Warsaw / 1926 | no specialization |

| First name and surname | Maiden name | Day, month of birth | Year of birth | Place of birth | Warsaw address (at the time of fillng the questionnaire) | Religion and nationality | | Place and year the studies were completed | | Specialization |
|---|---|---|---|---|---|---|---|---|---|---|
| Czarnożył Alicja | | 05.01 | 1912 | Łódź | 34/19 Świętojerska Street | j | p | Montpellier (France) | 1939 | no specialization |
| Czarnożył Leib | | 23.01 | 1869 | Kalisz | 34/6 Chłodna Street | j | p | Warsaw | 1895 | internist |
| Czernichow Luba | | 23.07 | 1905 | Brzozowiec | 11/5 Dzielna Street | j | p | Paris | 1931 | internist, pediatrician |
| Czerskier Fryda | | 15.03 | 1916 | Warsaw | 31/33 Nowolipki Street | j | p | Warsaw | 1939 | no specialization |
| Damensztejn Maria | | 14.12 | 1913 | Warsaw | 10/10 Waliców Street | j | p | Warsaw | 1937 | pediatrician |
| Dankowicz Herman | | 11.03 | 1909 | Warsaw | 45/30 Twarda Street | j | p | Warsaw | 1932 | internist |
| Datyner Edward Dawid | | 07.05 | 1910 | Warsaw | 42/3 Złota Street | j | p | Prague, Pavia and Milan (Italy) | 1930–33, 1933-37 | surgeon |
| Datyner Herman | | 20.05 | 1888 | Warsaw | 39 Jerozolimskie Avenue | j | p | Berlin | 1911 | urologist |
| Diament Awrugom | | 19.11 | 1904 | Koło | 69/17 Leszno Street | j | p | Vilnius | 1930 | no specialization |
| Dobryszycki Stefan | | 24.11 | 1894 | Warsaw | 65/7 Chmielna Street | j | p | Warsaw | 1923 | internist |
| Dobrzyński Marceli | | 10.07 | 1892 | Podgaje | 15/4 Pierackiego Street | r-c | p | Vienna | 1922 | dermatologist and venereologist |

| First name and surname | Maiden name | Day, month of birth | Year of birth | Place of birth | Warsaw address (at the time of fillng the questionnaire) | Religion and nationality | Place and year the studies were completed | Specialization |
|---|---|---|---|---|---|---|---|---|
| Drutman Adam | | 30.11 | 1901 | Warsaw | 60/20 Marszałkowska Street | j, p | Warsaw 1929 | gynecologist |
| Drutman Adam | | 29.01 | 1913 | Warsaw | 7/9 Nowy Zjazd Street | j, p | Bologna (Italy) 1937 | internist |
| Dynkiewicz Gilel | | 02.10 | 1898 | Łódź | 41/2 Nowolipki Street | j, p | Vilnius 1927 | neurologist |
| Dziewczepolski Adolf Abraham | | 16.02 | 1896 | Warsaw | 19/20 Nowolipki Street | j, p | Warsaw 1924 | no specialization |
| Edelist Maria | Rozenhaus | 19.02 | 1889 | Radashkovichy (now Belarus) | 16/12 Nowolipie Street | j, p | Kharkiv (now Ukraine) 1916 | pediatrician |
| Edelszein Adam | | 13.04 | 1881 | Warsaw | 21/3 Dzielna Street | j, p | Lviv 1910 | surgeon |
| Edelszein Zofia | | 06.12 | 1887 | Warsaw | 5/5 Ceglana Street | j, p | Geneva (Switzerland) 1914 | pediatrician |
| Ejnchorn Chaim Szulim | | 06.11 | 1910 | Warsaw | 32/2 Miła Street | j, p | Nancy (France) 1935 | internist |
| Ejzenberg Abram | | 29.11 | 1908 | Warsaw | 52/1 Nowolipie Street | j, p | Warsaw 1935 | no specialization |
| Elbinger Rywka Regina | | 15.05 | 1899 | Warsaw | 24/35 Muranowska Street | j, p | Warsaw 1931 | pediatrician |
| Eljasberg Michał | | 01.04 | 1891 | Jēkabpils (now Latvia) | 61 Wspólna Street | j, p | Warsaw 1914 | surgeon |

| First name and surname | Maiden name | Day, month of birth | Year of birth | Place of birth | Warsaw address (at the time of fillng the questionnaire) | Religion and nationality | | Place and year the studies were completed | | Specialization |
|---|---|---|---|---|---|---|---|---|---|---|
| Elkes Esther | Birger | 06.12 | 1888 | Grodno (now Belarus) | 49/1 Nowolipki Street | j | p | Montpellier (France) | 1912 | no specialization |
| Elwicz Stanisław Grzegorz | | 23.12 | 1870 | Warsaw | 81/11 Marszałkowska Street | r-c | p | Warsaw | 1896 | gynecologist and surgeon |
| **Endelman Bogumił (Ochrzanowski Stefan)** | | **26.01** | **1896** | **Warsaw** | **47/13 Hoża Street** | **r-c** | **p** | **Lviv** | **1921** | **urologist** |
| Endelman Jerzy Arnold | | 26.08 | 1913 | Warsaw | 2/1 Chłodna Street | j | p | Warsaw | 1937 | surgeon |
| Endelman Leon | | 05.11 | 1876 | Warsaw | 72/2 Chmielna Street | j | p | Warsaw | 1899 | ophthalmologist |
| Endelman Samuel Zygmunt | | 20.01 | 1873 | Kalisz | 16/16 Noakowskiego Street | j | p | Warsaw | 1894 | gynecologist |
| Epsztein Henryk | | 27.07 | 1894 | Warsaw | 23/21 Jerozolimskie Avenue | j | p | Warsaw | 1934 | gynecologist, surgeon |
| Erlich Bernard | | 24.09 | 1898 | Warsaw | 55 Chłodna Street | j | p | Warsaw | 1923 | gynecologist |
| Ettinger Zofia | Ginsburg | 04.08 | 1886 | Minsk (now Belarus) | 30/17 Polna Street | j | p | Moscow | 1916 | internist |
| Fajans Tadeusz | | 07.05 | 1905 | Warsaw | 83/5 Marszałkowska Street | r-c | p | Warsaw | 1931 | internist |

| First name and surname | Maiden name | Day, month of birth | Year of birth | Place of birth | Warsaw address (at the time of fillng the questionnaire) | Religion and nationality | Place and year the studies were completed | Specialization |
|---|---|---|---|---|---|---|---|---|
| Fajgenblat Janina Franciszka | Kon | 22.11 | 1905 | Łódź | 13/1 Elektoralna Street | j | p | Warsaw | 1931 | ophthalmologist |
| Fajgenblat Maksymilian | | 17.03 | 1896 | Warsaw | 3A Wspólna Street, apart. 10 | j | p | Warsaw | 1924 | internist |
| Fajgenblat Szymon | | 09.02 | 1900 | Warsaw | 13/1 Elektoralna Street | j | p | Warsaw | 1930 | ophthalmologist |
| Fajgienblat Ludwik Andrzej | | 05.06 | 1899 | Warsaw | 51/5 Leszno Street | r-c | p | Warsaw | 1930 | gynecologist |
| Fajncyn Zygmunt Symcha | | 18.03 | 1889 | Warsaw | 36/5 Leszno Street | j | p | Warsaw | 1920 | dermatologist and venereologist |
| Fajnzylber Chaim Moszek Henryk | | 18.03 | 1882 | Lublin | 48/4 Targowa Street | j | p | Odesa (now Ukraine) | 1911 | gynecologist |
| Fajwlewicz Izrael Izydor | | 27.09 | 1901 | Piotrków Tryb. | 9/89 Miła Street | j | p | Warsaw | 1926 | internist |
| Falkowska Roza Rebeka | Bernsztejn | 09.02 | 1899 | Daugavpils (now Latvia) | 16/30 Noakowskiego Street | j | p | Vilnius | 1927 | pediatrician |
| Falkowski Dawid | | 06.09 | 1896 | Veivirženai (now Lithuania) | 16/30 Noakowskiego Street | j | p | Strasbourg (now France) | 1922 | internist |
| Federman (Federman-Michalski) Michał Bolesław | | 11.04 | 1893 | Warsaw | 9/6 Zgoda Street | e-r | p | Zürich | 1919 | internist |

| First name and surname | Maiden name | Day, month of birth | Year of birth | Place of birth | Warsaw address (at the time of fillng the questionnaire) | Religion and nationality | | Place and year the studies were completed | | Specialization |
|---|---|---|---|---|---|---|---|---|---|---|
| Fedorowski Grzegorz | | 11.04 | 1901 | Warsaw | 157 Niepodległości Avenue | e-a | p | Warsaw | 1926 | factory doctor |
| Fedorowski Mojżesz | | 23.09 | 1873 | Zhytomyr (now Ukraine) | 12/3 Ks. Skorupki Street | j | p | Warsaw | 1898 | gynecologist |
| Feilchenfeld Zofia Sara | Rosenberg | 15.03 | 1890 | Pułtusk | 11 Zielna Street | j | p | London | 1917 | pediatrician |
| Feinstein Marek Markus | | 22.03 | 1910 | Warsaw | 41/29 Leszno Street | j | p | Warsaw | 1936 | internist |
| Feinstein Stanisław | | 01.12 | 1898 | Warsaw | 13/22 Zamenhofa Street | j | p | Warsaw | 1923 | internist |
| Fejgin Brandla Bronisława | | 13.11 | 1883 | Warsaw | 65/6 Kazimierzowska Street | j | p | Paris | 1914 | bacteriologist |
| Felhendler Jankiel Jakub | | 24.10 | 1897 | Łuków | 15/9 Leszno Street | j | p | Warsaw | 1923 | internist |
| **Fenigsztein (Fenigstein) Henryk** | | **12.05** | **1913** | **Warsaw** | **20 Wspólna Street** | **j** | **p** | **Warsaw** | **1937** | **pathologist** |
| Fenigsztein Bernard | | 21.01 | 1895 | Warsaw | 30/7 Żurawia Street | j | p | Warsaw | 1923 | internist |
| Ferber Szolem Wier Borys | | 03.07 | 1874 | Grodno | 39/5 Jerozolimskie Avenue | j | p | Warsaw | 1901 | laryngologist |

| First name and surname | Maiden name | Day, month of birth | Year of birth | Place of birth | Warsaw address (at the time of fillng the questionnaire) | Religion and nationality | Place and year the studies were completed | Specialization |
|---|---|---|---|---|---|---|---|---|
| Fernberg Adolf Abe | | 23.03 | 1897 | Warsaw | 16/9 Grzybowska Street | j p | Warsaw 1925 | internist gastrologist |
| Ferster Mendel | | 20.09 | 1902 | Pławno | 42/29 Muranowska Street | j p | Warsaw 1930 | internist, phtysiatrist |
| Ferszt Lejzer Leon | | 08.08 | 1890 | Warsaw | 9/7 Kupiecka Street (Majzelsa) | j p | Heidelberg (Germany) 1919 | internist |
| **Festensztadt Abram (Czesław Sobis)** | | **30.12** | **1896** | **Warsaw** | **16/21 Ceglana Street** | **o-c p** | **Warsaw 1926** | **pediatrician** |
| Filskraut Zofia | Goclaw | 13.01 | 1898 | Warsaw | 30/13 Nowolipki Street | j p | Warsaw 1927 | pediatrician |
| Finkelkraut Maurycy Markus | | 24.03 | 1864 | Warsaw | 26/2 Sienna Street | j p | Warsaw 1891 | laryngologist |
| Finkelstein Maurycy | | 17.05 | 1899 | Ivano-Frankivsk (now Ukraine) | 3/8 Pańska Street | j p | Lviv 1924 | gynecologist |
| Finkiel Josif Zamwel | | 15.03 | 1893 | Łódź | 52/5 Leszno Street | j p | Lviv 1925 | internist |
| Finkielsztejn Abram | | 26.07 | 1904 | Gąbin | 1/4 Pawia Street | j p | Frankfurt am Main (Germany) 1933 | no specialization |
| Finkielsztejn Felicja Pessa | | 17.10 | 1901 | Warsaw | 47/3 Stalowa Street | j p | Warsaw 1930 | internist |

| First name and surname | Maiden name | Day, month of birth | Year of birth | Place of birth | Warsaw address (at the time of fillng the questionnaire) | Religion and nationality | Place and year the studies were completed | Specialization |
|---|---|---|---|---|---|---|---|---|
| Finkielsztejn Leib Leon | | 14.05 | 1911 | Łódź | 12/10 Leszno Street | j | Vilnius 1937 | internist |
| Fiszhaut Zeldowicz Ludmiła | | 14.03 | 1905 | Warsaw | 139/8 Marszałkowska Street | j | Warsaw 1930 | neurologist |
| Fiszman Jakub | | 17.02 | 1885 | Płock | 11/5 Karmelicka Street | j | Basel (Switzerland) 1915 | internist |
| Flaksbaum Elżbieta | Berman | 07.04 | 1904 | Warsaw | 76 Złota Street | j | Lausanne (Switzerland) 1928 | ophthalmologist |
| Flamenbaum Liza | Słoń | 15.05 | 1896 | Białystok | 71/12 Złota Street | j | Warsaw 1927 | pediatrician |
| Flamenbaum Sender Moszek | | 04.05 | 1907 | Warsaw | 5/2 Karmelicka Street | j | Paris 1931 | laryngologist |
| Flancman Chaim Józef | | 31.03 | 1891 | Warsaw | 28/2 Świętojerska Street | j | Kraków 1919 | surgeon |
| Flattau Motek | | 17.04 | 1908 | Łódź | 29/12 Ogrodowa Street | j | Bologna (Italy) 1938 | no specialization |
| Flaum Jadwiga | Diekstein | 20.08 | 1890 | Warsaw | 53/4 Wspólna Street | r-c | Warsaw 1923 | ophthalmologist |
| Flejsyng Dawid | | 11.07 | 1911 | Żyrardów | 66/62 Pańska Street | j | Genoa (Italy) 1939 | no specialization |
| Fliderbaum Julian | | 11.05 | 1898 | St. Petersburg | 6/4 Leszno Street | j | St. Petersburg 1924 | interna |
| Fligel Łukasz Ludwik Łazarz | | 04.02 | 1908 | Łódź | 18/1 Śliska Street | j | Warsaw 1931 | surgeon |
| Floksztrumpf Sabina | | 20.05 | 1898 | Warsaw | 19/32 Prosta Street | j | Warsaw 1929 | pediatrician |

| First name and surname | Maiden name | Day, month of birth | Year of birth | Place of birth | Warsaw address (at the time of fillng the questionnaire) | Religion and nationality | | Place and year the studies were completed | Specialization |
|---|---|---|---|---|---|---|---|---|---|
| Florman Jakub | | 21.04 | 1906 | Dobrzyń | 15/24 Twarda Street | j | p | Montpellier (France) | 1935 | no specialization |
| Fogel Mojżesz Symche | | 28.01 | 1904 | Konin | 5/8 Lubeckiego Street | j | p | Warsaw | 1933 | internist, pediatrician |
| Fogelnest Sulamita Leja | | 17.10 | 1912 | Warsaw | 15A/16 Marszałkowska Street | j | p | Warsaw | 1934 | pediatrician |
| Folman Maryla | Orzeł | 31.12 | 1911 | Łódź | 29/25 Chłodna Street | j | p | Vienna | 1936 | pediatrician |
| Folman Paulina | Edelsburg | 13.04 | 1898 | Warsaw | 4/17 Chłodna Street | j | p | Warsaw | 1926 | pediatrician |
| Forbert Chil Henryk | | 09.04 | 1897 | Płock | 56/13 Leszno Street | j | p | Warsaw | 1925 | gynecologist |
| **Frajermauer Jakób** | | **13.04** | **1906** | **Częstochowa** | **44/25 Żelazna Street** | **j** | **p** | **Vilnius** | **1932** | **internist cardiologist** |
| Frakter Zofia Zlata Zoja | | 16.08 | 1912 | Ratne (now Ukraine) | 67/21 Nowolipki Street | j | p | Warsaw | 1937 | pediatrician |
| Frank Józef | | 04.04 | 1898 | Łódź | 13/15 Graniczna Street | j | p | Warsaw | 1928 | laryngologist |
| **Frant Hersz Nacham** | | **20.11** | **1903** | **Kalisz** | **99/23 Żelazna Street** | **j** | **p** | **Vilnius** | **1929** | **gynecologist** |
| Frejman Danuta | Strasman | 10.04 | 1907 | Warsaw | 32/15 Elektoralna Street | j | p | Paris | 1932 | internist |

| First name and surname | Maiden name | Day, month of birth | Year of birth | Place of birth | Warsaw address (at the time of filling the questionnaire) | Religion and nationality | | Place and year the studies were completed | Specialization |
|---|---|---|---|---|---|---|---|---|---|
| Frejwas Fanny | | 24.11 | 1910 | Vilnius | 34/2 Świętojerska Street | j | p | Vilnius 1934 | surgeon |
| **Frendler Czesława Cyrla** | **Fogiel** | **28.08** | **1887** | **Płock** | **6/6 Waliców Street** | **j** | **p** | **Odesa (now Ukraine) 1915** | **internist** |
| Frendler Johan | | 23.11 | 1913 | Warsaw | 14/37 Elektoralna Street | j | p | Warsaw 1939 | no specialization |
| Frendler Ludwika | | 21.02 | 1899 | Płock | 6/2 Solna Street | j | p | Warsaw 1926 | internist |
| Frendler Naftali Markus (or Anatol) | | 22.11 | 1887 | Płock | 6/6 Waliców Street | j | p | Kyiv 1914 | internist, gynecologist |
| Frenkiel Chaim Izaak Henryk | | 31.12 | 1894 | Warsaw | 42/8 Nalewki Street | j | p | Warsaw 1925 | ophthalmologist |
| Frenkiel Leonia | | 31.01 | 1915 | Warsaw | 21/12 Nowolipie Street | j | p | Warsaw 1938 | internist |
| Fridman Rywka | | 13.08 | 1905 | Zamość | 127 Leszno Street | j | p | Prague 1933 | no specialization |
| Friedman Hersch | | 14.02 | 1891 | Beleiv (now Ukraine) | 44/7 Chmielna Street | j | p | Kraków 1920 | internist, pediatrician, surgeon |
| Friedstein Gustaw | | 22.09 | 1893 | Łódź | 38/7 Sienna Street | j | p | Berlin 1921 | internist |
| Fryszberg Blima Bronisława | Firstenberg | 10.01 | 1884 | Płock | 30/4 Świętokrzyska Street | j | p | Berlin 1909 | ophthalmologist |
| Gabay Helena | Basenszpiler | 08.03 | 1886 | Warsaw | 28–30/27 Senatorska Street | j | p | Geneva (Switzerland) 1913 | gynecologist |

| First name and surname | Maiden name | Day, month of birth | Year of birth | Place of birth | Warsaw address (at the time of filling the questionnaire) | Religion and nationality | Place and year the studies were completed | | Specialization |
|---|---|---|---|---|---|---|---|---|---|
| Gabryjelew Mordka | | 18.12 | 1886 | Warsaw | 23/5 Złota Street | j | Warsaw | 1925 | internist |
| Gajer Czesław | | 30.12 | 1913 | Warsaw | 17/7 Prosta Street | j | Lyon (France) | 1939 | no specialization |
| Gajewska Janina | Milejkowska | 24.07 | 1913 | Warsaw | 34/4 Tamka Street | r-c | Warsaw | 1936 | internist |
| Gajst Izrael Icek | | 02.05 | 1894 | Kutno | 33 Ogrodowa Street | j | Kraków | 1930 | internist |
| Galewski Alfred | | 20.09 | 1903 | Warsaw | 4/9 Solna Street | e-r | Warsaw | 1928 | internist |
| Ganc (Radwański) Tadeusz | | 13.02 | 1897 | Pławno | 4A/11 Żurawia Street | e-r | Warsaw | 1926 | dermatologist and venereologist |
| Gantz Róża Maria (Grabowska Romana Maria, after the war, Gantz-Grabowska) | | 20.02 | 1895 | Kraków | 9A/7 Wilcza Street | r-c | Kraków | 1921 | ophthalmologist |
| Garfinkiel Jakób | | 17.11 | 1895 | Warsaw | 9/7 Ceglana Street | j | Warsaw | 1922 | internist, gynecologist |
| Gat Juda | | 27.06 | 1908 | Kalisz | 25/9 Dzielna Street | j | Vilnius | 1937 | internist |
| Geisler Józef | | 07.11 | 1886 | Włocławek | 41/23 Puławska Street | j | Munich (Germany) | 1916 | dematologist |
| Gelbard Aniela (Majewska Zofia) | | 13.01 | 1907 | Warsaw | 4/82 Słupecka Street | e-r | Warsaw | 1930 | neurologist |

| First name and surname | Maiden name | Day, month of birth | Year of birth | Place of birth | Warsaw address (at the time of fillng the questionnaire) | Religion and nationality | | Place and year the studies were completed | | Specialization |
|---|---|---|---|---|---|---|---|---|---|---|
| Gelbart Ajzyk | | 17.07 | 1882 | Piotrków | 28/24 6 Sierpnia Street | j | p | Kyiv | 1912 | internist, pediatrician |
| Gelbfisz Beniamin | | 12.07 | 1894 | Warsaw | 19/5 Senatorska Street | j | p | Bratislava | 1921 | dermatologist and venereologist |
| Gelbfisz Jakub | | 05.11 | 1895 | Warsaw | 27/2 Złota Street | j | p | Warsaw | 1923 | dermatologist and venereologist |
| Gelertner Bernard | | 16.09 | 1895 | Warsaw | 27/7 Leszno Street | j | p | Warsaw | 1926 | laryngologist |
| Gerkowicz Rafał | | 15.01 | 1894 | Warsaw | 25/4 Nowolipie Street | j | p | Bratislava | 1933 | no specialization |
| Gibiański Abram Abe | | 18.06 | 1873 | Warsaw | 16/14 Nowolipie Street | j | p | Warsaw | 1901 | internist |
| Gilde Siegfried | | 19.04 | 1905 | Szczecin | 95A/4 Żelazna Street | j | g | Berlin | 1929 | internist |
| Ginzberg Izaak | | 26.02 | 1896 | Warsaw | 48/24 Pawia Street | j | p | Warsaw | 1936 | internist |
| Ginzberg (or Ginsberg) Wolf Majer | | 28.02 | 1905 | Warsaw | 38/22 Nalewki Street | j | p | Paris | 1935 | no specialization |
| Ginzburg Bella | Ginsburg | 25.07 | 1891 | Luga (Russia) | 42/4 Wilcza Street | j | p | Kyiv | 1916 | dermatologist and venereologist |
| Ginzburg Abram Leon Lejba | | 17.12 | 1893 | Nieśwież | 35/4 Muranowska Street | j | p | Moscow | 1921 | gynecologist |

| First name and surname | Maiden name | Day, month of birth | Year of birth | Place of birth | Warsaw address (at the time of fillng the questionnaire) | Religion and nationality | | Place and year the studies were completed | | Specialization |
|---|---|---|---|---|---|---|---|---|---|---|
| Ginzburg Franciszka | Szpilman | 07.04 | 1898 | Warsaw | 35/3 Muranowska Street | j | p | Warsaw | 1925 | gynecologist |
| Gitler Tobias | | 13.02 | 1909 | Mazyr (now Belarus) | 34/2 Chłodna Street | j | p | Warsaw | 1935 | gynecologist |
| Gladsztern Szymon | | 27.10 | 1904 | Warsaw | 14/3 Złota Street | j | p | Warsaw | 1931 | gynecologist |
| **Glajchgewicht Uszer** | | **16.12** | **1906** | **Warsaw** | **56/1 Nowolipie Street** | **j** | **p** | **Warsaw** | **1934** | **internist** |
| Glass Boruch Bronisław | | 31.01 | 1874 | Mława | 18/5 Nowolipki Street | j | p | Warsaw | 1899 | infectious diseases |
| Glass Mieczysław | | 19.08 | 1897 | Warsaw | 72/18 Marszałkowska Street | j | p | Warsaw | 1922 | internist |
| Glauberman Morduch | | 13.06 | 1886 | Pinsk (now Belarus) | 26/6 Chłodna Street | j | p | Tartu (now Estonia) | 1915 | surgeon |
| Glauternik Haim | | 21.06 | 1905 | Kalisz | 2/8 Łucka Street | j | p | Padua (Italy) | 1929 | internist |
| Gleichgewicht Adolf | | 09.12 | 1907 | Warsaw | 74/31 Sienna Street | j | p | Geneva (Switzerland) | 1934 | radiologist |
| Gliksman Józef | | 22.11 | 1893 | Warsaw | 53/31 Nowolipki Street | j | p | Vilnius | 1931 | internist |
| Glozman Salomon | | 17.02 | 1890 | Kyiv | 37/5 Poznańska Street | j | p | Kyiv | 1917 | radiologist |

| First name and surname | Maiden name | Day, month of birth | Year of birth | Place of birth | Warsaw address (at the time of fillng the questionnaire) | Religion and nationality | | Place and year the studies were completed | | Specialization |
|---|---|---|---|---|---|---|---|---|---|---|
| Gold Helena | Waldman | 13.06 | 1898 | Łódź | 77/4 Leszno Street | j | p | Warsaw | 1928 | pediatrician |
| Gold Wolf Władysław | | 27.03 | 1896 | Słupca | 77/4 Leszno Street | j | p | Warsaw | 1925 | internist |
| Goldach Esther Anastazja | Schwartz | 15.05 | 1907 | Piotrków | 47/17 Wronia Street | j | p | Basel (Switzerland) | 1932 | internist |
| Goldband Izrael Mojżesz Marek | | 02.05 | 1913 | Warsaw | 13/4 Gęsia Street | j | p | Paris | 1936 | internist |
| Goldberg Anna Bronisława | | 08.09 | 1888 | Warsaw | 16/1 Zielna Street | r-c | p | Geneva (Switzerland) | 1912 | ophthalmologist |
| Goldberg Chaim Leib | | 11.01 | 1909 | Solec | 29/3 Nowolipki Street | j | p | Bordeaux (France) | 1936 | internist |
| Goldberg Chana Anna | | 12.04 | 1884 | Niasvizh (now Belarus) | 11/12 Mazowiecka Street | j | p | Bern (Switzerland) | 1914 | pediatrician |
| Goldberg Edward | | 12.07 | 1881 | Warsaw | 9 Zielna Street (16/1 Sienna Street) | j | p | Kazan (Russia) | 1932 | surgeon |
| Goldberg Henryk Dawid | | 21.11 | 1902 | Warsaw | 62 Złota Street | j | p | Warsaw | 1927 | internist |
| Goldberg Henryka Jadwiga | Neufeld | 25.10 | 1884 | Warsaw | 19/5 Wielka Street | r-c | p | Kazan (Russia) | 1916 | pediatrician |
| Goldberg Jadwiga | | 20.05 | 1890 | Warsaw | 16/1 Zielna Street | r-c | p | Warsaw | 1923 | bacteriologist |
| Goldberger Majlech | | 09.06 | 1908 | Łódź | 5/3 Orla Street | j | p | Prague | 1939 | no specialization |

| First name and surname | Maiden name | Day, month of birth | Year of birth | Place of birth | Warsaw address (at the time of fillng the questionnaire) | Religion and nationality | | Place and year the studies were completed | | Specialization |
|---|---|---|---|---|---|---|---|---|---|---|
| Goldberg-Górecki Julian Andrzej | | 31.05 | 1884 | Warsaw | 42/4 Hoża Street | r-c | p | Kyiv | 1910 | internist |
| **Golde Chaja Zlata Zofia** | **Żyżmorska** | **06.01** | **1882** | **Kaunas (now Lithuania)** | **24/1 Jerozolimskie Avenue** | **j** | **p** | **Bern (Switzerland)** | **1912** | **pediatrician** |
| Goldfarb Gita Gitel | | 14.04 | 1910 | Dubno | 18 Śliska Street | j | p | Florence (Italy) | 1937 | internist |
| Goldfarb Hersz | | 25.12 | 1905 | Siedlce | 31/1 Elektoralna Street | j | p | Vilnius | 1931 | internist |
| Goldflam Menachem Maks | | 20.08 | 1872 | Warsaw | 86/7 Marszałkowska Street | j | p | Warsaw | 1899 | dermatologist and venereologist |
| Goldlust Leon Szaja | | 27.06 | 1893 | Piotrków | 52/2 Nowolipki Street | j | p | Vienna | 1922 | internist |
| **Goldman Hersz** | | **16.05** | **1910** | **Warsaw** | **61/2 Sienna Street** | **j** | **p** | **Nancy (France)** | **1937** | **surgeon** |
| Goldman Maurycy | | 23.04 | 1908 | Piotrków | 36/9 Złota Street | j | p | Vilnius | 1931 | surgeon Dentist |
| Goldman Mieczysław | | 25.12 | 1897 | Warsaw | 24/9 Leszno Street | j | p | Warsaw | 1924 | internist |
| Goldstein Jan | | 18.02 | 1913 | Warsaw | 7/1 Ceglana Street | j | p | Warsaw | 1937 | surgeon |
| Goldstein Józef | | 13.07 | 1891 | Warsaw | 6/17 Nowiniarska Street | j | p | Kraków | 1920 | gynecologist |

| First name and surname | Maiden name | Day, month of birth | Year of birth | Place of birth | Warsaw address (at the time of fillng the questionnaire) | Religion and nationality | | Place and year the studies were completed | | Specialization |
|---|---|---|---|---|---|---|---|---|---|---|
| Goldszmid Szymon Menachem | | 01.05 | 1914 | Biała Podlaska | 6/15 Kurza Street | j | p | Bologna (Italy) | 1939 | no specialization |
| Goldszmidt Henryk (Korczak Janusz) | | 22.07 | 1878 | Warsaw | 8/4 Złota Street | j | p | Warsaw | 1905 | pediatrician |
| Goldsztajn Abram | | 18.01 | 1899 | Pabianice | 29/4 Zamenhofa Street | j | p | Warsaw | 1926 | no specialization |
| Goldsztein Chil Berek | | 14.04 | 1908 | Radom | 43A/2 Żelazna Street | j | p | Vilnius | 1928 | pediatrician |
| Goldsztein (or Goldstein) Berek | | 28.02 | 1900 | Piotrków | 38/6 Leszno Street | j | p | Warsaw | 1926 | no specialization |
| Goldsztein (or Goldsztajn, or Goldsztejn) Markus | | 17.08 | 1900 | Warsaw | 18/9 Majzelesa Street | j | p | Vilnius | 1933 | internist |
| Goldwasser Józef | | 07.08 | 1886 | Staszów | 11/11 Pawia Street | j | p | Tartu (now Estonia) | 1916 | internist |
| **Goliborska Teodozja** | **Gołąb** | **18.10** | **1899** | **Warsaw** | **60 Sienna Street** | **j** | **p** | **Warsaw** | **1926** | **bacteriologist** |
| Gordon Karpel | | 02.12 | 1874 | Ciechanowiec | 15/20 Karmelicka Street | j | p | Tartu (now Estonia) | 1902 | internist |

| First name and surname | Maiden name | Day, month of birth | Year of birth | Place of birth | Warsaw address (at the time of fillng the questionnaire) | Religion and nationality | | Place and year the studies were completed | | Specialization |
|---|---|---|---|---|---|---|---|---|---|---|
| Gordon Salomon | | 17.01 | 1894 | Warsaw | 11/10 Orla Street | j | p | Warsaw | 1923 | gynecologist |
| **Gotlib Albert Abram** | | **no data** | **1894** | **Włoszczowa** | **65A/4 Nowolipie Street** | - | - | **Vilnius** | **1926** | **gynecologist** |
| Gotlib Aron | | 10.09 | 1901 | Włoszczowa | 37/67 Nalewki Street | j | p | Vilnius | 1929 | internist |
| Gotlib Kazimierz Julian | | 14.02 | 1903 | Warsaw | 5/2 Cicha Street | r-c | p | Warsaw | 1928 | homeopath |
| Gottfryd Fabian | | 09.10 | 1880 | Kalisz | 42/5 Zielna Street | j | p | Kraków | 1908 | laryngologist |
| Grajwer Szymon | | 09.09 | 1909 | Warsaw | 30/2 Pawia Street | j | p | Geneva (Switzerland) | 1936 | surgeon |
| Grasberg Eluzor Jakób | | 15.02 | 1914 | Warsaw | 4/28 Pawia Street | j | p | Lyon (France) | 1937 | internist |
| Grauzam Albin | | 09.12 | 1909 | Kielce | 21/14 Sienna Street | r-c | p | Paris | 1925 | no specialization |
| Grodzieńska (or Dubrow-Grodzieńska) Irena | Tylko | 28.08 | 1906 | Warsaw | 4/3 Zielna Street | j | p | Warsaw | 1931 | internist |
| Grodzieńska Klara | Torończyk | 21.06 | 1897 | Warsaw | 24 Śliska Street | r-c | p | Warsaw | 1927 | internist |
| Grodzieński (Dobrowo) Michał | | 07.12 | 1875 | Warsaw | 81/3 Marszałkowska Street | j | p | Warsaw | 1900 | internist |
| Grodzieński Edward | | 04.10 | 1905 | Warsaw | 4/3 Zielna Street | j | p | Warsaw | 1929 | internist |
| Grodziński Hieronim | | 12.06 | 1902 | Warsaw | 10/12 Puławska Street | j | p | Warsaw | 1930 | internist, gynecologist |

| First name and surname | Maiden name | Day, month of birth | Year of birth | Place of birth | Warsaw address (at the time of fillng the questionnaire) | Religion and nationality | | Place and year the studies were completed | | Specialization |
|---|---|---|---|---|---|---|---|---|---|---|
| **Grojsblat Mojżesz** | | **12.10** | **1894** | **Warsaw** | **19/4 Żurawia Street** | **j** | **p** | **Warsaw** | **1925** | **internist, bacteriologist** |
| Groner Mojsze | | 18.08 | 1910 | Włocławek | 1/1 Ogrodowa Street | j | p | Bordeaux (France) | 1935 | no specialization |
| **Groniowski (Gruszczyński) Antoni** | | **15.08** | **1871** | **Warsaw** | **113/10 Marszałkowska Street** | **e-a** | **p** | **Warsaw** | **1896** | **dermatologist and venereologist** |
| Grosglik Józef | | 24.12 | 1897 | Warsaw | 44/11 Złota Street | j | p | Warsaw | 1925 | dermatologist and venereologist |
| Grosglik Zofia | Berkman | 08.09 | 1897 | Białystok | 44/11 Złota Street | j | p | Warsaw | 1923 | dermatologist and venereologist |
| Grycendler Stanisław | | 29.11 | 1897 | Warsaw | 29A/23 Wilcza Street | r-c | p | Warsaw | 1926 | gynecologist |
| Grynberg Chaim Izaak | | 10.07 | 1915 | Wymyślin | 36/23 Leszno Street | j | p | Genoa (Italy) | 1939 | no specialization |
| **Grynberg Zygmunt** | | **25.12** | **1903** | **Warsaw** | **15/2 Chłodna Street** | **j** | **p** | **Warsaw** | **1927** | **internist** |
| Grynblat Szmul | | 24.09 | 1895 | Łódź | 15/3 Graniczna Street | j | p | Warsaw | 1928 | internist |
| Gurfinkiel Róża | Efros | 23.09 | 1908 | Warsaw | 1/10 Rynkowa Street | j | p | Warsaw | 1936 | no specialization |
| Gutentag Stanisław | | 02.02 | 1866 | Warsaw | 92/4 Sienna Street | j | p | Warsaw | 1892 | pediatrician |

| First name and surname | Maiden name | Day, month of birth | Year of birth | Place of birth | Warsaw address (at the time of fillng the questionnaire) | Religion and nationality | Place and year the studies were completed | | Specialization |
|---|---|---|---|---|---|---|---|---|---|
| Gutman Łaja | | 27.12 | 1876 | Warsaw | 43/8 Mokotowska Street | - | Kharkiv (now Ukraine) | 1910 | analyst |
| Gutman Maria | Wolf | 04.10 | 1903 | Łódź | 9/5 Dzielna Street | j | Vilnius | 1929 | pediatrician |
| Hager Lejb | | 16.01 | 1915 | Warsaw | 25/26 Nowolipki Street | j | Bordeaux (France) | 1938 | internist |
| Hajman Jakub | | 10.10 | 1897 | Łódź | 12/7 Solna Street | j | Warsaw | 1927 | internist |
| Halbersztadt Józef | | 31.08 | 1912 | Warsaw | 38/7 Nowolipie Street | j | Warsaw | 1936 | surgeon |
| Halpern-Wieliczański Henryk | | 21.11 | 1903 | Łódź | 25/27 Złota Street | r-c | Warsaw | 1931 | internist, phthysiologist |
| Halperyn Necha Natalia | Pianko | 05.03 | 1900 | Warsaw | 28/5A Leszno Street | j | Vienna | 1928 | pediatrician |
| Halter Maria | | 26.03 | 1899 | Kalisz | 43/15 Krochmalna Street | j | Vilnius | 1931 | internist |
| Hanftwurzel Mieczysław | | 09.03 | 1908 | Warsaw | 18/58 Gęsia Street | j | Liege (Belgium) | 1938 | internist |
| Hartglas Janina | | 01.06 | 1888 | Biała Podlaska | 67/5 Leszno Street | j | St. Petersburg | 1914 | pediatrician |
| Hejman Włodzimierz | | 13.07 | 1904 | Warsaw | 25 Jerozolimskie Avenue | j | Warsaw | 1928 | internist |

| First name and surname | Maiden name | Day, month of birth | Year of birth | Place of birth | Warsaw address (at the time of fillng the questionnaire) | Religion and nationality | Place and year the studies were completed | Specialization |
|---|---|---|---|---|---|---|---|---|
| Heller Anna Chana Rywka | Braude | 06.01 | 1888 | Warsaw | 5/3 Szpitalna Street | j / p | Geneva (Switzerland), Zürich, Berlin / 1911 | pediatrician |
| **Heller Ari Leo** | | **27.07** | **1917** | **Warsaw** | **6–8/9 Śliska Street** | **j / p** | **Warsaw** / **1939** | **no specialization** |
| Heller Maurycy Mojżesz | | 15.12 | 1897 | Warsaw | 11A/5 Mylna Street | j / p | Warsaw / 1923 | urologist |
| Helman (after the war, Mintz) Emilia | Łaska | 24.06 | 1884 | Płock | 29A/3 Królewska Street | j / p | Warsaw / 1929 | internist |
| Hercberg Chaim Józef | | 06.11 | 1897 | Warsaw | 10 Pawia Street | j / p | Warsaw / 1923 | internist |
| Hercenberg Teofila Rachela | Flancer | 22.09 | 1899 | Warsaw | 24/7 Złota Street | j / ż | Warsaw / 1925 | internist, analysta |
| **Herman Eufemiusz** | | **29.09** | **1892** | **Tomaszów Maz.** | **6/3 Jasna Street** | **j / p** | **Lviv** / **1918** | **neurologist** |
| Hermelin Adolf Henryk | | 03.03 | 1896 | Warsaw | 23/3 Bielańska Street | j / p | Warsaw / 1923 | internist |
| Hermelinowa Berta | Heller | 23.01 | 1898 | Vawkavysk (now Belarus) | 23/3 Bielańska Street | j / p | Warsaw / 1923 | pediatrician |
| Herszenfus Perla | | 31.03 | 1917 | Warsaw | 6/37 Sierakowskiego Street | j / p | Lviv / 1941 | internist |

| First name and surname | Maiden name | Day, month of birth | Year of birth | Place of birth | Warsaw address (at the time of filling the questionnaire) | Religion and nationality | | Place and year the studies were completed | | Specialization |
|---|---|---|---|---|---|---|---|---|---|---|
| Herszfinkiel Jechiel | | 30.01 | 1896 | Czerków | 19/3 Nowolipki Street | j | p | Warsaw | 1923 | |
| Hertz Artur | | 22.03 | 1895 | Piotrków | 18/8 Sienna Street | j | p | Warsaw | 1925 | internist |
| Higier Henryk | | 13.01 | 1865 | Warsaw | 29 Królewska Street | j | p | Tartu (now Estonia) | 1890 | neurologist |
| Higier Stanisław | | 02.04 | 1894 | Warsaw | 18/30 Marszałkowska Street | r-c | p | Geneva | 1924 | neurologist, seksuolog |
| **Hindes Salomon Stanisław** | | **20.06** | **1894** | **Berestechko (now Ukraine)** | **34/1 Mokotowska Street** | **j** | **p** | **Kyiv** | **1916** | **ophthalmologist** |
| Hirsz Maksymilian | | 09.05 | 1877 | Lublin | 72/14 Marszałkowska Street | j | p | Warsaw | 1902 | dermatologist and venereologist |
| Hirszbajn Daniel | | 29.12 | 1895 | Warsaw | 6/25 Leszno Street | j | p | Warsaw | 1923 | internist and radiologist |
| Hirszbajn Stanisław Salomon | | 04.10 | 1893 | Warsaw | 16/2 Solna Street | j | p | Warsaw | 1923 | dermatologist and venereologist |
| **Hirszfeld Hanna Maria** | **Kasman** | **17.07** | **1884** | **Wilczkowice** | **27 Obrońców Street** | **r-c** | **p** | **Naples (Italy)** | **1916** | **pediatrician** |
| Hirszhorn Masza Sima | | 27.12 | 1880 | Słonim (now Belarus) | 29/15 Zielna Street | j | p | Paris | 1908 | bacteriologist, analyst, dermatologist and venereologist |

| First name and surname | Maiden name | Day, month of birth | Year of birth | Place of birth | Warsaw address (at the time of fillng the questionnaire) | Religion and nationality | Place and year the studies were completed | Specialization |
|---|---|---|---|---|---|---|---|---|
| Hochsinger Józef | | 06.08 | 1894 | Warsaw | 11 Elektoralna Street | j / p | Prague 1922 | internist cardiologist |
| **Holländer Alicja Ala (Jasińska Stefania)** | | **19.03** | **1883** | **Bochnia** | **no data** | **j / p** | **Zürich (Switzerland) 1921** | **psychiatrist** |
| Hufnagel Fejga | Charadeamo | 01.08 | 1898 | Vysokaje (now Belarus) | 38/14 Pawia Street | j / p | Warsaw 1926 | gynecologist |
| Hufnagel Kazimiera | Prechner | 09.06 | 1905 | Łódź | 21/23 Czerwonego Krzyża Street, apart. 15 | r-c / p | Warsaw 1930 | gynecologist |
| Hurwicz Natan | | 10.12 | 1907 | Łódź | 16/31 Ogrodowa Street | j / p | Paris 1934 | |
| Iberbein Mojżesz | | 06.04 | 1890 | Warsaw | 7/2 Karmelicka Street | j / p | Prague 1921 | pediatrician |
| **Jabłoński Józef** | | **05.06** | **1894** | **Warsaw** | **49/23 Marszałkowska Street** | **j / p** | **Warsaw 1925** | **laryngologist** |
| Jabłoński Leon | | 01.01 | 1902 | Warsaw | 25/5 Złota Street | j / p | Saratov (Russia) 1917 | gynecologist |
| Jacobi Mojżesz Chaim Marian | | 29.09 | 1913 | Łomża | 7/35 Elektoralna Street | j / p | Strasbourg (France) 1938 | surgeon |
| Jakobius Leonard | | 22.12 | 1912 | Tuchola | 42/8 Nalewki Street | j / p | Berlin 1937 | internist |

| First name and surname | Maiden name | Day, month of birth | Year of birth | Place of birth | Warsaw address (at the time of fillng the questionnaire) | Religion and nationality | | Place and year the stud-ies were completed | | Specialization |
|---|---|---|---|---|---|---|---|---|---|---|
| Jakubowicz Henryk | | 24.04 | 1866 | Warsaw | 54/6 Hoża Street | j | p | Warsaw | 1899 | internist |
| Jankielowicz Tolli | | 19.05 | 1912 | Łódź | 40/6 Nalewki Street | j | p | Warsaw | 1936 | internist |
| **Janower (after the war, Janowicz) Moszek** | | **24.09** | **1893** | **Warsaw** | **24/7 Złota Street** | **j** | **p** | **Warsaw** | **1925** | **internist, gynecologist** |
| Janowski Ilia | | 19.11 | 1904 | Skidzyel (now Belarus) | 28/9 Twarda Street | j | p | Vilnius | 1929 | internist |
| Jaszuński Michał | | 28.08 | 1914 | St. Petersburg | 78/5 Żelazna Street | j | p | Warsaw | 1938 | internist |
| Jawic Zusman | | 24.05 | 1893 | Baranów | 26/5 Muranowska Street | j | p | Warsaw | 1930 | internist |
| Jelenkiewicz Mira | Markson | 10.09 | 1898 | Warsaw | 22/29 Widok Street | r-c | p | Warsaw | 1926 | analyst |
| Jochelson Gitla | | 12.12 | 1885 | Vilnius | 12/26 Noakowskiego Street | j | p | Strasbourg (France) | 1912 | radiologist |
| Josefsberg Markus | | 26.03 | 1906 | Borysław | 39/6 Nowolipki Street | j | p | St. Petersburg | 1938 | no specialization |
| Judt Regina | | 08.09 | 1896 | Warsaw | 13/14 Śniadeckich Street | j | p | Kazan (Russia) | 1916 | dermatologist and venereologist |
| Justman Stanisław Samuel | | 06.05 | 1874 | Kalisz | 3/6 Poznańska Street | j | p | Warsaw | 1899 | neurologist |
| Kabacznik Leon | | 07.02 | 1891 | Moscow | 4/10 Komitetowa Street | j | p | Rostov (Russia) | 1920 | generalist |

| First name and surname | Maiden name | Day, month of birth | Year of birth | Place of birth | Warsaw address (at the time of fillng the questionnaire) | Religion and nationality | Place and year the studies were completed | Specialization |
|---|---|---|---|---|---|---|---|---|
| **Kachan Aleksander (Pacho Edward)** | | **03.04** | **1912** | **Warsaw** | **73/8 Marszałkowska Street** | **j** / **p** | **Warsaw** / **1937** | **no specialization** |
| Kachan Halina | Brylant | 20.06 | 1913 | Płock | 73/8 Marszałkowska Street | j / p | Warsaw / 1936 | internist and pediatrician |
| Kadysiewicz Leon (Kosiński Leon) | | 09.02 | 1891 | Radom | 46/4 Targowa Street | j / p | Jena (Germany) / 1918 | gynecologist, surgeon |
| Kahan Aleksander (Pacho Edward) | | 20.03 | 1898 | Warsaw | 38/4 Świętojerska Street | j / p | Warsaw / 1928 | internist and analyst |
| Kahan Chaja Helena | Słomnicka | 09.05 | 1904 | Warsaw | 19/4 Długa Street | j / p | Warsaw / 1929 | pediatrician |
| Kahan Dawid Hirsz | | 11.04 | 1912 | Warsaw | 19 Ogrodowa Street | j / p | Basel (Switzerland) / 1938 | neurologist |
| Kahan Izaak Józef | | 31.12 | 1905 | Warsaw | 40/8 Nalewki Street | j / p | Montpellier (France) / 1932 | surgeon dentist |
| Kahan Maria Lidia | | 14.03 | 1905 | Warsaw | 5/27 Nalewki Street | j / p | Warsaw / 1930 | pediatrician |
| Kahan Mieczysław | | 25.06 | 1878 | Zamość | 6/6 Żelaznej Bramy Square | j / p | Warsaw / 1900 | internist |
| Kahane Scheindla | Blumenstock | 23.05 | 1906 | Oświęcim | 18/10 Wawelberga Street | j / p | Brno (Czech Republic) / 1937 | internist |
| Kahanowicz Borys | | 07.11 | 1897 | Warsaw | 9/32 Przejazd Street | j / p | Warsaw / 1930 | laryngologist |

| First name and surname | Maiden name | Day, month of birth | Year of birth | Place of birth | Warsaw address (at the time of fillng the questionnaire) | Religion and nationality | Place and year the studies were completed | | Specialization |
|---|---|---|---|---|---|---|---|---|---|
| Kajzer Abram | | 26.11 | 1913 | Kielce | 17/94 Dworska Street | j p | Kraków | 1938 | surgeon |
| Kajzer Naftal | | 12.03 | 1907 | Łódź | 51A/3 Nowolipki Street | j p | Warsaw | 1930 | internist, pediatrician |
| Kandel Aron | | 29.04 | 1909 | Łódź | 32/3 Nowolipki Street | j p | Paris | 1934 | pediatrician |
| Kantor Salomon | | 21.12 | 1871 | Riga | 27/9 Nowolipki Street | j p | Tartu (now Estonia) | 1899 | dermatologist and venereologist |
| Karasz Henryk Hersz | | 31.06 | 1890 | Warsaw | 11/8 Mariańska Street | j p | Basel (Switzeland), Warsaw | 1924 | internist |
| Karbowska Paulina | Seidenbeutel | 07.08 | 1882 | Warsaw | 68/6 Piusa XI Street | j p | Kazan (Russia) | 1910 | laryngologist |
| Karbowski Mieczysław | | 24.04 | 1896 | Łomża | 49/3 Hoża Street | j p | Warsaw | 1924 | ophthalmologist |
| Karlsztat Mieczysław | | 25.12 | 1913 | Warsaw | 6/4 Lubeckiego Street | j p | Prague | 1937 | internist |
| Karsz Jefim | | 18.10 | 1906 | Brest (now Belarus) | 35/5 Muranowska Street | j p | Paris, Vilnius | 1938 | ophthalmologist |
| Katz (or Kac) Mendel | | 28.08 | 1896 | Brańsk | 27/5 Nowolipki Street | j p | Warsaw | 1923 | ophthalmologist |

| First name and surname | Maiden name | Day, month of birth | Year of birth | Place of birth | Warsaw address (at the time of fillng the questionnaire) | Religion and nationality | Place and year the studies were completed | Specialization |
|---|---|---|---|---|---|---|---|---|
| **Keilson Hela Helena Hinda Inda (Puławska Janina)** | | **26.06** | **1903** | **Szczuczyn** | **15/18 Graniczna Street** | **p** | **Warsaw** **1927** | **pediatrician** |
| Kenigsberg Dawid | | 12.10 | 1890 | Vilnius | 30/5 Chmielna Street | j p | Warsaw 1915 | dermatologist and venereologist |
| Kerz Abraham | | 13.11 | 1898 | Kobylanka | 21/3 Dzielna Street | j p | Kraków 1928 | internist, pediatrician |
| Kiejlson Abel Abe | | 24.02 | 1905 | Szczuczyn | 33/10 Warmińska Street | j p | Warsaw 1930 | internist |
| Kierszenblat Wigdor | | 17.02 | 1897 | Radom | 11/4 Mariańska Street | j p | Kraków 1928 | laryngologist |
| Kigiel Izaak | | 29.03 | 1890 | Sevastopol (now Russia) | 8/1 Leszno Street | j p | Odesa (now Ukraine) 1913 | surgeon |
| Kindler Dawid | | 27.01 | 1892 | Sokal | 29/7 Leszno Street | j p | Lviv 1917 | surgeon gynecologist |
| **Kinman (Majewska) Jadwiga Jenta** | **Hufnagel** | **01.01** | **1895** | **Wyszków** | **11/7 Elektoralna Street** | **j p** | **Warsaw** **1926** | **pediatrician** |
| Kipman Izabela | Endelman | 26.11 | 1897 | Warsaw | 37/3 Poznańska Street | r-c p | Warsaw 1923 | neurologist |

| First name and surname | Maiden name | Day, month of birth | Year of birth | Place of birth | Warsaw address (at the time of fillng the questionnaire) | Religion and nationality | | Place and year the studies were completed | | Specialization |
|---|---|---|---|---|---|---|---|---|---|---|
| Kipman Jerzy | | 07.07 | 1894 | Sosnowiec | 37/3 Poznańska Street | r-c | p | Warsaw | 1924 | gynecologist |
| **Kirjasefer Jerzy** | | **10.12** | **1911** | **Warsaw** | **29 Poznańska Street** | **j** | **p** | **Warsaw** | **1938** | **surgeon** |
| Kirszblum Rudolf | | 01.03 | 1899 | Warsaw | 6/5 Waliców Street | j | p | Paris | 1930 | internist |
| Kirszbraun Aleksander | | 30.12 | 1896 | Warsaw | 19/8 Wspólna Street | j | p | Warsaw | 1924 | pediatrician |
| Kirszenberg Zelik | | 13.06 | 1907 | Warsaw | 14/116 Elektoralna Street | j | p | Warsaw | 1935 | internist |
| Kiszycer (or Kiszygier) Grzegorz Girsz | | 15.07 | 1889 | Moscow | 7/12 Orla Street | j | p | Munich (Germany) | 1920 | internist |
| Klaczko Chana | Zeldowicz | 19.03 | 1888 | Sochaczew | 23/5 Złota Street | j | p | Kharkiv (now Ukraine) | 1914 | gynecologist |
| Klaczko Majer Nison | | 08.03 | 1884 | Sochaczew | 23/5 Złota Street | j | p | Kharkiv (now Ukraine) | 1914 | laryngologist |
| Klajer Rubin Roman | | 12.12 | 1897 | Warsaw | 2/15 Biała Street | j | p | Warsaw | 1924 | Surgeon |
| Klaperzak Jakub Pinchos | | 26.03 | 1903 | Warsaw | 41/9 Targowa Street | j | p | Lipsk | 1926 | pediatrician |
| Klein Fejga Mirla Felicja | Klejman | 21.02 | 1894 | Włodawa | 29/9 Pawia Street | j | p | Warsaw | 1925 | gynecologist |

| First name and surname | Maiden name | Day, month of birth | Year of birth | Place of birth | Warsaw address (at the time of fillng the questionnaire) | Religion and nationality | | Place and year the studies were completed | | Specialization |
|---|---|---|---|---|---|---|---|---|---|---|
| Klein Sara (or Stefania) | | 04.06 | 1900 | Włodawa | 36/34 Muranowska Street | j | p | Warsaw | 1927 | gynecologist |
| Kleinerman Samuel Ajzyk | | 25.06 | 1896 | Warsaw | 48/8 Niska Street | j | p | Warsaw | 1925 | internist, gynecologist |
| Klejmanowa Ewa | Cybulska | 02.06 | 1899 | Zakroczym | 18/17 Sienna Street | j | p | Warsaw | 1927 | pediatrician |
| Klejn Chaim | | 25.08 | 1896 | Warsaw | 24/6 Muranowska Street | j | p | Warsaw | 1924 | internist |
| Kleniec Eida Etel | Aronson | 17.10 | 1889 | Gritsevo (now Belarus) | 31/3 Złota Street | j | p | Paris | 1914 | pediatrician |
| **Kleszczelski Arno** | | **10.01** | **1899** | **Bielsk Podlaski** | **61/5 Leszno Street** | **r-c** | **p** | **Vienna** | **1928** | **urologist** |
| Knaster Ludwik | | 10.03 | 1868 | Warsaw | 44/3 Chmielna Street | j | p | Warsaw | 1891 | internist |
| Kocen Mieczysław | | 31.03 | 1896 | Łódź | 2/6 Tłomackie Street | j | p | Warsaw | 1925 | bacteriologist, hematologist |
| Koenigstein Ernestyna | Perlis | 22.07 | 1906 | Druskininkai (now Lithuania) | 4/16 Bielańska Street | j | p | Warsaw | 1930 | pediatrician |
| Kolin Michał | | 02.04 | 1896 | Trembowla | 62/11 Pańska Street | j | p | Vienna | 1931 | internist, pediatrician |
| Koliński Józef | | 25.04 | 1872 | Warsaw | 20/10 Sienna Street | j | p | Warsaw | 1900 | gynecologist |
| Kołb Celina Cyna | Rozengarten | 20.11 | 1899 | Warsaw | 44/3 Chłodna Street | j | p | Warsaw | 1926 | pediatrician |
| Kon Daniel | | 27.06 | 1909 | Łódź | 6/5 Orla Street | j | p | Vilnius | 1934 | neurologist, internist |
| Kon Stanisław | | 16.03 | 1879 | Łódź | 43/56 Koszykowa Street | j | p | Warsaw | 1901 | orthopaedist |

| First name and surname | Maiden name | Day, month of birth | Year of birth | Place of birth | Warsaw address (at the time of fillng the questionnaire) | Religion and nationality | | Place and year the studies were completed | | Specialization |
|---|---|---|---|---|---|---|---|---|---|---|
| Kon Isaj | | 27.07 | 1910 | Warsaw | 3/9 Alberta Street | j | p | Warsaw | 1938 | Surgeon |
| **Kon Jerzy (Stanisław Józef)** | | **17.09** | **1896** | **Kalisz** | **25/23 Widok Street** | **j** | **p** | **Warsaw** | **1923** | **dermatologist and venereologist** |
| **Kon (Kowalski) Mieczysław** | | **02.10** | **1894** | **Częstochowa** | **57/7 Sienna Street** | **j** | **p** | **Lviv** | **1921** | **internist** |
| Konstantyner Zysla | Bauninger | 12.04 | 1893 | Kraśnik | 6/10 Karmelicka Street | j | p | Warsaw | 1924 | Analyst |
| Kopciowski Aleksander | | 05.12 | 1893 | Łódź | 8/12 Teatralna Street | j | p | Vienna | 1924 | Internist |
| Kopersztych Dawid | | 12.02 | 1896 | Warsaw | 59/16 Targowa Street | j | p | Lviv | 1927 | Internist |
| Korman Jakub Dawid | | 17.02 | 1905 | Warsaw | 44/2 Muranowska Street | j | p | Warsaw | 1932 | Surgeon |
| Korman Kielman Klemens | | 09.11 | 1906 | Warsaw | 17/3 Nowolipki Street | j | p | Warsaw | 1938 | gynecologist |
| Korman Lejb Leon | | 14.04 | 1889 | Lublin | 22/4 Jagiellońska Street | j | p | Kazan (Russia) | 1918 | pediatrician, gynecologist |
| Kornberg Józef | | 17.12 | 1894 | Warsaw | 24/14 Senatorska Street | j | p | Warsaw | 1925 | dermatologist and venereologist |
| **Kosman Ezra Edward** | | **26.08** | **1910** | **Warsaw** | **5/12 Zamenhofa Street** | **j** | **p** | **no data** | **1933** | **internist** |

| First name and surname | Maiden name | Day, month of birth | Year of birth | Place of birth | Warsaw address (at the time of fillng the questionnaire) | Religion and nationality | Place and year the studies were completed | | Specialization |
|---|---|---|---|---|---|---|---|---|---|
| Krakowski Isaj Aleksander | | 27.07 | 1894 | Warsaw | 7/12 Wspólna Street | j | p | Warsaw | 1923 | neurologist |
| Krakowski Mieczysław | | 31.07 | 1887 | Warsaw | 23/4 Złota Street | r-c | p | Warsaw | 1913 | gynecologist |
| Kramsztyk Stefan | | 15.12 | 1877 | Warsaw | 18 Chłopickiego Street | e-r | p | Warsaw | 1903 | pediatrician |
| Krantz Ignacy | | 18.01 | 1877 | Warsaw | 22/22 Senatorska Street | j | p | Warsaw | 1901 | internist, analyst |
| Krel Moszek Aron | | 13.02 | 1887 | Lublin | 20/16 Elektoralna Street | j | p | Prague | 1922 | dermatologist and venereologist |
| Krenicki Izaak Ignacy | | 13/26.01 | 1874 | Vilnius | 37/3 Nowy Świat Street | j | p | Warsaw | 1898 | Internist |
| Krenicki Józef | | 10/23.12 | 1877 | Vilnius | 22/4 Zielna Street | j | p | Warsaw | | gynecologist |
| **Krongold Dawid** | | **22.06** | **1908** | **Warsaw** | **76/87 Leszno Street** | **j** | **p** | **Warsaw** | **1931** | **Internist** |
| Krongold Łaja Leokadia | | 10.02 | 1890 | Warsaw | 47/23 Wronia Street | j | p | Paris | 1910 | pediatrician |
| Kryński Abraham | | 25.11 | 1887 | Navahrudak (now Belarus) | 15/12 Leszno Street | j | p | Berlin | 1914 | dermatologist and venereologist |
| Krzewski-Liljenfeld Szymon Ludwik | | 24.11 | 1890 | Warsaw | 61 Wspólna Street | e-a | p | Lviv | 1924 | Internist |

| First name and surname | Maiden name | Day, month of birth | Year of birth | Place of birth | Warsaw address (at the time of fillng the questionnaire) | Religion and nationality | Place and year the studies were completed | | Specialization |
|---|---|---|---|---|---|---|---|---|---|
| Krzypow Bajnisz | | 29.05 | 1905 | Warsaw | 139/5 Marszałkowska Street | j | p | Paris | 1930 | Internist |
| Kurzman Izydor Jozef | | 15.03 | 1891 | Jarosław | 14/23 Solna Street | j | p | Vienna | 1915 | dermatologist and venereologist |
| Kustin Noe | | 24.09 | 1893 | Grodno (now Belarus) | 40/4 Muranowska Street | j | p | Warsaw | 1931 | analyst, internist |
| Lajchter Chil Hilary | | 22.11 | 1894 | Łódź | 19/23 Nowolipki Street | j | p | Warsaw | 1924 | dentist |
| Landau Abraham Abram Adam | | 27.02 | 1891 | Sokółka | 16 Muranowska Street | j | p | Moscow | 1916 | internist |
| Landau Eugenia | Bem | 17.11 | 1896 | Warsaw | 51 Koszykowa Street | - | p | Warsaw | 1927 | pediatrician |
| Landau Helena | Flatau | 20.01 | 1894 | Łódź | 1 Napoleona Square | r-c | p | Warsaw | 1928 | neurologist |
| Landau Henryk Jakub (Henryk Stypiński) | | 20.02 | 1898 | Tomaszów Maz. | 32/5 Zielna Street | j | p | Warsaw | 1925 | internist |
| **Landau Jerzy** | | **31.01** | **1895** | **Łódź** | **24/4 Puławska Street** | **e-r** | **p** | **Warsaw** | **1925** | **internist** |
| Lande Adam | | 12.12 | 1865 | Warsaw | 47/4 Złota Street | r-c | p | Warsaw | 1895 | internist |
| Landesman Maurycy | | 21.11 | 1911 | Nadwórna | 32/11 Sienna Street | j | p | Warsaw | | bacteriologist |

| First name and surname | Maiden name | Day, month of birth | Year of birth | Place of birth | Warsaw address (at the time of fillng the questionnaire) | Religion and nationality | | Place and year the studies were completed | | Specialization |
|---|---|---|---|---|---|---|---|---|---|---|
| Lando Boruch Bronisław | | 04.01 | 1907 | Warsaw | 4/8 Karmelicka Street | j | p | Vilnius | 1931 | surgeon |
| Landowski Julian | | 25.09 | 1885 | Przasnysz | 9/14 Złota Street | r-c | p | Halle (Germany) | 1920 | internist |
| **Landsberg Marceli Marek** | | **28.03** | **1890** | **Tomaszów Maz.** | **64/18 Leszno Street** | **j** | **p** | **Fribourg (Swtzerland)** | **1913** | **internist** |
| Landsberger Józef Henryk | | 14.07 | 1890 | Warsaw | 8/6 Ogrodowa Street | e-r | p | Warsaw | 1913 | internist |
| **Landstein Ignacy** | | **09.02** | **1871** | **Warsaw** | **61/4 Wspólna Street** | **e-a** | **p** | **Warsaw** | **1896** | **internist** |
| Lapidus Michał | | 31.01 | 1912 | Warsaw | 11/6 Dzielna Street | j | p | Warsaw | 1936 | analyst, internist |
| Lastman Hersz Chaskiel Henryk | | 20.12 | 1899 | Lublin | 5/15 Dzielna Street | j | p | Warsaw | 1930 | neurologist |
| **Laumberg Maksymilian** | | **18.01** | **1911** | **Warsaw** | **84/47 Leszno Street, 49/24 Pawia Street** | **j** | **p** | **Warsaw** | **1939** | **no specialization** |
| Leber Jakub Lajb | | 25.04 | 1899 | Piotrków | 15/6 Pawia Street | j | p | Warsaw | 1928 | internist, gynecologist |
| Lederman Symcha Herszon | | 15.07 | 1909 | Puławy | 11/19 Wierzbowa Street | j | p | Warsaw | 1935 | internist |

| First name and surname | Maiden name | Day, month of birth | Year of birth | Place of birth | Warsaw address (at the time of fillng the questionnaire) | Religion and nationality | Place and year the studies were completed | Specialization |
|---|---|---|---|---|---|---|---|---|
| **Leipuner Michał Mojżesz (Skowroński Feliks, pseudonym "Władysław")** | | **13.10** | **1911** | **Grójec** | **53/22 Elektoralna Street** | j **p** | **Warsaw** **1934** | **no specialization** |
| Lejpuner Izaak Icko | | 21.07 | 1874 | Suwałki | 14/4 Nowolipki Street | j p | Warsaw 1901 | internist |
| Leneman Bencjan | | 01.01 | 1911 | Warsaw | 12/3 Sosnowa Street | j p | Warsaw 1934 | gynecologist, surgeon |
| Leniewska Zofia Irena Izabella | Rundstein | 28.01 | 1906 | Wilmersdorf (Berlin) | 15/8 Bagatela Street | e-r p | Warsaw 1930 | pediatrician |
| **Leński Morduch Mordechaj** | | **23.11** | **1890** | **Warsaw** | **28 Miła Street** | j **u** | **Moscow** **1917** | **internist** |
| Lerner Markus | | 26.10 | 1897 | Częstochowa | 10/4 Piusa X Street | j p | Warsaw 1925 | pediatrician |
| **Lewendel Ewelina** | **Glocer** | **29.08** | **1900** | **Warsaw** | **9/24 Jerozolimskie Avenue** | j **p** | **Warsaw** **1926** | **pediatrician** |
| **Lewenfisz (Wojnarowski) Henryk Herszlik** | | **31.05** | **1891** | **Łódź** | **16/1 Solna Street** | - **p** | **Warsaw** **1922** | **laryngologist** |
| Lewenfisz Teofila | Marjanko | 26.08 | 1899 | Warsaw | 16/1 Solna Street | j p | Warsaw 1923 | pediatrician |
| Lewenstein Józef | | 16.03 | 1886 | Warsaw | 49/8 Wspólna Street | r-c p | Kyiv 1911 | internist |

| First name and surname | Maiden name | Day, month of birth | Year of birth | Place of birth | Warsaw address (at the time of fillng the questionnaire) | Religion and nationality | | Place and year the studies were completed | Specialization |
|---|---|---|---|---|---|---|---|---|---|
| Lewi Abram (Walewski Ryszard) | | 17.03 | 1906 | Kalisz | 13 Orla Street | j | p | Lviv 1940 | no specialization |
| Lewi Alfred | | 29.03 | 1899 | Łódź | 30/7 Zielna Street | j | p | Warsaw 1928 | no specialization |
| Lewin Henoch Henryk | | 25.12 | 1893 | Nowy Dwór | 12/27 Alberta Street | j | p | Warsaw 1922 | dermatologist and venereologist |
| Lewin Semion | | 04.03 | 1899 | Łódź | 22/5 Leszno Street | j | p | Warsaw 1927 | internist |
| Lewinson Julian | | 04.02 | 1900 | Warsaw | 7/11 Szczygła Street | j | p | Warsaw 1928 | radiologist |
| Lewinson Maria | Jozefów | 23.05 | 1889 | Bogusław | 13/1 Leszno Street | j | p | Kyiv 1914 | dermatologist gynecologist |
| **Libfeld Joel (Jędrzejewski Roman)** | | **06.02** | **1909** | **Warsaw** | **50/7 Ogrodowa Street** | **j** | **p** | **Warsaw 1939** | **surgeon** |
| Lichtenbaum Abram Lejb | | 21.11 | 1884 | Warsaw | 38/4 Poznańska Street | j | p | Geneva (Switzerland) 1920 | internist gastrologist |
| Lichtenbaum Natalia | Szpilfogel | 03.07 | 1887 | Wola Krysztoporska | 38/4 Poznańska Street | j | p | Berlin 1911 | pediatrician |
| Lichtenberg Izaak | | 09.06 | 1895 | Warsaw | 17/18 Przyokopowa Street | j | p | Warsaw 1922 | internist |
| Lifszyc Eljasz | | 07.11 | 1908 | Warsaw | 6/38 Waliców Street | j | p | Warsaw 1937 | neurologist |
| Lindenfeld Berta | | 26.05 | 1882 | Warsaw | 20/4 Sienna Street | j | p | Geneva (Switzeland) 1908 | ophthalmologist |

| First name and surname | Maiden name | Day, month of birth | Year of birth | Place of birth | Warsaw address (at the time of fillng the questionnaire) | Religion and nationality | | Place and year the studies were completed | | Specialization |
|---|---|---|---|---|---|---|---|---|---|---|
| Linke Jakób Majer Mieczysław | | 13.02 | 1892 | Włocławek | 85/15 Żelazna Street | j | p | Basel (Switzerland) | 1915 | dematologist and venereologist |
| Lipowska Sara Rossa | Krejnes | 29.11 | 1881 | Słutsk (now Belarus) | 60/15 Leszno Street | j | p | St. Petersburg | 1912 | internist, pediatrician |
| Lipszowicz Lew Leon | | 27.10 | 1897 | Warsaw | 64/47 Żelazna Street | j | p | Warsaw | 1926 | neurologist |
| Lipsztat Paweł Abraham | | 30.08 | 1903 | Warsaw | 109 Leszno Street | j | p | Warsaw | 1928 | |
| Lipszyc Gołda | Landau | 19.11 | 1903 | Działoszyn | 77/26 Leszno Street | j | p | Montpellier (France) | 1932 | pediatrician |
| Lipszyc Izrael Izaak | | 24.10 | 1881 | Płock | 24A/8 Żurawia Street | j | p | Tartu (now Estonia) | 1906 | pediatrician |
| Lipszyc Mieczysław Aleksander | | 22.01 | 1873 | Warsaw | 6/14 Książęca Street | e-a | p | Tartu (now Estonia) | 1898 | dentist |
| Litauer Marian | | 18.02 | 1907 | Łódź | 18/7 Rymarska Street | j | p | Paris | 1932 | surgeon |
| Litmanowicz Hersz Herszlik Henryk | | 09.03 | 1884 | Piotrków | 42/14 Złota Street | j | p | Kharkiv (now Ukraine) | 1910 | urologist |
| Liwszyc Iser | | 22.06 | 1910 | Pinsk (now Belarus) | 34/3 Pawia Street | j | p | Lausanne (Switzerland) | 1938 | no specialization |
| Liwszyc Józef | | 06.04 | 1902 | Warsaw | 10/4 Gęsia Street | j | p | Genoa (Italy) | 1927 | internist |

| First name and surname | Maiden name | Day, month of birth | Year of birth | Place of birth | Warsaw address (at the time of fillng the questionnaire) | Religion and nationality | | Place and year the studies were completed | | Specialization |
|---|---|---|---|---|---|---|---|---|---|---|
| Lobman Halina | | 16.10 | 1898 | Warsaw | 31/5 Wilcza Street | j | p | Warsaw | 1923 | internist |
| London Juda Jehuda Józef | | 04.08 | 1903 | Warsaw | 8/18 Żelaznej Bramy Square | j | p | Paris | 1932 | internist |
| Lubelczyk Eli | | 14.01 | 1896 | Miedzyrzec Podlaski | 36/25 Senatorska Street | j | p | Lviv | 1922 | radiologist |
| Luxenburg Stanisław Leopold | | 17.12 | 1903 | Warsaw | 17/16 Pierackiego Street | r-c | p | Warsaw | 1928 | internist |
| Łagunowski Walerian | | 20.12 | 1890 | Kansk (now Belarus) | 4 Chłodna Street | e-r | p | Warsaw | 1917 | dematologist, venereologist and internist |
| Łaska Anna | Abramowicz | 06.01 | 1886 | Płock | 29A/3 Królewska Street | j | p | Kazan (Russia) | 1910 | gynecologist |
| Łącka Anna | Rewucka | 20.08 | 1881 | Kamionka | 25/4 Chmielna Street | or-gr | | Paris | 1914 | pediatrician |
| Mackiewicz Paweł Pinchus | | 03.01 | 1894 | Wołkowysk | 13/14 Leszno Street | j | p | Rostov (Russia) | 1920 | laryngologist |
| Mackiewicz Zofia | Goldblum | 10.02 | 1903 | Piotrków | 8/10 Willowa Street, apart. 5 | e-a | p | Zürich (Switzerland) | 1930 | neurologist |
| **Makower (after the war, From) Emma Noemi** | **Wigdorowicz** | **24.11** | **1912** | **Warsaw** | **2/5 Chłodna Street** | **j** | **p** | **Warsaw** | **1937** | **dentist** |
| Makowski Józef | | 24.06 | 1891 | Mława | 26/5 Nowolipki Street | j | p | Warsaw | 1922 | pediatrician |

| First name and surname | Maiden name | Day, month of birth | Year of birth | Place of birth | Warsaw address (at the time of fillng the questionnaire) | Religion and nationality | | Place and year the studies were completed | | Specialization |
|---|---|---|---|---|---|---|---|---|---|---|
| Maliniak Izydor | | 19.04 | 1874 | Kraków | 18/142 Ujazdowskie Avenue | j | p | Warsaw | 1897 | internist |
| Maliniak Karolina | Schumann | 30.06 | 1883 | Mykolaiv (now Ukraine) | 32/12 Sienna Street | j | p | Zürich (Switzerland) | 1912 | house doctor |
| Mantin Izrael | | 29.08 | 1888 | Warsaw | 3/5 Marszałkowska Street | j | p | Halle (Germany) | 1915 | gynecologist |
| Margolis Perla Rywka | Lewi | 25.12 | 1901 | Zduńska Wola | 6/6 Solna Street | j | p | Warsaw | 1931 | gynecologist |
| Markusfeld Stanisław Abram | | 18.12 | 1864 | Warsaw | 23/35 Bracka Street | j | p | Warsaw | 1887 | dermatologist and venereologist |
| Marmor Salomon Bernard | | 18.07 | 1909 | Sucha Bielska | 35/12A Złota Street | j | p | Poznań | 1937 | gynecologist |
| Mastbaum Stanisław | | 19.11 | 1900 | Warsaw | 18/4 Wielka Street | j | p | Warsaw | 1926 | internist, pediatrician |
| Maszlanka Abram Moszek | | 20.05 | 1872 | Łódź | 59/5 Złota Street | j | p | Warsaw | 1899 | pediatrician |
| Matecki Władysław | | 10.09 | 1895 | Tomaszów | 10/3 Sosnowa Street | j | p | Warsaw | 1925 | psychiatrist |
| Mayzner Mojżesz Mojsze | | 09.07 | 1895 | Kowel | 2/3 Chłodna Street | j | p | Bratislava | 1921 | pediatrician |
| Mazur Albert Abram | | 11.06 | 1893 | Łódź | 5/11 Zimna Street | j | p | Warsaw | 1923 | laryngologist |

| First name and surname | Maiden name | Day, month of birth | Year of birth | Place of birth | Warsaw address (at the time of fillng the questionnaire) | Religion and nationality | | Place and year the studies were completed | | Specialization |
|---|---|---|---|---|---|---|---|---|---|---|
| Melzak Naftal | | 01.01 | 1896 | Warsaw | 11/7 Karmelicka Street | j | p | Warsaw | 1925 | internist |
| Mendelson Nochum Dawid | | 18.03 | 1893 | Haradzeya (now Belarus) | 73/25 Leszno Street | j | p | Bratislava | 1921 | internist |
| Merlender Michał | | 20.06 | 1896 | Płock | 52/21 Leszno Street | j | p | Warsaw | 1925 | gynecologist |
| Messing (Kwiatkowska) Anna Gustawa | | 08.03 | 1895 | Warsaw | 35/4 Nowy Świat Street | r-c | p | Warsaw | 1924 | dermatologist and venereologist |
| Mesz Frajda | Ratner | 16.03 | 1892 | Łaczwica-Sieńca | 18/18 Leszno Street | j | p | Geneva (Switzerland) | 1917 | gynecologist |
| Mesz Jadwiga | | 02.03 | 1906 | Warsaw | 55/13 Wilcza Street | j | p | Warsaw | 1930 | gynecologist |
| Mesz Stefania (Rygalska Irena Maria) | | 18.10 | 1912 | Warsaw | 14/13 Sienkiewicza Street | j | p | Warsaw | 1937 | no specialization |
| Miechowski Jakub | | 05.02 | 1904 | Ozorków | 8/9 Nowolipie Street | j | p | Geneva (Switzerland) | 1933 | internist |
| Miller Mendel Mieczysław | | 22.09 | 1900 | Warsaw | 24/2 Wilcza Street | j | p | Warsaw | 1926 | gynecologist |
| Minc Ludwik | | 12.02 | 1897 | Rypin | 89/16 Żelazna Street | j | p | Warsaw | 1926 | internist |
| Minc Zygmunt | | 22.12 | 1893 | Wola Stara | 15/8 Orla Street | j | p | Warsaw | 1926 | no specialization |
| Mindes Juliusz | | 02.12 | 1899 | Suwałki | 3/4 Kapucyńska Street | j | p | Vilnius | 1927 | laryngologist |

| First name and surname | Maiden name | Day, month of birth | Year of birth | Place of birth | Warsaw address (at the time of fillng the questionnaire) | Religion and nationality | Place and year the studies were completed | | Specialization |
|---|---|---|---|---|---|---|---|---|---|
| Mintz Tolla Tauba | Minc | 01.09 | 1901 | Mława | 31/48 Złota Street | j / p | Vilnius | 1928 | pediatrician, dentist |
| Miński German Leon | | 04.10 | 1882 | Suwałki | 6/9 Prusa Street | gr-k / p | Kharkiv (now Ukraine) | 1909 | internist |
| Mitelman Hirsz | | 05.12 | 1911 | Warsaw | 74/5 Żelazna Street | j / p | Warsaw | 1939 | gynecologist |
| Morgenstern Daniel | | 03.11 | 1911 | Koło | 34/98 Świętojerska Street | j / p | Montpellier (France) | 1935 | gynecologist |
| Morgenstern Józefa | Lanes | 29.12 | 1890 | Złazów | 9/10 Tatrzańska Street | j / p | Vienna | 1915 | gynecologist |
| Mosenkis Emilia | Grynberg | 13.08 | 1904 | Warsaw | 75 Jerozolimskie Avenue | j / p | Warsaw | 1926 | internist |
| Moszkowicz Benedykt | | 24.07 | 1883 | Warsaw | 14/22 Bagatela Street | j / p | Kazan (Russia) | 1912 | internist, pediatrician |
| Moszkowska Irena Maria | | 02.06 | 1910 | Warsaw | 17/8 Lwowska Street | r-c / p | Warsaw | 1935 | pediatrician |
| Mościsker Emma | | 18.06 | 1896 | Lviv | 4 Fredry Street, 3/4 Nowiniarska Street | j / p | Lviv | 1925 | laryngologist, speech therapist |
| Mozes Anna | Engel | 02.08 | 1911 | Warsaw | 1/10 Ogrodowa Street, 18/6 Wielka Street | j / p | Warsaw | 1934 | no specialization |
| Munwes (or Munwez) Jakub (or Jakób) | | 08.08 | 1894 | Warsaw | 21/7 Solna Street | j / p | Warsaw | 1925 | internist |

| First name and surname | Maiden name | Day, month of birth | Year of birth | Place of birth | Warsaw address (at the time of fillng the questionnaire) | Religion and nationality | | Place and year the studies were completed | | Specialization |
|---|---|---|---|---|---|---|---|---|---|---|
| Muszkat Natalia Julia | Lipsztat | 23.04 | 1908 | Warsaw | 10/9 Mariańska Street | j | p | Warsaw | 1932 | pediatrician |
| Muszkatblat Bolesław Perec | | 07.03 | 1892 | Warsaw | 43/5 Sienna Street | j | p | Lviv | 1922 | pediatrician |
| Nachtman Zelman (or Zygmunt) | | 14.11 | 1890 | Warsaw | 28/21 Sienna Street | r-c | p | Rostov (Russia) | 1917 | gynecologist |
| Nadel Henryk Chaim | | 21.09 | 1893 | Łódź | 85/5 Leszno Street | j | p | Wrocław | 1919 | internist |
| Nadel Izydor | | 13.01 | 1899 | Łódź | 7/4 Chłodna Street | j | p | Warsaw | 1928 | gynecologist |
| Naftali Salomea Sulamita | Stok | 02.04 | 1890 | Brest (now Belarus) | 56/3 Radzymińska Street | j | p | Paris | 1914 | pediatrician, ophthalmologist |
| Najman Abram | | 09.05 | 1911 | Warsaw | 52/50 Chłodna Street | j | p | Montpellier (France) | 1937 | internist |
| Najman Mieczysław | | 03.05 | 1913 | Warsaw | 13/8 Graniczna Street | j | p | Naples (Italy) | 1938 | analyst |
| Natan Feliks | | 12.09 | 1907 | Warsaw | 12 Walecznych Street | j | p | Zürich (Switzerland) | 1934 | surgeon |
| Neuding Paulina Hafta Perla | Szpilman | 06.08 | 1888 | Warsaw | 37/14 Poznańska Street | j | p | Geneva (Switzerland) | 1909 | neurologist |
| Neuman Izydor Mieczysław | | 29.08 | 1910 | Warsaw | 28/27 Długa Street | j | p | Warsaw | 1934 | internist |
| Nikielburg Aron | | 14.08 | 1910 | Łódź | 30/29 Nowolipki Street | j | p | Basel (Switzerland) | 1934 | pediatrician |

| First name and surname | Maiden name | Day, month of birth | Year of birth | Place of birth | Warsaw address (at the time of fillng the questionnaire) | Religion and nationality | | Place and year the studies were completed | Specialization |
|---|---|---|---|---|---|---|---|---|---|
| Nochlin Abraham Pinchos | | 06.05 | 1903 | Wołpa | 36/3 Nowolipki Street | j | p | Montpellier (France) 1931 | gynecologist |
| Nowomiast Sara | Śniadower | 03.10 | 1910 | Warsaw | 47/17 Krochmalna Street | j | p | Warsaw 1934 | internist |
| Olicki Michał | | 19.07 | 1908 | Warsaw | 1/12 Pańska Street, apart. 5 | j | p | Warsaw 1936 | surgeon |
| Openhejm Berek Bolesław | | 21.08 | 1894 | Warsaw | 75 Złota Street | j | p | Warsaw 1926 | internist |
| Oppenhejm Szmul Shmuel | | 18.10 | 1864 | Warsaw | 3/9 Żabia Street | j | p | Warsaw 1889 | laryngologist |
| Orliński Menasse Maks | | 22.10 | 1892 | Warsaw | 14 Wielka Street | j | p | Lyon (France) 1921 | neurologist |
| Orzech Chil Majer Mirosław | | 30.04 | 1889 | Warsaw | 33/7 Sienna Street | j | p | Zürich (Switzerland) 1913 | internist-gastrologist |
| Orzech Nessa Serla Natalia | Szenkier | 13.12 | 1887 | Warsaw | 33/7 Sienna Street | j | p | Zürich (Switzerland) 1913 | gynecologist |
| Ostrowski Mordko Eliasz | | 19.11 | 1870 | Tarashcha (now Ukraine) | 4/4 Karmelicka Street | j | p | Kraków 1898 | internist |
| Pakszwer Ryszard | | 14.04 | 1912 | Warsaw | 21/6 Wspólna Street | j | p | Kraków 1936 | internist |
| Papierny Kisiel Zus | | 11.08 | 1874 | Ostroh (now Ukraine) | 14/57 Elektoralna Street | j | p | Tartu (now Estonia) 1901 | internist gastrologist |

| First name and surname | Maiden name | Day, month of birth | Year of birth | Place of birth | Warsaw address (at the time of fillng the questionnaire) | Religion and nationality | Place and year the studies were completed | | Specialization |
|---|---|---|---|---|---|---|---|---|---|
| Pekielis Rubin | | 09.11 | 1896 | Warsaw | 142/5 Marszałkowska Street | j | p | Warsaw | 1925 | internist |
| Peltyn Bronisław | | 27.02 | 1868 | Warsaw | 39/6 Chłodna Street | r-c | p | Warsaw | 1894 | internist |
| **Penson Jakub (Lewandowski Jakub)** | | **23.04** | **1899** | **Płock** | **29 Sienna Street** | **j** | **p** | **Warsaw** | **1928** | **internist** |
| Penzon Izrael | | 10.03 | 1897 | Płock | 76/1 Targowa Street | j | p | Warsaw | 1924 | internist |
| Perelsztejn Szolom | | 04.11 | 1903 | Vilnius | 15/20 Karmelicka Street | j | p | Vilnius | 1931 | internist |
| Perl Jerzy Tadeusz | | 02.07 | 1902 | Warsaw | 52/4 Felińskiego Street | r-c | p | Warsaw | 1927 | gynecologist |
| Perlman Albert | | 29.05 | 1895 | Lviv | 21/6 Ceglana Street | - | p | Vienna | 1923 | internist |
| Perlmutter Stefania | Kranc | 24.10 | 1896 | Warsaw | 78/2 Wawelska Street | j | p | Warsaw | 1926 | pediatrician |
| Petersburg Mieczysław | | 12.11 | 1894 | Warsaw | 5/17 Złota Street, 6/56 Śliska Street | j | p | Warsaw | 1924 | internist |
| Pianko Irena Pesia | | 06.03 | 1898 | Warsaw | 7/18 Nowolipki Street | j | p | Vienna | 1926 | internist |
| Piekarski Jankiel | | 03.09 | 1914 | Warsaw | 20/9 Sienna Street | j | p | Rome | 1938 | orthopaedist |
| Piekielny Majer | | 23.10 | 1891 | Łódź | 67/35 Leszno Street | j | p | Moscow | 1919 | surgeon |

| First name and surname | Maiden name | Day, month of birth | Year of birth | Place of birth | Warsaw address (at the time of fillng the questionnaire) | Religion and nationality | | Place and year the studies were completed | | Specialization |
|---|---|---|---|---|---|---|---|---|---|---|
| Piekielny Symcha | | 24.02 | 1892 | Minsk (now Belarus) | 54/39 Leszno Street | j | p | Zürich (Switzerland) | 1917 | internist |
| Pik Juda Szaja | | 04.07 | 1907 | Zduńska Wola | 7/7 Pawia Street | j | p | Montpellier (France) | 1935 | internist |
| Pilipski Berko Bernard | | 28.01 | 1892 | Grodno (now Belarus) | 14/29 Waliców Street | j | p | Warsaw | 1927 | internist |
| Pinczewska Zofia | | 05.08 | 1899 | Łódź | 57/4 Chmielna Street | j | p | Warsaw | 1924 | gynecologist |
| Pinczewski Jakób Mordka | | 21.06 | 1893 | Kalisz | 43/56 Koszykowa Street | j | p | Warsaw | 1925 | neurologist |
| Pitzele Halina | | 13.04 | 1890 | Warsaw | 81/14 Marszałkowska Street | j | p | St. Petersburg | 1915 | pediatrician, house doctor |
| Pizmanter Stella | Dołkart | 20.08 | 1912 | Warsaw | 11/22 Mazowiecka Street | j | p | Warsaw | 1936 | no specialization |
| Plessner Jakub | | 22.01 | 1897 | Łódź | 21/4 Nowolipie Street | j | p | Giessen (Germany) | 1930 | internist |
| **Plockier (or Plocker) Leon (Szustowski Konstanty)** | | **23.12** | **1895** | **Łódź** | **25/2 Leszno Street** | **j** | **p** | **Basel (Switzerland)** | **1920** | **internist gastrologist** |

| First name and surname | Maiden name | Day, month of birth | Year of birth | Place of birth | Warsaw address (at the time of filling the questionnaire) | Religion and nationality | | Place and year the studies were completed | | Specialization |
|---|---|---|---|---|---|---|---|---|---|---|
| Plucer (or Pilicer) Jankiel | | 14.09 | 1889 | Łódź | 59/15 Sienna Street | j | p | Lausanne (Switzerland) | 1931 | internist |
| Płocki Juda | | 02.11 | 1891 | Kalisz | 11/11 Elektoralna Street | j | p | Lviv | 1925 | internist |
| Płońskier Estera Sara | Drabkin | 29.10 | 1896 | Łódź | 17/12 Poznańska Street | j | p | Lipsk | 1926 | pediatrician |
| Płońskier Moryc Markus | | 18.09 | 1896 | Płock | 20/3 Sienna Street | j | p | Warsaw | 1925 | pathologist |
| Polakiewicz Józef | | 07.10 | 1913 | Warsaw | 31/4 Leszno Street | j | p | Warsaw | 1939 | no specialization |
| Polakow Rozalia | | 23.10 | 1892 | Minsk (now Belarus) | 43/37 Żelazna Street | j | p | Kyiv | 1917 | ophthalmologist |
| Polisiuk Adolf Dawid | | 05.01 | 1907 | Złoczów | 34A/2 Chłodna Street | j | p | Vienna | 1932 | gynecologist |
| Poliszczukowa Renla | Avrutik | 15.02 | 1890 | Chişinău | 21/6 Koszykowa Street, 10/5 Nowolipki Street | j | p | Kharkiv (now Ukraine) | 1915 | internist, gynecologist |
| Pollak Kazimierz | | 05.03 | 1903 | Stare Brody | 7/46 3 Maja Street | r-c | p | Kraków | 1934 | surgeon, orthopaedist |
| Pomper Ewelina Chawa | Rosenthal | 07.01 | 1888 | Warsaw | 7/6 Zamenhofa Street | j | p | Paris | 1914 | internist |
| Poznański Nikodem | | 09.11 | 1909 | Warsaw | 49/3 Nowolipie Street | j | p | Warsaw | 1935 | internist |

| First name and surname | Maiden name | Day, month of birth | Year of birth | Place of birth | Warsaw address (at the time of filling the questionnaire) | Religion and nationality | Place and year the studies were completed | | Specialization |
|---|---|---|---|---|---|---|---|---|---|
| Pozner Icek Eisyk | | 07.04 | 1913 | Krzeszowice | 16/6 Dzielna Street | j / p | Bordeaux (France) | 1938 | no specialization |
| Praszkier Feliks Fiszel Zołme | | 16.05 | 1878 | Kłodawa | 35/7 Złota Street | j / p | Warsaw | 1903 | internist |
| Prawda Calel Jakub | | 17.01 | 1907 | Łódź | 4/3 Twarda Street | j / p | Paris | 1933 | internist cardiologist |
| Proszower Władysław | | 06.01 | 1898 | Warsaw | 17/7 Solna Street | j / p | Warsaw | 1924 | internist |
| Prussak Leon | | 14.09 | 1889 | Płock | 15/12 Leszno Street | j / p | Saratov (Russia) | 1915 | neurologist, psychiatrist |
| Prussakowa Salomea | Bau | 05.11 | 1889 | Siedliska | 15/12 Leszno Street | j / p | Kraków | 1918 | neurologist |
| Prywes Tola Teofila | Goldewajg | 09.06 | 1914 | Lublin | 20/13 Sienna Street | j / p | Florence (Italy) | 1937 | no specialization |
| Przedborski Jan Jonas Samuel | | 29.09 | 1885 | Kalisz | 51 Leszno Street | j / p | Kyiv | 1913 | pediatrician |
| **Przeworska Alicja** | **Glazer** | **04.10** | **1901** | **Łódź** | **47/10 Leszno Street** | **j / p** | **Warsaw** | **1927** | **pediatrician** |
| **Przeworski Bernard** | | **17.10** | **1901** | **Warsaw** | **47/10 Leszno Street** | **j / p** | **Warsaw** | **1928** | **gynecologist** |
| Pupko Szołom Samuel | | 28.08 | 1871 | Lida | 41/1 Leszno Street | j / p | Warsaw | 1899 | internist - pulmonologist, cardiologist |
| Rabinowicz Basza | Carkes | 14.04 | 1884 | Warsaw | 49/5 Nowolipie Street | j / p | St. Petersburg | 1914 | ophthalmologist |

| First name and surname | Maiden name | Day, month of birth | Year of birth | Place of birth | Warsaw address (at the time of fillng the questionnaire) | Religion and nationality | | Place and year the studies were completed | | Specialization |
|---|---|---|---|---|---|---|---|---|---|---|
| Rabinowicz Henryk | | 25.08 | 1894 | Łódź | 7/78 Miodowa Street | j | p | Warsaw | 1925 | internist |
| Rabinowicz Noj Wolf | | 23.09 | 1877 | Rivne (now Ukraine) | 49/5 Nowolipie Street | j | p | Kyiv | 1912 | internist |
| Rajcher Artur | | 08.08 | 1900 | Tomaszów Maz. | 261/9 Grochowska Street | j | p | Warsaw | 1938 | no specialization |
| **Rajchert Maurycy Salomon** | | **15.12** | **1898** | **Warsaw** | **12/4 Solna Street** | **j** | **p** | **Warsaw** | **1925** | **internist-gastrologist** |
| **Rajman Pesach Paweł** | | **20.04** | **1895** | **Warsaw** | **64/8 Targowa Street** | **j** | **p** | **Warsaw** | **1923** | **surgeon** |
| Rakowski Hersz Gerszko Henryk | | 01.07 | 1889 | Zambrów | 47/11 Leszno Street | j | p | Halle (Germany) | 1914 | internist |
| Rall-Szapiro Fejga Lea Fanny | | no data | 1887 | Chișinău | 15/9 Twarda Street | j | p | Kharkiv (now Ukraine) | 1915 | internist |
| **Rapaport (or Rapiport) Zelman** | | **27.08** | **1888** | **Warsaw** | **3/3 Zamenhofa Street** | **j** | **p** | **Warsaw** | **1913** | **surgeon** |
| Rappel Michał | | 14.04 | 1881 | Warsaw | 8/1 Daniłowiczowska Street | j | p | Kyiv | 1908 | pediatrician |
| Raszkes Bolesław | | 07.04 | 1901 | Warsaw | 43/38 Koszykowa Street | j | p | Warsaw | 1928 | dermatologist and venereologist |
| Raszkes Henryk Chaim | | 27.12 | 1875 | Vilnius | 18/41 Bracka Street | j | p | Warsaw | 1899 | gynecologist |

| First name and surname | Maiden name | Day, month of birth | Year of birth | Place of birth | Warsaw address (at the time of fillng the questionnaire) | Religion and nationality | Place and year the studies were completed | | Specialization |
|---|---|---|---|---|---|---|---|---|---|
| Ratner Izydor Jerzy | | 05.06 | 1910 | Warsaw | 17/29 Dworska Street | j | p | Warsaw | 1934 | internist |
| Rechtszaft Ozjasz | | 04.04 | 1899 | Lublin | 22/10 Leszno Street | j | p | Wrocław | 1914 | pediatrician |
| Regelman (or Redelman) Maurycy | | 14.01 | 1895 | Warsaw | 43/7 Chmielna Street | j | p | Warsaw | 1922 | dermatologist and venereologist |
| **Reicher Edward** | | **22.05** | **1900** | **Łódź** | **33/4 Chmielna Street** | **j** | **p** | **Warsaw** | **1926** | **dermatologist and venereologist** |
| **Reicher Eleonora (Gorecka or Kozłowska Barbara)** | | **29.09** | **1884** | **Warsaw** | **40/2 Polna Street (Franciscan Nun Cloister)** | **r-c** | **p** | **Bern (Switzerland)** | **1920** | **internist-rheuma- tologist** |
| Rein Józef | | 22.01 | 1916 | Zagórów | 16/29 Nowolipki Street | j | p | Poznań | 1939 | no specialization |
| Rejchman Pinkus Apolinary | | 27.11 | 1896 | Warsaw | 51/2 Złota Street | j | p | Warsaw | 1927 | internist |
| **Rejder Icek Ignacy (Romejko Kazimierz)** | | **20.06** | **1907** | **Rozhyshche (now Ukraine)** | **22/6 Leszno Street** | **j** | **p** | **Prague** | **1930** | **no specialization** |
| Rogoziński Piotr | | 18.06 | 1872 | Warsaw | 19/36 Prosta Street | j | p | Warsaw | 1988 | gynecologist |
| Romanowska Tamara | Kleckin | 19.02 | 1885 | Navahrudak (now Belarus) | 10/23 Noakowskiego Street | j | p | Moscow | 1911 | analyst |

| First name and surname | Maiden name | Day, month of birth | Year of birth | Place of birth | Warsaw address (at the time of fillng the questionnaire) | Religion and nationality | | Place and year the studies were completed | | Specialization |
|---|---|---|---|---|---|---|---|---|---|---|
| **Rosenberg Eta (Kamińska Wiktoria)** | **Krejndel** | **21.01** | **1897** | **Minsk (now Belarus)** | **14 Próżna Street, 2/11 Grzybowska Street** | **j** | **p** | **Vilnius** | **1926** | **pediatrician** |
| Rosenberg Jakób | | 28.12 | 1868 | Warsaw | 34/6 Złota Street | j | p | Warsaw | 1893 | dermatologist and venereologist |
| Rosental Antoni Tadeusz | | 23.07 | 1910 | Warsaw | 6/35 Leszno Street | j | p | Warsaw | 1937 | no specialization |
| **Rotbalsam (or Rom) Izrael (or Jurek)** | | **22.07** | **1909** | **Warsaw** | **23/18 Nowolipki Street** | **j** | **p** | **Warsaw** | **1932** | **dermatologist and venereologist** |
| Rotbard Daniel | | 31.05 | 1911 | Łódź | 61/5 Sienna Street | j | p | Warsaw | 1937 | internist |
| Rothaub Zygmunt | | 02.07 | 1886 | Warsaw | 11/12 Elektoralna Street | j | p | Fribourg (Switzerland) | 1913 | surgeon |
| Rotman Tadeusz | | 10.08 | 1910 | Kielce | 9/5 Dzielna Street | j | p | Vilnius | 1938 | internist |
| **Rotmil (Chmielewski) Stefan Jerzy** | | **31.05** | **1909** | **Warsaw** | **62/22 Hoża Street** | **j** | **p** | **Warsaw** | **1933** | **surgeon** |

| First name and surname | Maiden name | Day, month of birth | Year of birth | Place of birth | Warsaw address (at the time of fillng the questionnaire) | Religion and nationality | Place and year the studies were completed | Specialization |
|---|---|---|---|---|---|---|---|---|
| Szenicer-Rotstein (or Szenicer or Rotstein or Rotsztajnowa) Halina Franciszka | Kon | 03.03 | 1907 | Warsaw | 17 Dworska Street | j / p | Warsaw 1930 | dermatologist and venereologist |
| Rotsztadt Julian | | 14.02 | 1871 | Warsaw | 54/13 Chłodna Street | j / p | Kazan (Russia) 1902 | neurologist, physical therapist |
| Rozen (Rosen) Alicja | Neufeld | 23.09 | 1911 | Warsaw | 7/21 Ceglana Street | j / p | Warsaw 1939 | no specialization |
| Rozen Lewek | | 15.04 | 1899 | Warsaw | 61/38 Sienna Street | j / p | Nancy (France) 1930 | internist |
| Rozenbaum Abraham Chaim | | 15.11 | 1905 | Warsaw | 30/14 Franciszkańska Street | j / p | Paris 1933 | internist |
| Rozenbaum Helena | Goldman | 16.01 | 1894 | Warsaw | 14/1 Sienna Street | r-c / p | Warsaw 1923 | analyst |
| Rozenberg Jerzy | | 07.02 | 1899 | Warsaw | 50/49 Żelazna Street | j / p | Warsaw 1927 | internist |
| Rozenberg Łaja Łucja | Makower | 14.08 | 1906 | Łódź | 4/16 Ciepła Street | j / p | Paris 1931 | dermatologist and venereologist |
| Rozenberg Mordcha | | 13.07 | 1913 | Warsaw | 33 Dzielna Street | j / p | Genoa 1939 | no specialization |
| Rozenberg Nechuma Natalia | | 28.12 | 1902 | Opole Lub. | 29/6 Gęsia Street | j / p | Warsaw 1934 | gynecologist |

| First name and surname | Maiden name | Day, month of birth | Year of birth | Place of birth | Warsaw address (at the time of fillng the questionnaire) | Religion and nationality | | Place and year the studies were completed | | Specialization |
|---|---|---|---|---|---|---|---|---|---|---|
| Rozenberg Szmul Grejman Grzegorz | | 14.06 | 1889 | Łódź | 29/4 Leszno Street | j | p | Kazan (Russia) | 1915 | internist gastrologist |
| Rozenblat Jakub | | 06.04 | 1867 | Lublin | 19/4 Zielna Street | j | p | Kyiv | 1891 | school doctor, gynecologist |
| Rozenblit Aron Arkadiusz | | 25.05 | 1892 | Ołyka | 67/31 Leszno Street | j | p | Kyiv | 1917 | internist |
| Rozenblum Jakub | | 27.01 | 1895 | Białystok | 6/6 Zielna Street | j | p | Warsaw | 1930 | internist |
| **Rozenblum Zofia (after the war, Szymańska)** | | **25.06** | **1888** | **Łódź** | **3/4 Puławska Street** | **j** | **p** | **Paris** | **1915** | **pediatrician, neurologist** |
| Rozencwejg Dawid | | 11.05 | 1885 | Białystok | 8/28 Zielna Street | j | p | Jena (Germany) | 1910 | pediatrician |
| Rozenfeld Jakób | | 15.08 | 1904 | Warsaw | 18/4 Rymarska Street | j | p | Paris | 1931 | surgeon |
| Rozenszpir Abram | | 12.05 | 1908 | Lublin | 7/40 Ceglana Street | j | p | Montpellier (France) | 1933 | gynecologist |
| **Rozental Maurycy (Rosiński Antoni Marian)** | | **18.06** | **1893** | **Łódź** | **4/17 Moniuszki Street** | **r-c** | **p** | **Geneva** | **1919** | **gynecologist** |

| First name and surname | Maiden name | Day, month of birth | Year of birth | Place of birth | Warsaw address (at the time of fillng the questionnaire) | Religion and nationality | | Place and year the studies were completed | Specialization |
|---|---|---|---|---|---|---|---|---|---|
| Rozental Samuel Stanisław | | 15.08 | 1909 | Rypin | 95/28 Marszałkowska Street | j | p | Warsaw 1934 | neurologist |
| **Rozental Zofia** | | **07.09** | **1899** | **Warsaw** | **22/12 Chłodna Street** | **j** | **p** | **Warsaw 1927** | **interna** |
| Rozenwurcel Róża | | 16.11 | 1903 | Warsaw | 38/9 Szeroka Street | j | p | Warsaw 1926 | internist |
| Rubaszew Icchok Nuchym (or Ignacy) | | 03.05 | 1892 | Warsaw | 13/24 Graniczna Street | j | p | Warsaw 1925 | internist, pediatrician |
| Rubinlicht Mordka Mieczysław | | 13.02 | 1894 | Warsaw | 24/24 Chłodna Street | j | p | Lausanne (Switzerland) 1929 | internist |
| Rubinraut Leon Aleksander | | 01.10 | 1896 | Warsaw | 6 Chmielna Street | r-c | p | Warsaw 1930 | psychiatrist |
| Rubinrot Salomon Stanisław | | 06.05 | 1875 | Warsaw | 3 Tłomackie Street | j | p | Warsaw 1901 | surgeon, radiologist |
| Rubinstein Borys Benedykt | | 04.10 | 1899 | Warsaw | 38/40 Nowolipie Street | j | p | Warsaw 1927 | internist |
| Rubinstein Izrael Michał Chaim | | 05.06 | 1897 | Warsaw | 101/11 Żelazna Street | j | p | Warsaw 1923 | internist |
| Rubinsztein Mojżesz Mordcha | | 01.03 | 1899 | Warsaw | 31/3 Smocza Street | j | p | Warsaw 1925 | gynecologist |

| First name and surname | Maiden name | Day, month of birth | Year of birth | Place of birth | Warsaw address (at the time of fillng the questionnaire) | Religion and nationality | | Place and year the studies were completed | | Specialization |
|---|---|---|---|---|---|---|---|---|---|---|
| Rundsztein Moszek | | 01.01 | 1900 | Łódź | 22/32 Widok Street | j | p | Warsaw | 1930 | gynecologist |
| Rundsztejn Teodozja | Jakubowicz | 06.11 | 1899 | Warsaw | 22/32 Widok Street | j | p | Warsaw | 1929 | pediatrician |
| Rybak Szołom | | 12.05 | 1909 | Białystok | 3/3 Poznańska Street | j | p | Vilnius | 1936 | urologist |
| Rywlin Jakób | | 28.04 | 1895 | Kyïv | 49/5 Elektoralna Street | j | p | Warsaw | 1925 | dermatologist and venereologist |
| Sajetowa Noma | Cukier | 13.09 | 1898 | Radom | 66/3 Wolska Street | j | p | Warsaw | 1922 | internist, pediatrician |
| **Salamon Mojżesz** | | **01.01** | **1891** | **Stawiski, Kolneński district** | **15/11 Nalewki Street** | **j** | **p** | **Kharkiv (now Ukraine)** | **1919** | **bacteriologist, analyst** |
| Salman Eugenia | | no data | 1892 | Słonim | 13/3 Nowolipie Street | j | p | St. Petersburg | 1918 | pediatrician |
| Sarna Symcho | | 07.12 | 1909 | Grajewo | 46/4 Targowa Street | j | p | Warsaw | 1936 | internist |
| Schoenman Hipolit | | 26.05 | 1889 | Tomaszów Maz. | 6/8 Górskiego Street | j | p | Kazan (Russia) | 1917 | dermatologist and venereologist |
| Schumert Flora | Dobrzyńska | 03.04 | 1911 | Łódź | 26/15 Wielka Street | j | p | Bologna (Italy) | 1937 | no specialization |
| Schwalbe Sarra(h) | Roller | 11.11 | 1897 | Wizniesieńsk | 49 Gęsia Street | j | p | Odesa (now Ukraine) | 1922 | dermatologist and venereologist, cosmetologist |

| First name and surname | Maiden name | Day, month of birth | Year of birth | Place of birth | Warsaw address (at the time of fillng the questionnaire) | Religion and nationality | Place and year the studies were completed | | Specialization |
|---|---|---|---|---|---|---|---|---|---|
| Seidenbeutel Zdzisław | | 26.05 | 1900 | Warsaw | 11/12 Warecka Street | j | Warsaw | 1929 | internist |
| **Sellig Gusta** | Aberdam | **31.05** | **1896** | **Krystynpol** | **29/7 Leszno Street** | **j** | **Lviv** | **1923** | **court doctor, pediatrician** |
| **Sellig Leopold (Zoliński Jan)** | | **03.02** | **1897** | **Lviv** | **29/7 Leszno Street** | **j** | **Lviv** | **1923** | **radiologist** |
| Ser Izaak | | 16.10 | 1908 | Łódź | 20/8 Nowolipie Street | j | Strasbourg (France) | 1932 | internist |
| Serejska Perla | | 25.11 | 1890 | Warsaw | 9/13 Warecka Street | j | Tartu (now Estonia) | 1917 | analyst |
| **Sieradzka Irena** | | **14.10** | **1908** | **Warsaw** | **73/8 Złota Street** | **j** | **Warsaw** | **1933** | **internist** |
| Sieradzki Stanisław | | 17.06 | 1895 | Warsaw | 30/5 Wilcza Street | j | Warsaw | 1925 | dermatologist and venereologist |
| Sierota Salomea Chaja Sura | | 05.07 | 1885 | Warsaw | 30/2 Świętojerska Street | j | Brno (Czech Republic) | 1914 | internist and pediatrician |
| Silberstein Salomea | Katz | 26.07 | 1886 | Przsanysz | 44/5 Chłodna Street | j | Tartu (now Estonia) | 1916 | ophthalmologist |
| **Simchowicz Tauba Tola** | Mendelsburg | **23.05** | **1883** | **Warsaw** | **27/4 Złota Street** | **j** | **St. Petersburg** | **1916** | **pediatrician** |
| Sirota Lewi Lejwi | | 01.06 | 1893 | Odesa | 16/2 Solna Street | j | Warsaw | 1926 | internist |
| **Skotnicki Arkadiusz Andrzej** | | **27.02** | **1896** | **Warsaw** | **11/16 Elektoralna Street** | **r-c** | **Warsaw** | **1923** | **gynecologist** |

| First name and surname | Maiden name | Day, month of birth | Year of birth | Place of birth | Warsaw address (at the time of fillng the questionnaire) | Religion and nationality | Place and year the studies were completed | | Specialization |
|---|---|---|---|---|---|---|---|---|---|
| Skórnik Salomon | | 22.12 | 1906 | Kalisz | 31/45 Mokotowska Street | j | p | Vilnius | 1931 | medical practitioner |
| Sochaczewski Dawid | | 12.11 | 1911 | Warsaw | 12/13 Nowolipie Street | j | p | Bologna (Italy) | 1936 | surgeon orthopaedist |
| **Sołowieczyk Józef** | | **14.04** | **1902** | **Warsaw** | **80/1 Nowolipie Street** | **j** | **p** | **Warsaw** | **1930** | **internist** |
| Sołowiejczyk Orko Andrzej | | 20.10 | 1865 | Warsaw | 80/1 Nowolipie Street | j | p | Warsaw | 1893 | surgeon |
| Somach Ruchla | Inhorn | 07.01 | 1888 | Warsaw | 11/9 Elektoralna Street | j | p | Geneva (Switzerland) | 1910 | ophthalmologist |
| Sonnenberg-Bergson Heinrich Henryk | | 30.08 | 1888 | Tomaszów Maz. | 20/36 Chłodna Street | j | p | Lipsk | 1912 | gynecologist |
| **Spielman Karol (Załęski Piotr)** | | **23.01** | **1892** | **Warsaw** | **28/30 Senatorska Street, apart. 36** | **j** | **p** | **Warsaw** | **1922** | **internist -phtysiatrist** |
| Spielrein Elżbieta | Kurchin | 29.12 | 1890 | Warsaw | 19/7 Wielka Street | j | p | Zürich (Switzerland) | 1914 | pediatrician |
| Srebrny Symcha Zygmunt | | 09.12 | 1860 | Warsaw | 9/6 Widok Street | j | p | Warsaw | 1885 | laryngologist |
| Srebrowicz Chaja Zlata Helena | | 16.05 | 1889 | Wysokie Maz. | 9/3 Warecka Street | j | p | Tartu (now Estonia) | 1916 | neurologist, internist |

| First name and surname | Maiden name | Day, month of birth | Year of birth | Place of birth | Warsaw address (at the time of fillng the questionnaire) | Religion and nationality | Place and year the studies were completed | Specialization |
|---|---|---|---|---|---|---|---|---|
| Stabholz Henryk | | 20.06 | 1882 | Warsaw | 17/1 Dworska Street | j / p | Odesa (now Ukraine) / 1907 | surgeon |
| Stabholz (or Sztabholc) Ludwik Marceli (Desidewicz Bolesław) | | 10.11 | 1911 | Warsaw | 17/1 Dworska Street | j / p | Warsaw / 1939 | no specialization |
| Stein Józef | | 27.03 | 1904 | Warsaw | 17/78 Dworska Street | e-a / p | Warsaw / 1928 | pathologist |
| Sterling Bronisława | Turkus | 12.05 | 1889 | Warsaw | 29/31 Sienna Street | r-c / p | Geneva (Switzerland) / 1920 | ophthalmologist |
| Sterling Władysław | | 18.01 | 1877 | Warsaw | 1/12 Boduena Street | j / p | Warsaw / 1901 | neurologist |
| Stiller Feliks | | 10.12 | 1889 | Radom | 7/8 Smocza Street | j / p | Warsaw / 1928 | dermatologist and venereologist |
| Stopnicka Marta Janina | Wizel | 28.04 | 1897 | Warsaw | 20/14 Jerozolimskie Avenue | r-c / p | Warsaw / 1923 | pediatrician |
| Strykowska Róża Rojza | Lebensohn | 28.12 | 1884 | Łódź | 34/4 Żelazna Street | j / p | Erlangen (Germany) / 1914 | internist |
| Stückgold Abram | | 10.10 | 1890 | Warsaw | 39A/10 Chłodna Street | j / p | Warsaw / 1920 | surgeon |

| First name and surname | Maiden name | Day, month of birth | Year of birth | Place of birth | Warsaw address (at the time of fillng the questionnaire) | Religion and nationality | | Place and year the studies were completed | | Specialization |
|---|---|---|---|---|---|---|---|---|---|---|
| Stückgold (or Sztykgold) Chaskiel Hillary | | 20.05 | 1892 | Warsaw | 34/32 Muranowska Street | j | p | Warsaw | 1926 | internist |
| Stückgold Władysław | | 03.05 | 1893 | Warsaw | 3/9 Solna Street | j | p | Warsaw | 1923 | pediatrician |
| **Stupaj Jakób Aron** | | **12.06** | **1889** | **Gąbin** | **18/142 Krasińskiego Street** | **j** | **p** | **Berlin** | **1917** | **ophthalmologist** |
| Suchotin Borys | | 14.10 | 1891 | Viazma (Russia) | 10/3 Franciszkańska Street | j | p | Moscow | 1918 | internist and pediatrician |
| Suchowczycki Eliezer | | 09.04 | 1897 | Brest (now Belarus) | 10 Prózna Street | j | p | Lviv | 1926 | surgeon |
| Sulkes Jakub | | 18.07 | 1900 | Piotrków Tryb. | 32/26 Sienna Street | j | p | Warsaw | 1928 | pediatrician |
| **Szachnerowicz Anna Jehudit (Wójcik Paulina)** | **Hochberg** | **18.11** | **1904** | **Warsaw** | **38/5 Muranowska Street** | **j** | **p** | **Warsaw** | **1931** | **pediatrician** |
| Szarogroder Ludwik | | 12.07 | 1897 | Kielce | 44/2 Sienna Street | j | p | Kraków | 1925 | internist |
| Szejnberg Jakób Aron | | 09.07 | 1893 | Warsaw | 3 Solna Street | j | p | Warsaw | 1921 | gynecologist |
| Szejnfajn Irena | Ajbeszyc | 15.01 | 1911 | Warsaw | 34/26 Nowy Świat Street | j | p | Warsaw | 1937 | surgeon, pediatrician |

| First name and surname | Maiden name | Day, month of birth | Year of birth | Place of birth | Warsaw address (at the time of fillng the questionnaire) | Religion and nationality | Place and year the studies were completed | | Specialization |
|---|---|---|---|---|---|---|---|---|---|
| Szejnman Michał Mszulom | | 13.06 | 1912 | Moscow | 17/97 Dworska Street | j | p | Warsaw | 1936 | internist |
| Szejnman Mieczysław Robert | | 22.11 | 1901 | Warsaw | 33/4 Ogrodowa Street | j | p | Warsaw | 1928 | internist and pediatrician |
| **Szenicer (Kurowska) Halina** | | **09.02** | **1907** | **Warsaw** | **23/49 Miodowa Street** | **r-c** | **p** | **Warsaw** | **1933** | **gynecologist** |
| Szenicer Stanisław | | 04.01 | 1905 | Warsaw | 23/49 Miodowa Street | r-c | p | Warsaw | 1929 | surgeon |
| **Szenkier Dawid (Mazurek Tadeusz)** | | **15.02** | **1886** | **Moscow** | **6 Pawia Street** | **-** | **p** | **Basel (Switzerland)** | **1911** | **urologist** |
| Szenkier Nikodem Nussen Nik | | 02.02 | 1895 | Warsaw | 3/15 Boduena Street | j | p | Warsaw | 1922 | gynecologist |
| **Szenwic Wilhelm (Sowiński Włodzimierz)** | | **01.12** | **1892** | **Płock** | **27/11 Królewska Street** | **r-c** | **p** | **Berlin** | **1917** | **gynecologist** |
| Szer Moszek Mojzesz Icek | | 12.02 | 1903 | Annopol | 34/10 Chmielna Street | j | p | Paris | 1934 | no specialization |
| Szer Rojza Rozalia Róża | | 28.12 | 1891 | Mława | 26/8 Żurawia Street | j | p | Warsaw | 1923 | ophthalmologist |

| First name and surname | Maiden name | Day, month of birth | Year of birth | Place of birth | Warsaw address (at the time of fillng the questionnaire) | Religion and nationality | | Place and year the studies were completed | | Specialization |
|---|---|---|---|---|---|---|---|---|---|---|
| Szereszewska Eugenia Enia | Holcman | 15.11 | 1897 | Medzhybizh (now Ukraine) | 6/18 Pawia Street | j | p | Paris | 1912 | pediatrician |
| Szerman Joel Julian | | 12.11 | 1897 | Lublin | 11/14 Elektoralna Street | j | p | Vilnius | 1934 | gynecologist |
| Szlifsztejn Jozef | | 05.09 | 1895 | Warsaw | 11/4 Nowolipie Street | j | p | Warsaw | 1925 | |
| Szmirgeld Abram Icek | | 23.01 | 1882 | Głowno | 14/11 Próżna Street | j | p | Kharkiv (now Ukraine) | 1910 | neurologist and psychiatrist |
| Sznajderman Adam | | 24.02 | 1909 | Radom | 17 Dworska Street | j | p | Warsaw | 1939 | internist |
| Sznajderman Ignacy Icchak | | 17.08 | 1896 | Radom | 41/12 Sienna Street | j | p | Warsaw | 1924 | neurologist |
| Szoor Henryk Hersz | | 10.12 | 1895 | Warsaw | 31/6 Żelazna Street | j | p | Warsaw | 1927 | internist |
| Szor Szlama | | 22.02 | 1911 | Łódź | 22/3 Wielka Street | j | p | Bratislava | 1938 | no specialization |
| Szour Michał | | 29.04 | 1892 | Warsaw | 7/4 Zielna Street | j | p | Kyiv | 1934 | internist |
| Szpecht Blima | | 25.03 | 1902 | Warsaw | 5/56 Brzeska Street | j | p | Warsaw | 1930 | pediatrician |
| Szpigelman Mieczysław | | 17.05 | 1912 | Warsaw | 29A/25 Królewska Street | j | p | Warsaw | 1937 | no specialization |
| Szpinak Adolf | | 13.09 | 1893 | Warsaw | 61/4 Leszno Street | j | p | Warsaw | 1924 | pediatrician |
| Sztajnkalk Zelman Zygmunt | | 06.07 | 1872 | Warsaw | 17/6 Nowolipki Street | j | p | Warsaw | 1898 | pediatrician, internist |

| First name and surname | Maiden name | Day, month of birth | Year of birth | Place of birth | Warsaw address (at the time of fillng the questionnaire) | Religion and nationality | Place and year the studies were completed | Specialization |
|---|---|---|---|---|---|---|---|---|
| Szteinsapir Azrjel Zelig Zelko | | 10.07 | 1880 | Rajgród | 31/12 Elektoralna Street | j / p | Kyiv 1910 | internist |
| Sztokhamer Szymon | | 19.01 | 1912 | Warsaw | 21/3 Złota Street | j / p | Lyon (France) 1938 | bacteriologist, hygienist |
| Sztokman Rozenblum Abram Fajwel | | 14.03 | 1894 | Warsaw | 47/9 Żelazna Street | j / p | Bratislava 1923 | gynecologist |
| Sztycer Hersz (or Herman) Lejzor | | 06.02 | 1896 | Warsaw | no data | j / p | Lviv 1929 | gynecologist |
| Szwalbe Mendel Menachem | | 13.12 | 1895 | Berdychiv (now Ukraine) | 49 Gęsia Street | j / p | Odesa (now Ukraine) 1922 | dermatologist and venereologist |
| Szwalberg Izrael | | 15.02 | 1884 | Warsaw | 9/4 Ordynacka Street | j / p | Moscow 1913 | gynecologist |
| Szwarcenberg Kazimierz | | 15.03 | 1880 | Warsaw | 25/4 Wielka Street | j / p | Tartu (now Estonia) 1908 | ophthalmologist |
| Szwarcman Józef | | 20.10 | 1878 | Krasnopol | 48/7 Złota Street | j / p | Rostov (Russia) 1917 | pediatrician |
| Szyfrys Ajzyk Lejba | | 29.08 | 1896 | Torczyn | 8/31 Nowiniarska Street | j / p | Warsaw 1922 | internist, neurologist |
| Szyk Naum | | 25.05 | 1898 | Warsaw | 10/10 Rymarska Street | j / p | Warsaw 1924 | internist |
| Szymel Tila | Halberszstadt | 17.11 | 1898 | Warsaw | 30/6 Nowolipie Street | j / p | Warsaw 1927 | bacteriologist analyst |
| Świeca Salomon | | 23.07 | 1914 | Warsaw | 9 Gocławska Street | j / p | Warsaw 1938 | surgeon |

| First name and surname | Maiden name | Day, month of birth | Year of birth | Place of birth | Warsaw address (at the time of fillng the questionnaire) | Religion and nationality | | Place and year the studies were completed | | Specialization |
|---|---|---|---|---|---|---|---|---|---|---|
| Świstocki Zusman | | 16.02 | 1906 | Warsaw | 55/8 Sienna Street | j | p | Warsaw | 1933 | internist-pulmonologist |
| Tadelis Józef | | 25.11 | 1911 | Gąbin | 20/66 Ogrodowa Street | j | p | Warsaw | 1939 | no specialization |
| Taube Sara | Kotler | 18.08 | 1888 | Węgrów | 9/11 Długa Street | j | p | St. Petersburg | 1914 | gynecologist |
| Taubenfeld Teofila Aniela | Kraushar | 22.08 | 1911 | Warsaw | 16/18 Krakowskie Przedmieście Street, apart. 28 | r-c | p | Warsaw | 1936 | bacteriologist |
| Tauman Fala | | 20.02 | 1911 | Warsaw | 5/28 Walicόw Street | j | p | Paris | 1935 | internist |
| Teichner Izydor | | 28.02 | 1889 | Żarnowiec | 22/7 Twarda Street | j | p | Wrocław | 1918 | gynecologist |
| Temczyn Mejsze | | 05.08 | 1909 | Pinsk (now Belarus) | 6/6 Ciepła Street | j | p | Warsaw | 1938 | surgeon |
| Temerson Stanislaw | | 08.02 | 1903 | Radom | 34/5 Żelazna Street | j | p | Warsaw | 1928 | internist |
| Temerson Herman Hersz | | 17.04 | 1884 | Płock | 27/4 Sienna Street | j | p | Moscow | 1911 | gynecologist |
| Temkin Maria | | 17.09 | 1884 | Warsaw | 45/7 Hoża Street | j | p | St. Petersburg | 1911 | internist, analyst |
| Tempelhof Mira (Mery) | Mejnster | 06.03 | 1912 | Łόdź | 17 Dworska Street | - | p | Warsaw | 1935 | surgeon |
| Tencer Jόzef | | 04.03 | 1899 | Radom | 30/1 Elektoralna Street | j | p | Warsaw | 1925 | laryngologist |
| Tenenbaum Ezriel | | 21.03 | 1892 | Piotrkόw Tryb. | 24 Gęsia Street | j | p | Krakόw | 1924 | laryngologist |

| First name and surname | Maiden name | Day, month of birth | Year of birth | Place of birth | Warsaw address (at the time of fillng the questionnaire) | Religion and nationality | Place and year the studies were completed | Specialization |
|---|---|---|---|---|---|---|---|---|
| Tenenbaum Jerzy | | 20.03 | 1910 | Łódź | 6/17 Orla Street | j | p | Warsaw | 1935 | internist pulmonologist |
| Thursz Dawid | | 13.03 | 1883 | Warsaw | 11/15 Warecka Street | j | p | Kharkiv (now Ukraine) | 1906 | gynecologist |
| Tiefenbrunn Benon | | 14.02 | 1891 | Pisarzowice | 9/22 Moniuszki Street | r-c | p | Vienna | 1918 | internist |
| Tombak Jakub | | 28.09 | 1895 | Warsaw | 24/7 Sienna Street | j | p | Vilnius | 1928 | interna, pediatrician |
| Tonenberg Leon | | 10.11 | 1889 | Warsaw | 32/3 Elektoralna Street | j | p | Zürich (Switzerland) | 1915 | surgeon |
| Trachtenherc Naftali Naftul Herc | | 07.10 | 1883 | Nemyriv (now Ukraine) | 5/19 Mławska Street | j | p | Kyiv | 1912 | internist |
| Trepman Jechiel | | 26.02 | 1894 | Warsaw | 28/3 Nowolipki Street | j | p | Warsaw | 1927 | dermatologist and venereologist |
| **Tuchendler Antoni** | | **02.02** | **1873** | **Warsaw** | **6/8 Królewska Street** | **e-r** | **p** | **Tartu (now Estonia)** | **1897** | **internist gastrologist** |
| Tuchendler Maksymilian | | 11.01 | 1874 | Warsaw | 44/21 Belwederska Street | j | p | Tartu (now Estonia) | 1900 | dermatologist and venereologist |
| **Tursz (or Thursz, then Tuszyński) Mojżesz Mieczysław** | | **16.02** | **1910** | **Warsaw** | **5/19 Miła Street** | **j** | **p** | **Warsaw** | **1935** | **internist phtysiatrist** |

| First name and surname | Maiden name | Day, month of birth | Year of birth | Place of birth | Warsaw address (at the time of fillng the questionnaire) | Religion and nationality | | Place and year the studies were completed | | Specialization |
|---|---|---|---|---|---|---|---|---|---|---|
| Tylbor Rubin Roman | | 25.12 | 1895 | Warsaw | 18/20Muranowska Street, apart. 1 | j | p | Warsaw | 1925 | internist |
| Tyras Zygfryd | | 25.07 | 1912 | Piotrowice | 17/10 Ceglana Street | j | p | Bratislava | 1937 | gynecologist |
| Ukraińczyk Ludwika Rywka | Rosenwasser | 16.05 | 1887 | Warsaw | 22/6 Chłodna Street | j | p | Paris | 1914 | gynecologist |
| Uryson Akiwa Akiba | | 31.12 | 1894 | Łódź | 28/6 Twarda Street | j | p | Warsaw | 1924 | internist |
| Urzdański Salomon Szloma | | 21.12 | 1877 | Turzec | 4/9 Chłodna Street | j | p | Warsaw | 1903 | internist |
| Wachs Jerzy | | 01.09 | 1893 | Łódź | 4 Pańska Street | j | p | Vienna | 1924 | internist |
| Wajnbaum Alina | Gelbard | 06.04 | 1905 | Częstochowa | 9/8 Ceglana Street | e-a | p | Warsaw | 1924 | microbiologist |
| Wajnbaum Józef | | 12.08 | 1902 | Warsaw | 29/6 Złota Street | r-c | p | Warsaw | 1929 | internist |
| Wajnsztok Samuel Szlama | | 10.02 | 1897 | Płock | 15/2 Orla Street | j | p | Warsaw | 1925 | internist-cardiologist |
| Wajntraub Szloma Salomon | | 14.08 | 1885 | Siedlce | 66 Leszno Street | j | p | Strasbourg (France) | 1914 | dermatologist and venereologist |
| Wajsberg Efraim | | 28.08 | 1906 | Bielsk Podlaski | 4/3 Zielna Street | j | p | Warsaw | 1931 | dermatologist and venereologist |
| Wajshoff Herszlik | | 24.06 | 1886 | Piotrków Tryb. | 4/5 Leszno Street | j | p | Saratov (Russia) | 1915 | internist |
| Wajsman Lejbus Leon | | 08.05 | 1871 | Radom | 39/3 Chłodna Street | j | p | Warsaw | 1896 | internist |
| Wajsman Noemi | | 14.03 | 1909 | Suwałki | 39/3 Chłodna Street | j | p | Vilnius | 1934 | pediatrician |

| First name and surname | Maiden name | Day, month of birth | Year of birth | Place of birth | Warsaw address (at the time of fillng the questionnaire) | Religion and nationality | | Place and year the studies were completed | | Specialization |
|---|---|---|---|---|---|---|---|---|---|---|
| Waks Łaja | | 05.01 | 1901 | Warsaw | 3/5 Waliców Street | j | P | Warsaw | 1926 | no specialization |
| **Waksman Bernard** | | **28.11** | **1909** | **Warsaw** | **2/7 Przebieg Street** | **j** | **P** | **Warsaw** | **1937** | **internist** |
| Walfisz Artur | | 27.06 | 1894 | Warsaw | 9/3 Hoża Street | j | P | Warsaw | 1925 | internist phtysiatrist |
| **Waller Szmul Stanisław** | | **26.05** | **1904** | **Płock** | **3/6 Przejazd Street** | **j** | **P** | **Warsaw** | **1930** | **surgeon** |
| Warmbrum Izaak Icek Izrael | | 17.10 | 1901 | Tomaszów Maz. | 31/2 Elektoralna Street | j | P | Warsaw | 1928 | surgeon |
| Waserman Hanna | Hufnagel | 10.07 | 1892 | Warsaw | 75 Jerozolimskie Avenue | j | P | Warsaw | 1922 | internist, pediatrician |
| Waserman Henryk Marian | | 10.12 | 1896 | Warsaw | 75 Jerozolimskie Avenue | j | P | Warsaw | 1925 | internist |
| Wasersztejn Abraham | | 13.02 | 1899 | Warsaw | 20/5 Twarda Street | j | P | Warsaw | 1939 | no specialization |
| Wasserman Jakub | | 01.01 | 1912 | Kalisz | 11/5 Dzielna Street | j | P | Vilnius | 1938 | laryngologist |
| Wasserthal Jakób Ignacy | | 01.11 | 1874 | Częstochowa | 9/31A Żabia Street | r-c | P | Graz (Austria) | 1898 | internist |
| Wdowińska Antonina | Berger | 22.08 | 1897 | Lviv | 7/15 Jerozolimskie Avenue | j | P | Vienna | 1932 | dentist |
| **Wdowiński Dawid** | | **25.02** | **1895** | **Będzin** | **7/15 Jerozolimskie Avenue** | **j** | **P** | **Brno (Czech Republic)** | **1925** | **neurologist** |
| Weinberg Izaak Icek | | 12.04 | 1886 | Łódź | 55/21 Sienna Street | j | P | Tartu (now Estonia) | 1915 | internist |

| First name and surname | Maiden name | Day, month of birth | Year of birth | Place of birth | Warsaw address (at the time of fillng the questionnaire) | Religion and nationality | Place and year the studies were completed | Specialization |
|---|---|---|---|---|---|---|---|---|
| Weinberg Perec | | 12.06 | 1899 | Warsaw | 9/5 Marjańska Street | j / P | Montpellier (France) 1928 | gynecologist, internist |
| Weisblat Julian | | 16.07 | 1863 | Warsaw | 142/10 Marszałkowska Street | j / P | Warsaw 1888 | analyst |
| **Werebajczyk Róża** | **Szajn** | **28.04** | **1900** | **Warsaw** | **48/18 Chłodna Street** | **j / P** | **Warsaw 1926** | **pediatrician** |
| Werksztel Aron Adolf | | 02.01 | 1901 | Warsaw | 50 Leszno Street | j / p | Warsaw 1929 | internist |
| Wertheim Aleksander Jerzy | | 21.08 | 1872 | Warsaw | 75/9 Jerozolimskie Avenue | e-r / p | Tartu (now Estonia) 1896 | surgeon |
| Wiener Betty | | 02.01 | 1894 | Berlin | 109 Leszno Street | j / g | Berlin 1918 | pediatrician |
| **Wiener Zbigniew** | | **02.09** | **1913** | **Warsaw** | **34/88 Świętojerska Street** | **j / p** | **Warsaw 1939** | **no specialization** |
| Wiernikowski Wolf | | 21.09 | 1901 | Warsaw | 21/4 Dzielna Street | j / p | Vilnius 1929 | generalist |
| Wiesen Władysław | | 16.10 | 1908 | Warsaw | 15/25 Grzybowska Street | j / p | Warsaw 1933 | internist |
| **Wilk Maria Bronisława (Wojciechowska Bronisława)** | **Goldman** | **10.12** | **1901** | **Łódź** | **53/5 Wspólna Street** | **j / p** | **Warsaw 1927** | **ophthalmologist** |

| First name and surname | Maiden name | Day, month of birth | Year of birth | Place of birth | Warsaw address (at the time of fillng the questionnaire) | Religion and nationality | | Place and year the studies were completed | | Specialization |
|---|---|---|---|---|---|---|---|---|---|---|
| **Wilk Seweryn (Wilczyński Stefan)** | | 26.06 | 1896 | **Węgrów** | **63/6 Wspólna Street** | j | p | **Warsaw** | **1922** | surgeon |
| Wilner Samuel | | 07.07 | 1892 | Łuków | 16 Hoża Street | j | p | Prague | 1919 | internist |
| Winawer Artur Aron | | 16.02 | 1869 | Warsaw | 18 Ujazdowskie Avenue | j | p | Tartu (now Estonia) | 1897 | internist |
| Witenberg Leokadia | | 10.01 | 1900 | Warsaw | 6/6 Leszno Street | j | p | Warsaw | 1926 | ophthalmologist |
| Włodawer Julian Judka | | 16.09 | 1889 | Warsaw | 3/7 Żabia Street | r-c | p | Kyiv | 1926 | internist phtysiatrist |
| Wohl Rachela | Garfinkel | 27.12 | 1888 | Suwałki | 31/46 Królewska Street | j | p | Geneva | 1914 | internist |
| Wohl Ichaskil | | 15.06 | 1895 | Brzozdowce | 3/5 Ogrodowa Street | j | p | Vienna | 1926 | internist |
| Wojdysławska Elżbieta Maria | Litauer | 18.01 | 1899 | Zgierz | 20/1 Dygasińskiego Street | r-c | p | Warsaw | 1926 | neurologist |
| Wolf Ludwik | | 01.08 | 1887 | Karlsburg | 12/1 Widok Street | j | p | Lviv | 1926 | internist, neurologist |
| Wolf Mojsiej Maurycy | | 30.09 | 1900 | Warsaw | 8/1 Teatralna Street | j | p | Warsaw | 1925 | internist, neurologist, |
| Wolińska Tauba Laja | Rozenberg | 24.11 | 1910 | Łódź | 3/8 Orla Street | j | p | Prague | 1936 | internist |

| First name and surname | Maiden name | Day, month of birth | Year of birth | Place of birth | Warsaw address (at the time of fillng the questionnaire) | Religion and nationality | Place and year the studies were completed | | Specialization |
|---|---|---|---|---|---|---|---|---|---|
| Woliński Abram Icchok | | 17.05 | 1910 | Łódź | 3/8 Orla Street | j | p | Prague | 1936 | internist |
| Zaks Łazarz Abram | | 15.01 | 1893 | Warsaw | 13/6 Graniczna Street | j | p | Geneva | 1921 | pediatrician |
| Zalcman Henryk | | 13.02 | 1904 | Warsaw | 43/26 Jerozolimskie Avenue | j | p | Warsaw | 1928 | internist |
| **Zamenhof (Zaleska) Wanda** | **Frenkiel** | **19.07** | **1893** | **Warsaw** | **6/3 Teatralna Street** | **j** | **p** | **Warsaw** | **1921** | **ophthalmologist** |
| Zamenhof Irena | | 29.10 | 1915 | Warsaw | 6/8 Stawki Street | j | p | Warsaw | 1939 | no specialization |
| Zamenhof Zofia | | 13.12 | 1889 | Kowno | 3/17 Ogrodowa Street | j | p | Lausanne (Switzerland) | 1913 | internist, pediatrician |
| Zand Natalia | Zylberblast | 28.03 | 1883 | Warsaw | 18/14 Ujazdowskie Avenue | j | p | Geneva | 1907 | neurologist |
| Zarchi Berko | | 03.09 | 1885 | Ulla | 31/5 Leszno | j | p | Tartu (now Estonia) | 1915 | gynecologist |
| Zarchi Maria | Żarnower | 14.02 | 1889 | Warsaw | 31/5 Leszno Street | j | p | Tartu (now Estonia) | 1915 | internist |
| Zaurman Stanisław | | 01.01 | 1900 | Warsaw | 15/5 Orla Street | j | p | Warsaw | 1926 | laryngologist |
| Zimmerman Aleksander Uszer | | 24.02 | 1875 | Warsaw | 11/5 Twarda Street | j | p | Warsaw | 1901 | internist |

| First name and surname | Maiden name | Day, month of birth | Year of birth | Place of birth | Warsaw address (at the time of filling the questionnaire) | Religion and nationality | | Place and year the studies were completed | | Specialization |
|---|---|---|---|---|---|---|---|---|---|---|
| Zirler Maksymilian | | 20.01 | 1897 | Rohatyń | 18/9 Noakowskiego Street | j | p | Vienna | 1924 | ophthalmologist |
| Złotowska Stefania | | 24.02 | 1897 | Warsaw | 11/9 Elektoralna Street | j | p | Warsaw | 1928 | bacteriologist, analyst |
| Zuckerwar Godfried Gustaw Gedalia | | 09.11 | 1894 | Warsaw | 9/4 Warecka Street | j | p | Warsaw | 1922 | dermatologist and venereologist |
| Zusman Henryk | | 06.12 | 1896 | Tomaszów Maz. | 36/4 Jerozolimskie Avenue | j | p | Warsaw | 1926 | dermatologist and venereologist |
| Zusman Pesach Lejb | | 18.04 | 1897 | Korzec | 43/5 Nowolipki Street | j | p | Warsaw | 1926 | internist |
| **Zweibaum (Zakrzewski) Kazimierz** | | **11.11** | **1918** | **Warsaw** | **6/24 Chłodna Street** | **j** | **p** | **Lviv (now Ukraine)** | **1941** | **no specialization** |
| Zweigbaum Marek Maksymilian | | 24.02 | 1855 | Warsaw | 22/6 Zielna Street | r-c | p | Warsaw | 1878 | gynecologist |
| Zylberbart Rozalia Ewelina | Gesundheit | 27.11 | 1888 | Warsaw | 57/5 Nowolipie Street | j | p | Bern (Switzerland) | 1911 | no specialization |
| **Żyłkieiwcz Józef (Syłkiewicz Kazimierz)** | | **11.06** | **1904** | **Warsaw** | **125/8 Marszałkowska Street** | **r-c** | **p** | **Warsaw** | **1932** | **laryngologist** |
| Żyw Izaak | | 06.07 | 1899 | Łódź | 25/9 Hoża Street | j | p | Vilnius | 1932 | surgeon |

# Appendix 4

# List of Jewish Doctors Moved from the Warsaw Ghetto to the Łódź Ghetto in 1941/1942

This is the list of doctors that were moved from the Warsaw Ghetto to the Łódź Ghetto in 1941 or 1942. Amongst these were doctors who had worked in Łódź before the war.

1. Czarnożył Alicja
2. Eljasberg Michał
3. Geist Izrael
4. Goldwasser Józef
5. Hartglass Janina
6. Kleszczelski Arno
7. Lewi Alfred
8. Mazur Albert
9. Moszkowicz Benedykt
10. Nekricz Majer Izaak
11. Nikielburg Aron
12. Rubinstein Salomon
13. Ser Izaak
14. Świder Zdzisław

# Appendix 5

# Schedule of Pharmacies Overseen by the Pharmacy Department of the *Judenrat*

This schedule was found in the *Jewish Newspaper* (*Gazeta Żydowska*), June 5, 1942. In the third column the names of employees that were identified have been added.

| Pharmacy Number | Address | Employees |
|---|---|---|
| 1 | 51 Nowolipki Street | |
| 2 | 10 Grzybowski Square | |
| 3 | 12 Mariańska Street | |
| 4 | 60 Niska Street | |
| 5 | 30 Leszno Street | |
| 6 | 28 Nalewki Street | |
| 7 | 12 Franciszkańska Street | |
| 8 "Północna" | 20 Dzika (Zamenhofa) Street | Zofia Gressowa |
| 9 | 33 Śliska Street | |
| 10 | 21 Karmelicka Street | |
| 11 | 35 Elektoralna Street | |
| 12 | 27 Grzybowska Street | |
| 13 | 34 Twarda Street | Izaak Sereth |
| 14 | 46 Twarda Street | |
| 15 | | |
| 16 | | |
| 17 | 23 Dzika (Zamenhofa) Street | |
| 18 | 57a Gęsia Street | |

# Appendix 6

# A List of Pharmacies Overseen by the Pharmacy Department of the *Judenrat* in the Ghetto in September 1942

This list is based on Jolanta Adamska, Janina Kazmierska, and Ruta Sakowska, eds., *Tak było . . . Sprawozdania z warszawskiego getta 1939–1943* (Warsaw: ZPPU ZETPRESS, 1988), 52–62.

| Pharmacy number | Address | Employees |
|---|---|---|
| 1 | 22 Gęsia Stret, at the corner of Zamenhofa Street, then moved to 44 Muranowska Street | Łaja Leonia Grynbergowa, Ola Iskolska-Kacenelenbogenowa, Józef Zandberg, Stefania Zandberg |
| 2 | 30 Zamenhofa Street | |
| 3 | 60 Niska Street | |

# Appendix 7

# List of Doctors who Saved Jews in Warsaw in 1939–1945

These names were collected by Maria Ciesielska in 2014 as part of research work on rescuers within the framework of a project initiated by the Jewish Historical Institute, Warsaw. The stories of the Righteous among the Nations are recorded at Sprawiedliwi.org: https://sprawiedliwi.org.pl/pl/ historie-pomocy, as well as in Yad Vashem's online database: http://db.yadvashem.org/righteous/search.html?language=en.

|    | Surname and first name | Year of receiving the Righteous among the Nations medal |
|----|------------------------|----------------------------------------------------------|
| 1  | Aleksandrowicz Leszek  |      |
| 2  | Bacia Kazimierz        |      |
| 3  | Balicka Jadwiga        | 1985 |
| 4  | Bando Anna             | 1984 |
| 5  | Baziak Tadeusz         |      |
| 6  | Białecki Stanisław     |      |
| 7  | Boryszewski Sergiusz   |      |
| 8  | Burakowska Alicja      | 1983 |
| 9  | Charemza Tadeusz       | 2012 |
| 10 | Dryjski Józef          |      |
| 11 | Ferens Tadeusz         | 1985 |

| 12 | Franio Zofia | 1971 |
| 13 | Garlicka Zofia | |
| 14 | Grocholski Stanisław | |
| 15 | Grzanowska (first name unknown) | |
| 16 | Hruzewicz Jerzy | |
| 17 | Kanabus Feliks | 1965 |
| 18 | Kanabus Irena | 1995 |
| 19 | Kapuściński Stanisław | |
| 20 | Kaszubski Tadeusz | |
| 21 | Kawataradze (née Worobiewa) Halina | 2003 |
| 22 | Kozłowski Kazimierz | |
| 23 | Kozubowski Adam | 2013 |
| 24 | Krajewska Janina | |
| 25 | Kubiak Józef | |
| 26 | Kurowska Aleksandra | |
| 27 | Litwin Franciszek | 1997 |
| 28 | Lityński Michał | 1984 |
| 29 | Loth Edward | 1996 |
| 30 | Makuch Wanda | 1994 |
| 31 | Mantel-Kłosińska Maria | 1995 |
| 32 | Meyer Adam | |
| 33 | Michałek-Grodzki Stanisław | |
| 34 | Michałowicz Mieczysław | |
| 35 | Niemirowska-Mikulska Anna | 2004 |
| 36 | Niemirowski Jerzy | 2004 |
| 37 | Ojrzanowska Maria | 1981 |
| 38 | Olesiński (or Oleszyński) Ignacy | |
| 39 | Paluch Emil | |
| 40 | Pągowska Janina | |
| 41 | Piotrowska Alicja | 1972 |
| 42 | Popowski Stanisław | 1991 |

| 43 | Przerwa-Tetmajer Alina | |
|----|------------------------|------|
| 44 | Puszet-Piechowska Janina | 1996 |
| 45 | Radlińska Janina | 1985 |
| 46 | Rajewska Ewa | 1978 |
| 47 | Raszeja Franciszek | 2000 |
| 48 | Rogala Marianna | 1987 |
| 49 | Rostkowski Ludwik | 1997 |
| 50 | Rowińska Aleksandra | 1987 |
| 51 | Rutkiewicz Jan | 1994 |
| 52 | Semerau-Siemianowski Mściwój | |
| 53 | Skonieczny Wacław | |
| 54 | Stępniewski Tadeusz | 1994 |
| 55 | Strojecki Lech | 1983 |
| 56 | Szmurło Jan | |
| 57 | Szymoński Karol Bożydar | 1981 |
| 58 | Śwital Stanisław | |
| 59 | Tarłowska Ludwika | 1966 |
| 60 | Trojanowski Andrzej | |
| 61 | Tylicki Mieczysław | |
| 62 | Tyszkówna Zofia | |
| 63 | Wacek Szczepan | |
| 64 | Walter Magdalena | 1978 |
| 65 | Wesołowski Stefan | |
| 66 | Węckowski Kazimierz | |
| 67 | Widerman Maria | |
| 68 | Wiechno Wojciech | 1984 |
| 69 | Wieliczański Henryk | 1981 |
| 70 | Wierzbowska Maria | |
| 71 | Więckowski Kazimierz | 1989 |
| 72 | Wolff Helena | |
| 73 | Ziębowa Kazimiera | 1978 |
| 74 | Żeligowska-Szulcowa Janina | |

# Appendix 8

# Photographs of Selected Doctors and Nurses

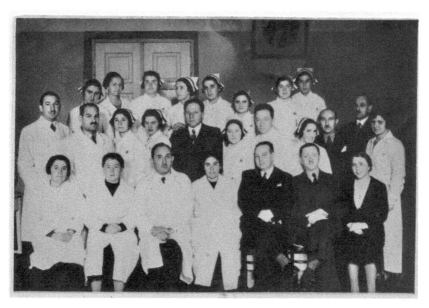

The graduates of the third year of the Nursing School with the teaching staff and administrative employees in December 1934. In the photograph, sitting in the first row from the left: second is Dr. Natalia Szpilfogel-Lichtenbaum, third, Dr. Mieczysław Seidman, fourth, Dr. Anna Braude-Heller, fifth, Henryk Kroszczor, and seventh, Dr. Jadwiga Hufnagel-Kinman. Standing in the middle row from the left: second, Dr. Aleksander Kirschbraun, fifth, Dr. Abram Festensztadt, seventh, Dr. Aleksander Owczarek, ninth, Dr. Adolf Piltz. Standing in the top row, second from the left is Dr. Zofia Gocław-Filskraut. The photograph comes from the archive of the Ghetto Fighters' House, Israel.

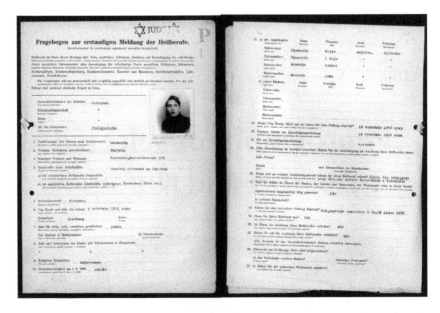

The first and second pages of the questionnaire for the initial registration of medical professions (*Fragebogen zur erstmaligen Meldung der Heilberufe*), which was filled out by doctors, nurses, and other medical personnel during the German occupation with the aim of being registered and authorised to perform medical duties. State Archives, Sygn. 1227.

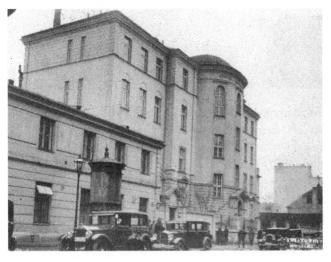

The Bersohn and Bauman Hospital by Sienna Street in Warsaw, November 1930. The photograph comes from the National Digital Archive (Code: 1-C-683-1).

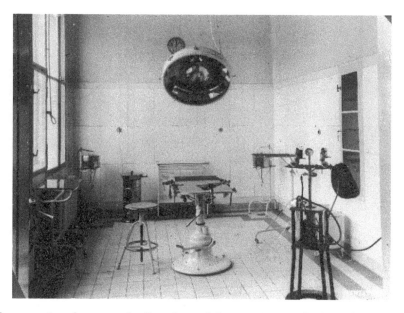

The operating theatre at the Bersohn and Bauman Hospital, November 1930. The photograph comes from the National Digital Archive (Code: 1-C-683-3).

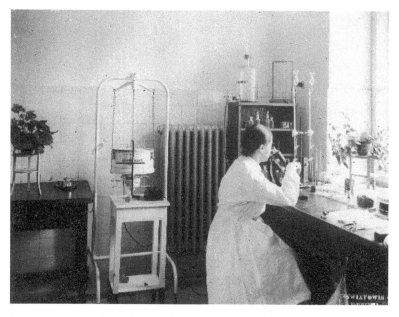

The laboratory at the Bersohn and Bauman Hospital, November 1930. The photograph comes from the National Digital Archive (Code: 1-C-683-5).

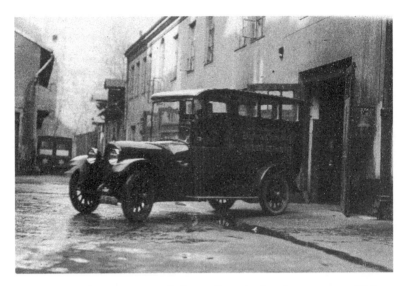

The departure of a Warsaw ambulance from its headquarters on 58 Leszno Street, March 1926. The photograph comes from the National Digital Archive (Code: 1-C-804-1).

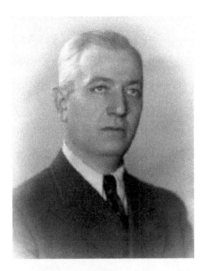

Dawid Amsterdamski (1895–1943), surgeon, in the ghetto was head physician at the surgical department at the Czyste Hospital. The photograph comes from the Main Medical Library Archives.

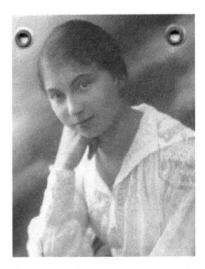

Róża Amzel (?–1943?), bacteriologist, worked with Prof. Ludwika Hirszfeld in the Czyste Hospital laboratories. The photograph comes from the Warsaw University Archives.

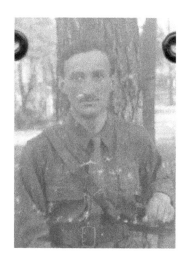

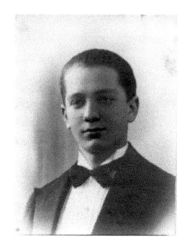

Emil Apfelbaum (1890–1946), cardiologist. In the ghetto he worked in the Czyste Hospital as well as in the hospital at 6 Gęsia Street. He led the medical research on hunger and was a lecturer at the ghetto medical school. Apfelbaum crossed over to the Aryan side where he hid under the false name Kowalski. He died of a heart attack in 1946. The photograph comes from the Warsaw University Archives.

Zdzisław Askanas (1910–1974), internist. He took part in the September campaign for which he received the Cross of Valour. In the ghetto he worked for TOZ's infirmary as well as a doctor assigned to the Jewish work units and took part in hunger research. Askanas crossed over to the Aryan side in March 1943 and worked for the Central Welfare Council. In 1954 he received the title of a professor of medicine. The photograph comes from the Warsaw University Archives.

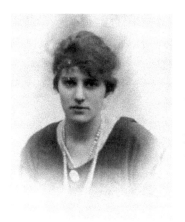

Ida Iza Asz (1900–?), a doctor in physical therapy who was a head physician at the Czyste Hospital and also worked in the hospital at 6 Gęsia Street. The photograph comes from the Warsaw University Archives.

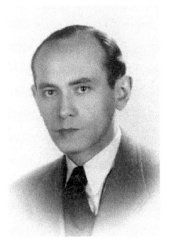

Jeszaja Bejles (1901–1942?), was a doctor at the Wolski Hospital. He was arrested on the Aryan side and imprisoned at the Gęsia Prison where he worked as a prison doctor. The photograph comes from the Main Medical Library Archives.

Alter Artur Ber (1908–1977), a veterinary and medical doctor, took part in the September campaign and was a prisoner of war. On returning to Warsaw, he worked in the Old Order Hospital and taught physiology. He worked in the Płońsk Ghetto from July 1941 where he was sent with his wife Irena. In December 1942 the couple managed to escape from a train bound for Auschwitz and hid in Warsaw under the false name Borowski in the Miecznikowski apartment. He took part in the Warsaw Uprising. After the war, he had teaching posts in Lublin and Łódź and was the first chairman of the Polish endocrinology society. He emigrated to Israel in 1956. The photograph comes from the Warsaw University Archives.

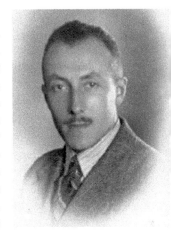

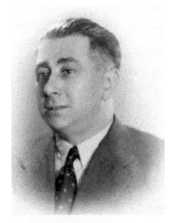

Władysław Bezberg (1893–?), a gynaecologist, worked at the Jewish Old Order Hospital and at an association for the support of poor midwives. The photograph comes from the Main Medical Library Archives.

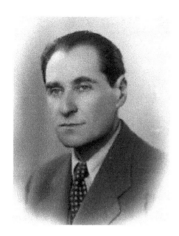

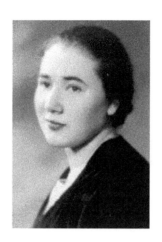

Owsiej Bieleński (1884–1943?) was a pulmonologist and a phtysiatrist. He was head of department at the Czyste Hospital. The photograph comes from the Main Medical Library Archives.

Adina Blady-Szwajger (after the war, Świdowska, 1917–1993), paediatrician, worked at the Bersohn and Bauman Hospital from March 1940. Adina and other doctors gave a lethal dose of morphine to their young patients when the Nazis arrived at the hospital. She crossed over to the Aryan side in January 1943, worked as a courier for ZOB, and took part in the Warsaw Uprising. After the war she worked as a paediatrician in Łódź. The photograph comes from the Ghetto Fighters' House archive, Israel.

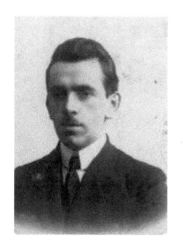

Lejba Leon Blacher (1894–1942) was an internist who worked at the Second Cathedral and Disease Clinic at the Warsaw University before the war. He took part in hunger research in the ghetto and was murdered in Treblinka. The photograph comes from the archives of the Warsaw University.

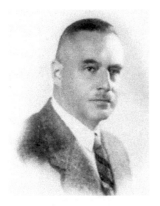

Izaak Ignacy Borkowski (1888–1943), surgeon. In the ghetto, he was the head physician at the third surgery department of the Czyste Hospital. The photograph comes from the Main Medical Library Archives.

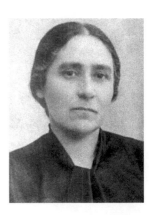

Anna Chana Riwka Braude-Heller (1888–1943), pediatrician, was the head doctor and director of the Bersohn and Bauman Hospital. She worked at the hospital at 6 Gęsia Street until its liquidation and died during the Ghetto Uprising refusing opportunities to leave the ghetto. She did smuggle her son and his family out of the ghetto to the Aryan side. The photograph comes from Yad Vashem's archive (Code 5027/951).

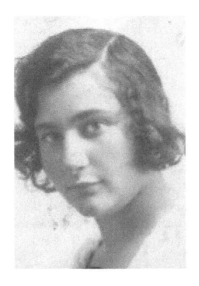

Alina Brewda (1905–1988), gynecologist. She worked in Dr. Endelman's private midwifery as well as the Czyste Hospital. In the ghetto she had her own private midwifery. In April 1943 she was sent to Majdanek Concentration Camp and then in July to Auschwitz where she was asked to take part in sterilization experiments, which she refused. She was evacuated to the Ravensbrück and Neustadt-Glewe Concentration Camps. After the war she emigrated to the United Kingdom. The photograph comes from the Warsaw University Archives.

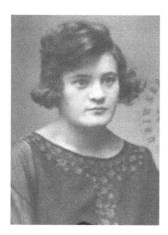

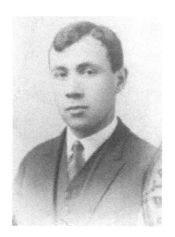

Regina Rywka Elbinger (1899–1943), pediatrician. In the ghetto she headed up the department for children suffering from spotted typhus at the Bersohn and Bauman Hospital. She took part in hunger research. She worked in the hospital at 6 Gęsia Street until its liquidation and died during the Ghetto Uprising. The photograph comes from the Warsaw University Archives.

Szymon Fajgenblat (1900–1943), ophthalmologist. In the ghetto he worked at the Czyste Hospital as well as at a private clinic and with TOZ. He took part in hunger research relating to its impact on eyesight. In summer 1942, he crossed over to the Aryan side with his wife Janina, who was also an ophthalmologist. He returned though to the ghetto for the Uprising and died there. On hearing the news of the death of her husband, Janina committed suicide. The photograph comes from the Warsaw University Archives.

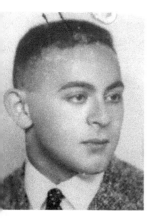

Henryk Fenigsztein (1913–1993), anatomopathologist. He took part in the September campaign and was a prisoner of war till April 1940. In the ghetto, he worked at the Czyste Hospital and conducted 3,000 autopsies with 500 relating to the hunger research. He also taught anatomy and pathology at the ghetto medical school. He hid in the bunker with his wife Ala till April 21, 1943, when he managed to bribe a Nazi officer with his stamp collection to avoid being sent to Treblinka. Whilst his wife was murdered in Lublin in November 1943, Henryk managed to survive work camps and five concentration camps. After the war he briefly worked in Munich before emigrating to Canada and specializing in psychiatry. The photograph comes from the Warsaw University Archives.

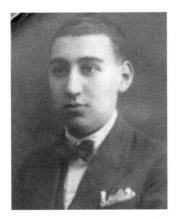

Jerzy Fryszman (1904–1976), urologist, worked at the Czyste Hospital and in a private urologist practice at 4 Tłomacka Street owned by his father. He spent the war in the Rivne district, where he escaped to with his family before being recruited by the Red Army and subsequently the Polish Army, and was demobilized with the rank of a major in 1947. He was a founding member of the Polish Urology Association. The photograph comes from the Warsaw University Archives.

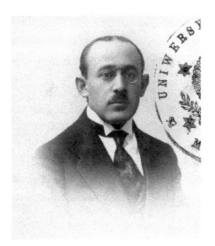

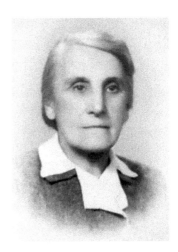

Aron Glasman (after the war, Artur Galewicz), (1892–circa 1960) was an urologist who worked at the Czyste Hospital and was imprisoned by the Nazis. After the war he worked for the Ministry of Public Security. The photograph comes from the Warsaw University Archives.

Chaja Zlata Zofia Golde-Żyżmorska (1882–1959), pediatrician, worked in Warsaw after the war, where she was an acclaimed children's doctor. The photograph comes from the archive of the Joanna Lasserre family.

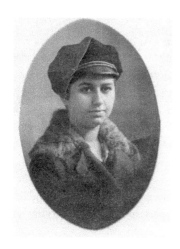 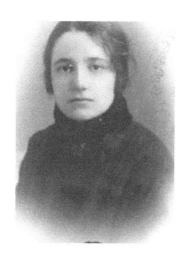

Halina Goldsztajn (born Kon, 1900–?), was a doctor of internal medicine who worked at the Czyste Hospital and specialized in gastrology.

Teodozja Goliborska (1899–1992) worked as the head of the laboratory at the Bersohn and Bauman Hospital and took part in hunger research. She crossed over to the Aryan side and was a courier for the ZOB. She survived the Warsaw Uprising and with the help of Dr. Świtala was led out a hide-out on 43 Promyka Street safely. She emigrated to Melbourne after the war where she worked as a doctor. The photograph comes from the Warsaw University Archives.

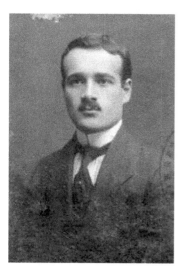

Mojżesz Grojsblat (1894–1942/1943), doctor, internist, and bacteriologist. Worked at the Czyste Hospital and lectured at the ghetto medical school. His final position was at the Gęsia Street hospital. The photograph comes from the Warsaw University Archives.

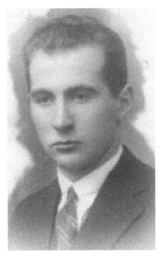

Henryk Halpern-Wieliczański (1903–1996), internist. During the war he lived on the Aryan side where he worked in the underground helping Jews that were hiding. He was arrested by the Gestapo and imprisoned in Pawiak Prison, from where he was sent to Majdanek (where he worked with an AK underground network) and subsequently Auschwitz Concentration Camp. He survived the war and settled in Łódź where he was an assistant professor at the Medical Academy. The photograph comes from the Warsaw University Archives.

Arie Leo Heller (1917–2008), doctor, son of Dr. Anny Braude-Heller. Worked at the Bersohn and Bauman Hospital and crossed over to the Aryan side, where he survived the war. The photograph comes from the Main Medical Library Archives.

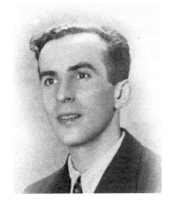

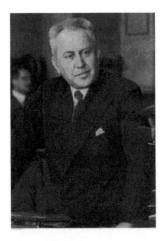

Ludwik Hirszfeld (1884–1954), professor of bacteriology and immunologist, was the co-discoverer of the inheritance of ABO blood types. In the ghetto he was the head of the Medical Council of the *Judenrat*. He fled the ghetto with his family in 1943 and became director of the Institute for Medical Microbiology at Wrocław and dean of the medical faculty in 1945 where he taught until his death in 1954. The photograph comes from the National Data Archives of 1933.

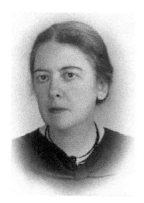

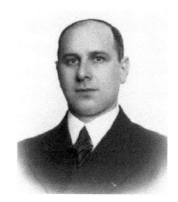

Hanna Hirszfeld (1884–1964), pediatrician. In the ghetto was the head physician in the infants department. The photograph comes from the Main Medical Library Archives.

Józef Jabłoński (1894–?), laryngologist, surgeon. In the ghetto he was the head physician of the laryngology department of the Czyste Hospital. The photograph comes from the Main Medical Library Archives.

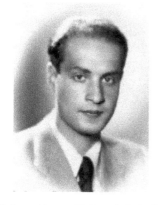

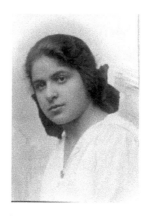

Adam Abram Kajzer (1913–?), surgeon. In the ghetto he worked in the surgical department of the Czyste Hospital. The photograph comes from the Main Medical Library Archives.

Helena Hinda Keilson (1903–?), pediatrician. Worked at the Bersohn and Bauman Hospital and the Sanatorium Medema in Miedzeszyn and as a doctor at the orphanage at 7 Grzybowska Street. Her husband, Władysław, died in Katyń. She was head of internal medicine at the hospital in the ghetto. She crossed over to the Aryan side after surviving the January 1943 deportations and used the false name Janina Puławska. But she was arrested on April 22, 1943, and imprisoned in Pawiak Prison before being sent to Auschwitz. Shortly after the war she emigrated to Sweden. The photograph comes from Warsaw University Archives.

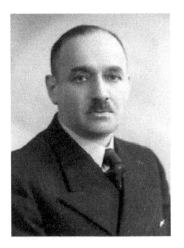

Dawid Kenigsberg (1890–?), dermatologist and venereologist. Worked at the Czyste Hospital as the head physician. The photograph comes from the Main Medical Library Archives.

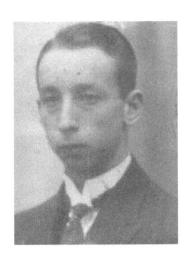

Ludwik Koenigstein (1904–1944), surgeon and laryngologist, worked at the Czyste Hospital. He took part in the Warsaw Uprising and was shot on August 30 on Miodowa Street in unexplained circumstances. The photograph comes from the Warsaw University Archives.

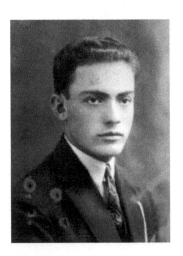

Symcha Herszon Lederman (1909–1943), internist. In the ghetto, he worked at the Czyste Hospital. The photograph comes from the archives of Prof. Avi Ohry.

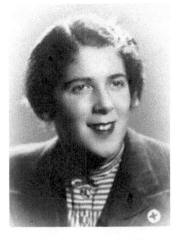

Noemi Makower (1912–2015), surgeon, worked at the surgery department of the Czyste Hospital. The photograph comes from the Main Medical Library Archives.

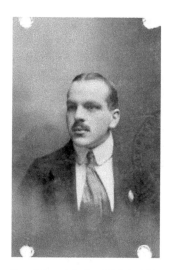

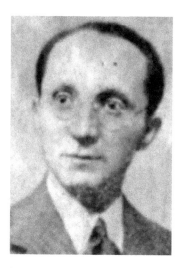

Stanisław Markusfeld (1864–1943), dermatologist, head physician in the skin and venerological department of the Czyste Hospital. According to one report, he and his wife Felicia committed suicide jumping out of the fourth floor of a building during the *Grossaktion*. The photograph comes from the Warsaw University Archives.

Izrael Milejkowski (1887–1943), dermatologist, head of the Health Department of the *Judenrat* and of the Hospital Department of the Jewish Medical Council in the ghetto. He initiated the hunger studies in the ghetto and the ghetto medical school. He was deported to Treblinka in January 1943. The photograph comes from the Ghetto Fighters' House archive, Israel.

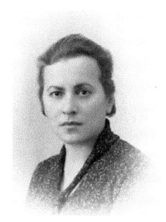

Tolla Mintz (1901–1942), dentist, worked at the Włodzimierza Medema Sanatorium in Miedzeszyn. She and her the children in her care were deported to Treblinka in 1942 after she declined the opportunity to escape. The photograph comes from the Main Medical Library Archives.

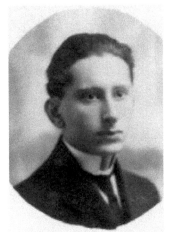

Jakób Munwes (1914–1943), internist and head physician at the Czyste Hospital and a lecturer at the ghetto medical school, was arrested and taken as a hostage to Pawiak Prison in July 1942. On release, he worked in the hospital at 6 Gęsia Street and hid in the hospital bunkers till May 1943 before being murdered in Treblinka. The photograph comes from the Warsaw University Archives.

Jakub Penson (1899–1971), internist. In the ghetto he was the head physician in the typhus department in the Czyste Hospital. After the war he became a professor of nephrology and worked as rector of the Medical Academy in Gdańsk. The photograph comes from the Main Medical Library Archives.

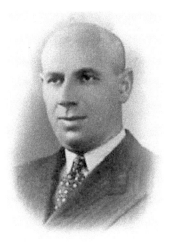

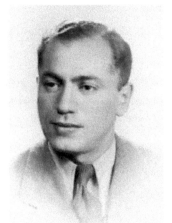

Jankiel Piekarski (1914–?), surgeon, worked in the surgery department of the Czyste Hospital. The photograph comes from the Main Medical Library Archives.

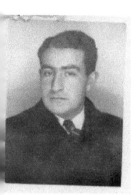

Adolf Polisiuk (1907–1943?), gynecologist, worked in the gynaecology department of the Czyste Hospital. In the ghetto worked at hospital on 6 Gęsia Street before crossing over to the Aryan side in May 1943, where he wrote his memoirs, which were provided to the Jewish Institute after the war. He did not survive the war and died in unexplained circumstances. The photograph comes from the Warsaw University Archives.

Kazimierz Pollak (1903–1942), surgeon. In the ghetto he worked as an emergency ambulance doctor. The photograph comes from the Main Medical Library Archives.

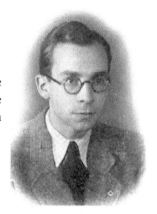

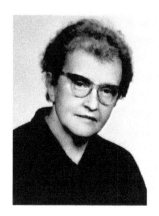

Dr. Janina Natalia Radlińska (1903–1996), was recognized as a Righteous among the Nations on September 10, 1985. During the German occupation, Janina Radlińska worked in the surgical ward of the Infant Jesus Hospital and the Omega clinic on Jerozolimskie Avenue in Warsaw. She participated in fifteen ear-and-nose operations as well as undertaking urological procedures to reverse the effects of circumcision. She hid Jews in her apartment and after the Uprising left Warsaw with one of these Jews, Czesława Frendler, who subsequently emigrated to the United States. Janina Radlińska was credited with having led two of Dr. Halina Szenicer-Rotstein's four children out of the ghetto, saving their lives.

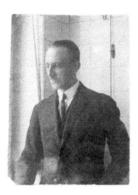

Franciszek Paweł Raszeja (April 2, 1896, Chełmno—July 21, 1942, Warsaw) was a Polish orthopaedic physician and a professor at Poznań University before the war. He was killed on July 21, 1942, while visiting a patient in the Warsaw Ghetto. The photograph comes from the family collection of his daughter, Professor B. Raszei-Wanic.

Bolesław Raszkes (1901–1942?), dermatologist. In the ghetto he worked at the Czyste Hospital and took part in the hunger research. According to Dr. Rotbalsam, he died on the Aryan side, and according to Edward Kossoy, he fought in the Warsaw Uprising. The photograph comes from the Warsaw University Archives.

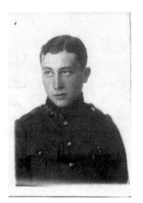

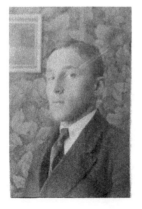

Edward Reicher (1900-1975) was a dermatologist and venereologist. Before the war he worked in Łódź but he escaped the Łódź Ghetto to Warsaw and survived the war. The photograph comes from the Warsaw University Archives.

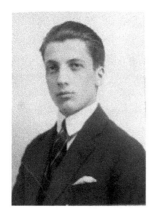

Izrael Jurek Rotbalsam (1909–?) was a dermatologist and venereologist. He worked at the Bersohn and Bauman Hospital and took part in the hunger research. From January 1943 he hid on the Aryan side but after two months decided to return to the ghetto where he worked at the hospital at 6 Gęsia Street. In April 1943 he was sent to Treblinka but was chosen there as "fit for work" to go to Majdanek and subsequently to Buchenwald and Mauthausen. After the war he emigrated to Palestine and worked as a doctor in Tel Aviv. The photograph comes from the Warsaw University Archives.

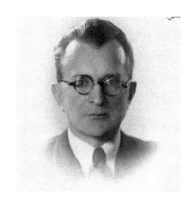

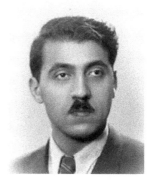

Wacław Skonieczny was a Polish Catholic doctor who was appointed the administrator of the Bersohn and Bauman hospital. He helped Jews, saving amongst other Dr. Dora Keilson. The photograph comes from the Main Medical Library Archives.

Dawid Sochaczewski (1911–?), surgeon. In the ghetto he worked in the surgery department of the Czyste Hospital. The photograph comes from the Main Medical Library Archives.

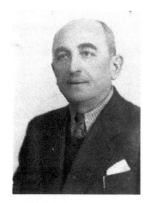

Henryk Stabholz (1882–1941), surgeon and director of the Czyste Hospital. The photograph comes from the Main Medical Library Archives.

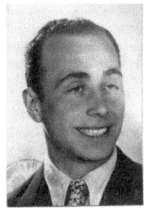

Ludwik Stabholz (1911–2007), doctor and anatomist, worked at the Czyste Hospital. He lectured at the ghetto medical school. Professor Edward Loth helped him move across to the Aryan side after April 1943. After working in a military hospital in Gdańsk, he emigrated to Israel with his wife in 1950 and worked as a doctor in Tel Aviv. The photograph comes from the Warsaw University Archives.

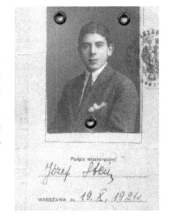

Józef Stein (1904–1943), anatomopathologist, director of the Czyste Hospital. He took part in hunger research. He was at the hospital at 6 Gęsia Street until its liquidation in May 1943, after which he was murdered in Treblinka. The photograph comes from the Warsaw University Archives.

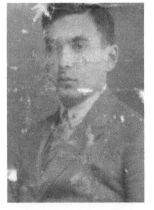

Izaak Szachnerowicz (1896–1940), gynaecologist, worked at the department of women's illnesses at the Czyste Hospital. He was arrested in January 1940 as part of the Kotta Affair and shot in Palmiry. The photograph comes from the Warsaw University Archives.

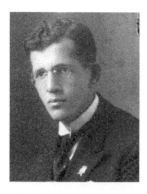

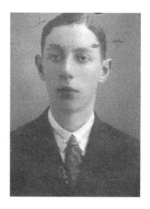

Mieczysław Szejnman (1901–1943) was a specialist in internal medicine who took part in the hunger research and was Professor Hirszfeld's assistant. He left the ghetto before the Uprising but was arrested by the Gestapo and murdered. The photograph comes from the Warsaw University Archives.

Michał Szejnman (1912–1942), was a doctor at the Czyste Hospital. He took part in the hunger disease research and died of hunger in the ghetto. Photograph comes from the Warsaw University Archives.

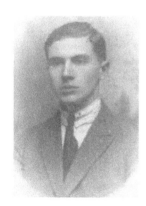

Stanisław Szenicer (1905–1944), surgeon. In the ghetto, he worked in the surgery department of the Czyste Hospital at 1 Leszno Street and lectured at the ghetto medical school. With the help of his colleague from his medical studies, Dr. Andrzej Trojanowski, he received false documents and stayed in Stoczek nad Bugiem as a hospital attendant. He participated in operations to reverse circumcisions. He committed suicide before the end of the war. The photograph comes from the Warsaw University Archives.

Halina Szenicer-Rotstein (1907–1942), dermatologist and venereologist, was a physician at the Czyste Hospital. She worked with nurse Fryd in a wooden cabin on the *Umschlagplatz* during the Great Deportation and took on responsibilities at the Stawki Street hospital before voluntarily surrendering her "life ticket" and going with her patients to her death in Treblinka on September 12, 1942. The photograph comes from the Main Medical Library Archives.

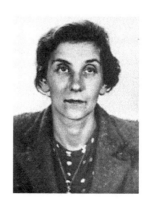

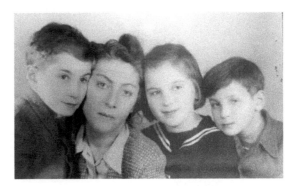

Dr. Halina Szenicer (Kurowska) was a gynecologist who escaped the Warsaw Ghetto with the assistance of Dr. Trojanowski (who also helped her mother and her brother Stanisław Szenicer to escape). She is credited with leading two of the four children of Dr. Halina Szenicer-Rotstein out of the ghetto, saving their lives. The photograph shows three of the four children with Dr. Szenicer after the war. The photograph comes from the Rowiński family photograph collection.

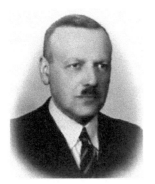

Wilhelm Szenwic (1892–?), urologist. In the ghetto he was the head physician in the urology department of the Czyste Hospital. The photograph comes from the Main Medical Library Archives.

Ignacy Sznajderman (1896–1942), neurologist from the Czyste Hospital. He worked at the Jewish community's infirmary and TOZ's infirmary. He took his son and went to the *Umschlagplatz* for deportation to Treblinka in August 1942. The photograph comes from the Warsaw University Archives.

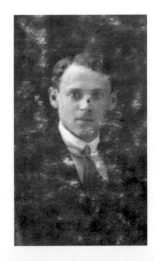

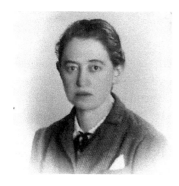

Natalia Szpilfogel-Lichtenbaum (1887–1942?) worked at the internal medicine infirmary belonging to the Bersohn and Bauman Hospital as well as the health center belonging to the Society of Friends of Children and managed the Medem Sanatorium in Miedzeszyn. The photograph comes from the Main Medical Library Archives.

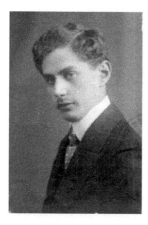

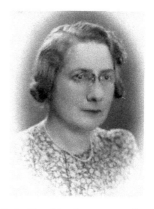

Adolf Szpinak (1893–1944), a pediatrician, was killed during the Warsaw Uprising. The photograph comes from the Warsaw University Archives.

Maria Temkin (1884–1942), internist, medical analyst, managed the analytical laboratories at the Bersohn and Bauman Hospital. The photograph comes from the Main Medical Library Archives.

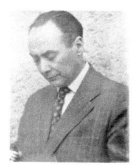

Dr. Natan Trachtenherc (1910–1991) was a doctor who worked during the war in Białystok. The photograph was made after the war in Poland and comes from his daughter Anna Trachtenherc.

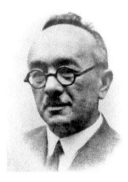

Dr. Naftul Trachtenherc (1883–1942) was a dermatologist and venereologist who worked in the refugee centres in the Warsaw Ghetto and died in Treblinka. The photograph comes from his grand-daughter Anna Trachtenherc.

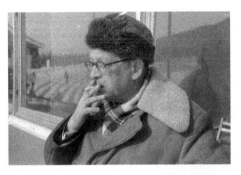

Dr. Trojanowski was a member of the Consensus Committee of Democratic and Socialist doctors, which sought to help their Jewish colleagues with money, false papers and hideouts and he was one of the most active members of the medical unit attached to Żegota. Dr. Trojanowski's home on 127 Marszałkowska Street was a haven for Jews. Many Jews owe their lives to Dr. Trojanowski including the Szenicers as well as the children of Dr. Halina Szenicer-Rotstein. Dr. Trojanowski sought to enhance Jews' safety on the Aryan side by carrying out about fifty ear-and-nose operations as well as surgery that sought to reverse the effects of circumcision. Trojanowski was awarded the status of a Righteous among the Nations by Yad Vashem in 1966. The photograph comes from Ewa Trojanowska, his daughter.

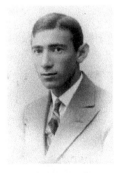

Mojżesz Mieczysław Tursz (or Thursz, 1910–1995), doctor, phtysiatrist, worked at TOZ's infirmary at Gęsia Street. Zenon and Irena Kanabus helped him cross to the Aryan side with his wife Irena. He then participated in the Warsaw Uprising at a field hospital in Żoliborz. He emigrated to Paris after the war. The photograph comes from the Warsaw University Archives.

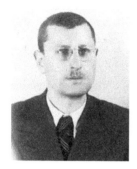

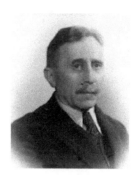

Szmul Stanisław Waller (1904–?), surgeon. Worked at the Czyste Hospital. The photograph comes from the Main Medical Library Archives.

Aleksander Wertheim (1872–1942), surgeon, in the ghetto, worked in the surgical department at the Czyste Hospital. The photograph comes from the Main Medical Library Archives.

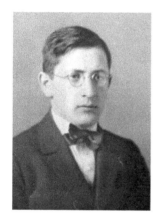

Dawid Wdowiński (1895–1970), doctor of nervous diseases and psychiatry, worked at the Czyste Hospital. He was head of the Political Bureau of the Jewish Military Union. He took part in the Warsaw Uprising. He was sent to Majdanek and then to another camp in the Lubelski region. After the war he emigrated to the United States. The photograph comes from the Warsaw University Archives.

Seweryn Wilk (1896–?), surgeon. In the ghetto, he headed the surgery department at the Bersohn and Bauman Hospital. The photograph comes from the Main Medical Library Archives.

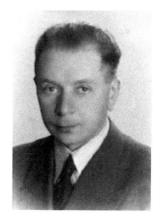

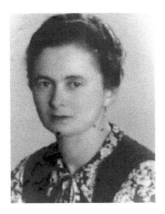

Maria Wilkowa (1901–?), ophthalmologist. In the ghetto, she was the head physician in the ophthalmology department of the Czyste Hospital. The photograph comes from the Main Medical Library Archives.

Ichaskil Wohl (1895–1943), internist, head physician of the Czyste Hospital. The photograph comes from the Main Medical Library Archives.

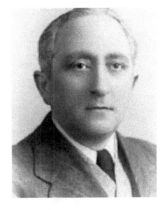

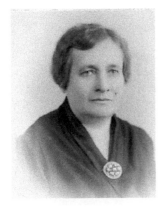

Zofia Zamenhof (December 13, 1889–probably August 1942) worked at the Czyste Hospital in the internal medicine department and decided to accompany her patients to Treblinka in August 1942. The photograph comes from the Main Medical Library Archives.

# Appendix 9

# List of Teachers of Medicine in the Ghetto

| Name | Subject of teaching | Date of birth and death if known | What happened to her/him if known |
|---|---|---|---|
| Amzel Róża | bacteriology, serology | 1904–1943 | died on the Aryan side |
| Apfelbaum Emil | internal diseases, cardiology | 1890–1946 | died after the war |
| Barow Piotr | internal diseases | 1898–? | from July 1941 worked as doctor in *Stalag* in Grodno |
| Bejles Jeszaja Isaj | infectious diseases | 1901–? | shot in the ghetto |
| Ber Alter Pałtych | physiology | 1908–? | fought in the Warsaw Ghetto Rebellion under the name of Borowski |
| Bieleński Owsiej | internal diseases, pulmonology | 1888–1943 | probably died in Trawniki camp or in Majdanek |

| | | | |
|---|---|---|---|
| Borenstein Paweł | parasitology, biology | ?–1942 | died in Treblinka death camp |
| Braude-Hellerowa Anna | pediatrics | 1888–1943 | died on the territory of the ghetto |
| Brokman Henryk | pediatrics | 1886–1976 | died after the war |
| Cunge Mieczysław | histology, embryology | 1908–1942 | died on the territory of the ghetto or in Treblinka |
| Fejgin Bronisława | bacteriology | 1893–1943 | died on the territory of the ghetto |
| Fenigsztein Henryk | descriptive and pathological anatomy | 1913–1993 | died after the war |
| Fliederbaum Julian | internal diseases | 1898–1943 | together with his family committed suicide in the ghetto |
| Gelbard Aniela | neurology | 1907–1997 | died after the war |
| Gold B. | disinfection and disinfestation | no information | no information |
| Grojsblat Mojżesz | internal and infectious diseases | 1894–1942 or 1943 | died on the territory of the ghetto |
| Grynberg Maria | physiological chemistry | 1903–1942 | died in Treblinka death camp |
| Heller Arie Leo | human nutrition | 1917–2008 | crossed to the Aryan side |
| Herman Eufemiusz | neurology | 1892–1985 | crossed to the Aryan side |
| Herszenkrug Mieczysław | descriptive anatomy | no information | no information |

| | | | |
|---|---|---|---|
| Hirszfeld Hanna | pediatrics | 1884–1964 | crossed to the Aryan side |
| Hirszfeld Ludwik | bacteriology, serology | 1884–1954 | crossed to the Aryan side |
| Jelenkiewicz Lucjan or Józef | physiology | 1897–1942 | no information |
| Karbowski Mieczysław | ophthalmology, eye physiology | 1896–1942 | died in Treblinka death camp |
| Kenigsberg Dawid | dermatology | 1890–? | no information |
| Kon (Kohn) Mieczysław | epidemiology, social medicine | 1884–1942 | died in Treblinka death camp |
| Landsberg Marceli | no information | 1890–? | no information |
| Lewenfisz Henryk | laryngology, physiology of the system of hearing | 1889–1965 | died after the war |
| Makower Henryk | microbiology and infectious diseases | 1904–1964 | crossed to the Aryan side |
| Mesz Natan | radiology | 1875–1944 | died following the Warsaw Ghetto Rebellion |
| Milejkowski Izrael | hygiene | 1887–1943 | died in Treblinka death camp |
| Munwes Jakób | internal diseases | 1894–1943 | died in a hideout on the territory of the ghetto |
| Penson Jakub | internal diseases, nephrology | 1899–1971 | died after the war |
| Przedborski Jan Jonas | pediatrics | 1885–1942 | died in Auschwitz concentration camp |

| | | | |
|---|---|---|---|
| Rosenblum Zofia | childcare | 1888-1978 | died after the war |
| Stabholz Ludwik | descriptive anatomy | 1917–2007 | crossed to the Aryan side |
| Stein Józef | pathological anatomy | 1904–1943 | died in Treblinka death camp |
| Sterling Władysław | neuropsychiatry | 1877–1943 | died on the Aryan side |
| Szenicer Stanisław | surgery, first aid | 1905–1944 | committed suicide on the Aryan side |
| Szenwic Wilhelm | gynecology | 1892–1955 | changed his name to Włodzimierz Sowiński and survived the war |
| Świeca Salomon | disinfection and disinfestation | 1914–1943 | committed suicide on the way to Majdanek |
| Waksman Bernard | internal diseases | 1909–? | died after the war |

# Index

CPSIA information can be obtained
at www.ICGtesting.com
Printed in the USA
LVHW030308070322
712497LV00001B/3